Being a Counselor
Directions and Challenges

Being a Counselor
Directions and Challenges

Jeannette A. Brown
University of Virginia

Robert H. Pate, Jr.
University of Virginia

Brooks/Cole Publishing Company
Monterey, California

Brooks/Cole Publishing Company
A Division of Wadsworth, Inc.

©1983 by Wadsworth, Inc., Belmont, California 94002. All rights reserved.
No part of this book may be reproduced, stored in a retrieval system, or transcribed,
in any form or by any means—electronic, mechanical, photocopying, recording, or otherwise—
without the prior written permission of the publisher, Brooks/Cole Publishing Company,
Monterey, California 93940, a division of Wadsworth, Inc.

Printed in the United States of America
10 9 8 7 6 5 4 3 2

Library of Congress Cataloging in Publication Data
   Main entry under title:
   Being a counselor.

   Bibliography: p.
   Includes index.
   1. Counseling. 2. Counseling—Vocational guidance.
I. Brown, Jeannette A., [date]. II. Pate, Robert H.
BF637.C6B338   1983   158'.3   82-20764
ISBN 0-534-01261-2

Subject Editor: *Claire Verduin*
Manuscript Editor: *Rephah Berg*
Production Editors: *Joan Marsh, Jane Stanley*
Interior Design: *Katherine Minerva*
Cover Design: *Lori Hughes*
Typesetting: *Instant Type, Monterey, California*

PREFACE

Departments of counselor education have experienced many programmatic changes in recent years. This book is a response to the multiple needs and differential concerns of professional counselors-in-training for human service agencies, rehabilitation, and higher education, as well as school settings. It is a text for the introductory required course. It provides an introduction to the profession of guidance, counseling, and student personnel administration by addressing those aspects of professional preparation that are common to all the differing areas of specialization by presenting counseling as a profession rather than a work setting.

The text examines (1) historical and philosophical foundations; (2) professional evolution and organizational affiliations, (3) legal and ethical considerations, and (4) the role and functions of professional counselors in a variety of work settings. Also examined are current issues and their implications for the profession of counseling. All the material in the text is new. Each of the authors is an acknowledged expert on the topic of the solicited manuscript.

Part 1 of the text traces the development of counseling services in the United States with reference to the philosophical, sociological, economic, and technological influences that shaped the professional counselor's identity. The evolution of the professional organizations representing professional counselors is traced as well. Critical analyses of legal and ethical considerations are presented and discussed.

Part 2 discusses professional preparation and identifies skills critical to professional counselor competence. Each of these skills is defined theoretically but also pragmatically.

Part 3 examines the variety of developmental stages represented in the counselees with whom professional counselors work. The uniqueness of each population is identified, and the implications of these various life stages for counselor behavior are examined. In addition, in each chapter a practicing counselor describes the role and functions of counselors: (1) what the counselor does, (2) what hours the counselor keeps, and (3) what rewards—present/future and intrinsic/extrinsic—exist. The life-style, activities, competencies, and compensations of on-the-job professional counselors in different work settings are presented.

Part 4 is a synthesis of the entire text. Tentative hypotheses generated by the various chapter authors are postulated, to provoke student involvement. It is an action-oriented exercise for students to deal with, and attempt resolutions of, the critical issues influencing the professional future of guidance, counseling, and student personnel administration.

Throughout there is a simplicity of writing style and a concern for practicality. Not only are the "why" and the "what" addressed, but there is a continuing concern with "how" the presented concepts can be applied. Each chapter concludes with a series of group-oriented, situational problem-solving quizzes requiring students to derive practical applications for the previously presented material.

Professional counselors have a high regard for effective helping relationships. Our own regard for this concept has been greatly enhanced by this particular project. Help was provided tirelessly and without complaint or compromise. We are particularly indebted to the many on-the-job counselors whose combined insights and suggestions provided not only the substance of the statements attributed to them but direction for our planning of the entire text.

We acknowledge with gratitude the contribution of numerous colleagues and friends. We extend special thanks to the students who reviewed drafts of the manuscript and provided valuable suggestions, and to the student assistants in the University of Virginia Department of Counselor Education for their help. We are also grateful to a number of reviewers who studied drafts of this manuscript and made many helpful suggestions for improvements. They include Edward S. Beck of Pennsylvania State University and president of the American Mental Health Counselors Association, Dr. Robert M. Bollet, of University of Central Florida, Dr. Robert W. Cash of California State University at Long Beach, Dr. William A. Lewis of University of Missouri at Kansas City, and Dr. Ronald E. Smith of Portland State University.

Finally, we express sincere appreciation to Karen Owings Clifford, whose dependability and never-failing good humor were vital to our completion of this project.

Jeannette A. Brown
Robert H. Pate, Jr.

CONTENTS

PART 1 THE COUNSELOR OF THE 1980s 1

1 *Professional Identity: Crisis or Challenge?* 3   PATE

Definitions and Explications 4
    A Counselor is . . . Conventionally 4
    A Counselor is . . . Professionally 6
    The Professionalization of Counselors 8
    The American Personnel and Guidance Association 11
    Related Occupations 12
Diversities, Commonalities, and Opportunities 16
    It's Not Where We Do It 16
    It's the Way We Do It 16
    Who Needs Us 19
Perspectives for the '80s 21
Summary 23
Now It's Your Turn 24
References 24

2 *The Law and the Counselor* 26   SWANSON

An Emerging Profession 27

vii

The Counselor and the Law: Ethical Standards 31
Statutory Law—Acts of the Legislature 32
    Privileged Communication Statutes 32
    Other Statutes 33
The Common Case Law 36
    Confidentiality and Recordkeeping 37
    The Good Faith Doctrine 37
    Constitutional Rights 38
    Perspectives for the '80s 39
    Summary 40
    Now It's Your Turn 40
    References 44

3   *Ethics and the Counselor 47*   SWANSON

Incompetent and Unethical Behavior 49
    Incompetent Behavior 49
    Unethical Behavior 50
Ethical Codes 53
The Counselor's Ethical Orientation 55
Ethical Decision Making 57
Perspectives for the '80s 59
Summary 59
Now It's Your Turn 60
Questions for Discussion 61
References 62

PART 2   THE WORK OF THE COUNSELOR 63

4   *Individual Counseling 66*   BOYD

Conversation, Counseling, and Psychotherapy 67
    Conversation and Counseling 68
    Psychotherapy and Counseling 70
Three Categories of Individual Counseling 72
    Developmental Counseling 73
    Career Counseling 75
    Personal Adjustment Counseling 76
    Categories and Counseling Practice 77

Case Example 78
Three Approaches to Counseling 83
- *Client-Centered Counseling 84*
- *Rational-Emotive Counseling 85*
- *Behavioral Counseling 87*

Perspectives for the '80s 89
Summary 91
Now It's Your Turn 91
References 92

5 Group Counseling 95   COREY

Group Counseling for Special Populations 96
- *Children 96*
- *Adolescents 96*
- *Adults 97*
- *The Elderly 98*

Some General Goals and Purposes of Groups 98
Advantages of Group Counseling 99
Evolution and Development of a Group 100
- *Where to Begin: Formation of the Group 100*
- *Announcing a Group and Recruiting Members 101*
- *Screening and Selecting Members 101*
- *Some Practical Considerations in Group Formation 102*
- *Conducting a Pregroup Session 104*

Stage 1—Initial Stage: A Time for Orientation and Exploration 105
- *Characteristics of the Initial Stage 106*
- *Ways of Creating Trust during the Initial Stage 107*
- *Helping Members Define Goals 108*
- *Major Member Functions and Possible Problems 109*
- *Major Leader Functions 109*

Stage 2—The Transition Stage: Learning to Deal With Conflict 110
- *Characteristics of the Transition Stage 110*
- *Learning to Recognize and Deal with Conflict 111*

Stage 3—The Working Stage 112
Stage 4—The Final Stage: Consolidation and Termination 114
Postgroup Issues: Follow-Up and Evaluation Procedures 115
- *Conducting Follow-Up Interviews 116*

x　CONTENTS

   Encouraging Contact With Other Members 116
   Arranging A Follow-Up Group Session 116
   Ways of Carrying One's Learning Further 117
 A Commentary on the Group Leader's Competence 117
   Determining One's Own Level of Competence 117
   Some Paths toward Becoming a Qualified Group Leader 118
   Some Dimensions of the Education and Training of
   Group Counselors 118
 Perspectives for the '80s 120
 Summary 121
 Now It's Your Turn 121
 References and Suggested Readings 122

6　Consulting 124　　BROWN

 Why Counselors Consult 125
 Definitions and Approaches 126
   Provision 127
   Prescription 127
   Mediation 127
   Collaboration 128
 A Critical Analysis 129
   Societal Considerations 129
   Professional Considerations 130
   Reconsiderations 130
 Practical Considerations 133
 Perspectives for the '80s 137
   Educational Goals and Objectives 138
   Social Goals and Objectives 139
   Economic Goals and Objectives 141
 Summary 142
 Now It's Your Turn 142
 References and Suggested Readings 145

7　Assessment and Information Giving 147　　PATE

 Assessment, Information Giving, and Counseling 148
 Environmental Information 153
   Career Information 153
   Educational Information 153
   Informational Materials 154
 Assessment Information 155

What Counselors Must Know about Assessment 157
Standardized Tests and Inventories 157
Other Assessment Devices 159
Reliability and Validity 160
Errors of Difference and Prediction 161
Social, Ethical, and Legal Issues 162
Perspectives for the '80s 167
Summary 169
Now It's Your Turn 170
References 171

8 Research and Evaluation 173   LaFLEUR

Ways of Knowing and Understanding 174
Authority 174
Experience 175
Methods of Reaching Conclusions 176
Deductive Reasoning 176
Inductive Reasoning 177
The Scientific Method 177
Methods of Research and Evaluation 178
Historical 178
Case Study 179
Survey 180
Participant Observer 181
Experimental 181
Data Sources in Research and Evaluation 182
Observational Data 182
Questionnaires and Inventories 182
Use of Statistics in Research and Evaluation 184
Perspectives for the '80s 185
Summary 188
Now It's Your Turn 189
References 190

PART 3   THE CLIENTS OF THE COUNSELOR 191

9 Children 195   FRANKS

A Historical Overview 195
Theories of Human Development 196

Piaget and Cognitive Development 196
Erikson and Emotional and Development 198
Kohlberg and Moral Development 199
Havighurst and Developmental Tasks 199
Implications for Counseling 200
Individual Counseling 201
Group Counseling 201
Classroom Group Guidance 201
Consultation 201
Referral Services 203
Perspectives for the '80s 203
Changes in Family Structure 203
Rights of Children 203
Needs of Exceptional Children 203
Summary 204
Now It's Your Turn 204
References and Suggested Readings 205

10 Adolescents 207   FUHRMANN

Adolescence: A Cultural Phenomenon 208
Development in Adolescence 209
Current Cultural Effects 211
Tasks of Adolescence 212
Cognitive Development: Jean Piaget 213
Psychological Development: Erik Erikson 216
Moral Development: Lawrence Kohlberg 218
Adolescent Concerns: The Counselor's Role 221
Perspectives for the '80s 223
Summary 226
Now It's Your Turn 227
References 228

11 Adults 230   WORTH

Developmental Issues 232
Early Adulthood 233
Achieving Intimacy 235
Becoming Autonomous 236
The Thirties Transition 239

　　　　Settling Down 239
　　　　The Midlife Transition 240
　　Middle Adulthood 242
　　　　Biological Changes 243
　　　　Achieving Generativity 243
　　　　Other Issues of Middle Adulthood 243
　　Women and Men as Clients 244
　　　　The Male Client 244
　　　　Women as Clients 246
　　Work Settings 247
　　　　Higher Education 247
　　　　Community Agencies 248
　　Perspectives for the '80s 248
　　Summary 249
　　Now It's Your Turn 250
　　References 251

12 The Elderly 253　　GROBE

　　Stereotyping, Expectancy, and Learned Helplessness 254
　　　　Stereotyping 254
　　　　The Expectancy Phenomenon 255
　　　　Learned Helplessness 255
　　Biomedical Myths 256
　　　　The Myth of Poor Health 256
　　　　The Myth of Sexual Incompetence 257
　　Psychosocial Myths 258
　　　　Myth: Intellectual Deterioration Is Inevitable 258
　　　　Myth: Learning Ability Declines 259
　　　　Myth: Remarriage Is a Mistake 259
　　Socioeconomic Myths 260
　　　　The Myth of Nonproductivity 260
　　　　The Myth of the Golden Years 261
　　　　The Myth That Their Needs Are Few 262
　　Implications for Counseling Older Adults 263
　　　　Retirement 263
　　　　Physical and Emotional Decompetence 264
　　　　Dying 265
　　　　Marriage and Remarriage 265
　　　　Sex and Sexuality 266

Institutionalization 266
Adaptations to Retirement: Life Enhancement 267
   Leisure 268
   Education 269
   Rehirement (Reemployment) 271
Perspectives for the '80s 272
Summary 274
Now It's Your Turn 274
References 276

13 Special Populations 279   GRESSARD/HUME

Deviance 280
   Reactions of Society 281
   Reactions of the Stigmatized 282
Physically Disabled and Retarded 283
   Counselor Settings 285
   Counselor Role 286
   Counselor Competencies 287
Alcoholics 288
   Counselor Settings 289
   Counselor Role 290
   Counselor Competencies 291
Other Substance Abusers 292
   Counselor Settings 293
   Counselor Competencies 294
Offenders 295
   Counselor Settings 296
   Counselor Role 297
   Counselor Competencies 299
Perspectives for the '80s 299
   Rehabilitation 300
   Alcoholism 300
   Drug Abuse 301
   Offenders 301
Summary 302
Now It's Your Turn 302
References 303

PART 4 THE DECISIONS OF THE COUNSELORS 305

14 *Practical Exercises* 307   BROWN

Sarah 308
- Exercise #1 309
- Exercise #2 310
- Exercise #3 312

Our Gang 312
- Exercise #4 314
- Exercise #5 315

Final Report 316
- Exercise #6 316
- Exercise #7 320
- Exercise #8 321

Timothy 322
- Exercise #9 322

The Convention 326
- Exercise #10 326

References 329

Appendix A Professional Organizations of Interest to Counselors 330

Appendix B Ethical Standards American Personnel and Guidance Association 337

Appendix C Ethics Committee Virginia Counselors Association Responsibilities and Procedures 345

Appendix D Regulations of Virginia Board of Professional Counselors 350

Appendix E Regulations of Virginia Board of Behavioral Science 360

Appendix F APGA Convention Registration Materials Detroit Michigan, 1982 363

Appendix G 1983 APGA Convention Call for Content Programs 368

Name Index 375

Subject Index 378

PART 1

The Counselor of the 1980s

The counselor of the 1980s is unlike any other who previously claimed the title—and rightly so. All counselors, regardless of their time and place, share the same rich heritage of change and diversity. Responsiveness to societal change is a hallmark of influential professions, and counselors claim membership in this elite community of professionals. Our historical evolution is testimony to such concerned dedication.

Not only have counselors served society and its differing cultural amalgamations, economic changes, and industrial innovations, but they have also sought new ways to serve each of society's individual members. These latter efforts, depending on the time, have ranged from analyzing and prescribing to supporting and designing new modes of learning opportunities. However counselors perceived their mission and its most effective interpretation, paramount in their evolution was a concern for professionalism in their service.

In Chapter 1 Robert H. Pate, Jr., discusses the diversity and contradiction in the professional counselor's history and evolution. Pate discusses not merely the counselor's variety of work settings and definitions but also the common focus and dedication of all counselors regardless of their specialized concerns. Pate furthermore presents a critical analysis of the criteria for determining professional status. In Chapter 1 the reader is addressed not merely philosophically and theoretically but also pragmatically. In discussing career opportunities for professional counselors, Pate presents a systematic approach for identifying and predicting employment needs as these relate to a variety of work settings. In addition, the history of the American Personnel and Guidance Association is traced, and the societal changes and professional tensions that influenced its evolution are identified. APGA's multiple divisions, reflecting its membership diversity, are of critical importance to students preparing for careers as professional counselors. Professionalism requires affiliation with, and active participation in, professional organizations on the local, state, regional, and national levels. Of equal importance is contribution to professional meetings and publications.

Chapter 2, by Carl W. Swanson, is an analytical review of the rights and privileges accorded to, as well as the limitations and constraints imposed by law on, professional counselors. Swanson provides a concise and practical review and interpretation of the legal regulations that govern the work of the counselor. He discusses the counselor's right to practice as defined by differing certification and/or licensure regulations as well as the rights of counselees. Regardless of the topic being discussed, Carl Swanson provides his readers with both an understanding of the issue and an analysis of its implications. Swanson's practical approach to the law and its meaning for professional counseling make this chapter a unique professional contribution.

Chapter 3, also by Carl Swanson, examines counselor behavior as it has consequences for the profession as well as the counselee. Swanson provides a historical review of professional codes and describes the specific ethical codes of professional counselors. He does not limit his discussion of ethical behavior to counselor interactions with professional colleagues; noncounselor colleague interactions are also discussed. Swanson's major thesis is that because self-regulation is the hallmark of all professions, it seems to follow that ethical codes, regulations, and standards will exert only minimal influence in the absence of *self-imposed* codes of behavior.

Part 1 is an effort to introduce you to your profession. It is relatively young and has few claims to established tradition or legal sanctions. It is, consequently, a profession capable of being influenced and shaped by all those who want to share our challenges and contribute to our professional future. A serious consideration of the information, ideas, and issues presented in this section is a necessary first step to accepting our invitation to become professional counselors.

CHAPTER *1*

Professional Identity: Crisis or Challenge?

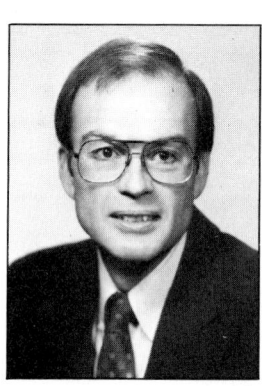

Robert H. Pate, Jr.
Robert H. Pate, Jr., is professor and chair of counselor education at the University of Virginia. He has been active regionally and nationally in the counselor education program accreditation movement. He was the first licensed professional counselor in Virginia to receive the specialty designation Research Counselor.

One of the behaviors of conventioneers is the wearing of badges. At a recent convention of the American Personnel and Guidance Association (APGA), the national organization representing professional counselors, badges were in abundance. One of the more popular was the one handed out by a major division of APGA, the National Vocational Guidance Association. In bold print the badge announced "I'm Available" and then, in smaller print, "for career guidance."

Although the popularity of the button may have had more to do with its suggestiveness than with its basic truth, counselors are available to all sorts of people with all sorts of needs for help. A nationally syndicated religious television program, *The 700 Club,* offers the services of counselors to those who call a toll-free number. Advertisements in a leading national newsmagazine tell how a 700 Club counselor prevented a caller from committing suicide. For those who do not watch television, a similar phone-in counseling service is offered to listeners of a Southern Baptist Convention radio program. Most local communities have one or more organizations of "hot line" counselors who stand by telephones to respond to callers with a variety of concerns. In addition to the telephone counselors who are available to those in various kinds of distress, there are real estate counselors, insurance counselors, and even a popular brand of bathroom scale, the Beauty Counselor. Many schools and colleges have organized programs of peer counseling services in which students meet some of the counseling needs of their peers. "Yes, but I'm not interested in being that kind of counselor, I want to be a professional counselor." What *are* professional counselors, and what distinguishes them from other kinds of counselors?

Definitions and Explications

Definitions can be tedious, but this exploration was designed to provide a foundation for your introduction to the profession of counseling.

A Counselor Is . . . Conventionally

So, what *is* a counselor, and how do professional counselors differ from all those other counselors? You will find little help in conventional dictionaries. The definitions offered for the word *counselor* are typically limited to givers of advice and attorneys. One exception is that for a camp counselor. The verb *counsel,* however, is defined to include processes with which professional counselors more closely identify. These definitions introduce the quality of discussion, as opposed to advice giving. Only an unabridged dictionary (Random House, 1971) provides a definition of *counselor* that would properly describe the persons who can appropriately be labeled professional counselors. However, that definition is so broad as to encompass most, if not all, of the previously mentioned varieties of counselors.

Conventional dictionaries cannot be relied on for occupational definitions. That was not their purpose. One of the more appropriate sources for definitions of *counselor* is the 1977 *Dictionary of Occupational Titles* (DOT). The DOT, a publication of the U. S. Department of Labor, Employment and Training Administration, provides definitions of 20,000 occupational titles. The DOT provides a base title and sometimes alternate titles for each defined occupation and includes the following definition of the base title *counselor* under the group "Occupations in Psychology."

Counsels individuals and provides group educational and vocational guidance services: Collects, organizes, and analyzes information about individuals through records, tests, interviews, and professional sources, to appraise their interests, aptitudes, abilities, and personality characteristics, for vocational and educational planning. Compiles and studies occupational, educational, and economic information to aid counselees in making and carrying out vocational and educational objectives. Refers students to placement service. Assists individuals to understand and overcome social and emotional problems. May engage in research and follow-up activities to evaluate counseling techniques. May teach classes [p. 48].

Alternate titles are *guidance counselor, vocational adviser,* and *vocational counselor.*

The DOT definition of *counselor* indicates that the term may be designated according to area of activity. Additional base-title definitions are provided for director of counseling, director of guidance in public schools, residence counselor, and vocational-rehabilitation counselor. However, the essential aspects of the counseling component of all the titles are included in the definition of *counselor* quoted above.

Another source for "official" descriptions of occupations is also a federal government publication. *The Occupational Outlook Handbook* (OOH) is a biennial publication of the Bureau of Labor Statistics to provide information about the employment outlook for major occupations. The OOH is a major source of information for career counselors and provides, for each occupation included, descriptions of the nature of the work; training, other qualifications, and advancement; employment outlook; earnings and working conditions; and sources of additional information.

In the current OOH (1980), the chapter "Occupations in Counseling," included in the section "Social Service Occupations," is introduced by the following paragraph.

> At some point in their lives most people seek advice or assistance for personal, education, or vocational problems. These problems may be relatively minor, such as a conflict in a student's class schedule, or may involve serious emotional or physical disabilities. Regardless of the problem, counselors often are the ones to whom people turn for help [p. 435].

The OOH chapter is divided into a discussion of four counseling specialties:

> *School counselors* are the largest counseling group. They are primarily concerned with the personal, social, and educational development of students.
> *Rehabilitation counselors* help persons with physical, mental, or social handicaps to become productive individuals.
> *Employment counselors* advise people—the unemployed or unskilled for example—who cannot find a job and/or have problems in career choice and planning.

College career planning and placement counselors help college students examine their own interests, abilities, and goals; explore career alternatives; and make and follow through with a career choice [p. 435].

The definitions and descriptions provided in the two federal publications are not completely consistent. For example, the DOT lists "counselor" under occupations in psychology, whereas the OOH lists Counseling Occupations in a section entitled "Social Work Occupations." More important than the structural distinctions are the substantive differences. The OOH discussion of the rehabilitation counselor reflects a newer and more widely endorsed view of the rehabilitation counselor and rehabilitation clients than does the DOT definition of vocational-rehabilitation counselor. The DOT and OOH do provide a solid basis for our contention that the title "counselor" should refer to a specific occupation, as opposed to the idea that a person who discusses financial investments with clients, for example, is a counselor.

We accept the notion that many people "counsel" if that term is defined simply as a verb meaning "to advise or discuss with" but contend that the term *counselor* should refer to persons whose occupation is to provide professional assistance to individuals who have vocational, educational, or personal problems. The modifier *professional* is suggested by the DOT classification of counselor as a "professional, technical, and managerial" occupation. The concept is important because we may be forced to accept the reality that in the semantic sense many counsel but in the professional sense few are counselors.

A Counselor Is . . . Professionally

Professions have certain generally recognized characteristics. Before discussing them, one final definitional consideration should be mentioned. You will learn that the term *professional counselor* has a legal meaning in some states, but the following consideration of the meaning ascribed to, and expectations held for, professional counselors will not be restricted to legal interpretations. The term *professional counselor* is limited to persons who have specialized training (a minimum of a master's degree in counseling), who subscribe to the professional Code of Ethics of the American Personnel and Guidance Association or a similar professional code, and who view counseling as a vocation—an occupation to which they are committed.

The term *professional* may seem redundant when coupled with *counselor* but the terms *counselor* and *counsel* are used so commonly that the modifier is necessary. Unfortunately, alternative terms conveying level of training and expertise, similar to *bookkeeper* and *accountant,* do not exist. The term *adviser* would be more appropriate for many who use the title *counselor,* because just as all who keep books are not accountants, neither are all who advise counselors. The need for some distinction for those who are in fact professional counselors is further demonstrated by the frequent use of such terms as *peer counselor* and *paraprofessional counselor* in the publications of professional associations. As students preparing to be professional counselors, you expect your graduate training program to result in professional status. But what does it mean to be a professional? What are the essential elements of a profession?

Greenwood (1966) states, "Succinctly put, all professions seem to possess: (1) systematic theory, (2) authority, (3) community sanction, (4) ethical codes, and (5) a culture" (p. 10). Greenwood cautions that occupations cannot be classified as either professional or not professional; rather, all are on a continuum relative to each of the criteria. Moore (1970) proposes (1) full-time occupation, (2) commitment to a calling, (3) formalized organization, (4) specialized education, (5) service orientation, and (6) autonomy as characteristics of a profession. Like Greenwood, Moore suggests that occupations are on a continuum, or scale, relative to each of the characteristics of professions he has suggested.

The question whether counseling is a profession has been explored by Dunlop (1969) and Shevlin (1968), using criteria developed on the basis of work by McCully (1962) in which he proposed 11 criteria for a profession. Ritchie (1978) has condensed McCully's 11 criteria into three: legal recognition, training standards, and an enforceable code of ethics. One of Ritchie's recommendations was that counselors must achieve changes in each of the three areas if they are to attain uncontested professional status.

A detailed exploration of the professional status of counselors is not possible here, but a foundation for our consideration of counseling as a profession is necessary. The attributes and characteristics suggested by Greenwood and Moore were selected because any occupation can be placed on a continuum relative to the factors they have proposed.

On the basis of Greenwood's attributes of a profession, counselors appear to be well toward the professional end of the scale, compared with occupations in general. Part 2 of this book, "The Work of the Counselor," indicates that counselors do base their work on *systematic theory* about human behavior. The debate about whether counseling is an art or a science will continue, but few professions are based solely on systematic theory. A comparison of counselors' acceptance as *authority* with the degree of acceptance of other professionals would require a complex empirical investigation, but we do know that counselors are accepted by students and increasingly by parents, teachers, and adult counselees as authorities in the sense that the counselor is a source of help. Because counselors do not want to give expert advice, they have not worked to establish themselves as authorities in the traditional sense.

Moore's six characteristics of a profession add other dimensions. We find counselors clearly on the professional end of all but one of these continua. We do not dispute that some fully qualified volunteers do provide part-time counseling services. Counseling is, however, a legitimate *full-time occupation*. Counselors do have a sense of vocation and a *commitment to a calling*. We recognize that some people who receive graduate training in counselor education programs do not become counselors because they entered the training program for other reasons than to become counselors.

The current trend toward two-year graduate training programs for entry-level counselors will go far to establish a distinction between those who want some level of human relations training and those who have a commitment to a career field. The characteristic of *formalized organization* is similar to Greenwood's "culture." The organizations that provide formalized organization and culture for counselors are discussed in the section that follows. Counselors do have *specialized education:* preparation is in graduate programs. The American Personnel and Guidance Association (APGA) has endorsed and adopted the proposals of its Association for Counselor Education and Supervision (ACES) that counselor education programs be accredited by the professional association. The accreditation will be by the Council for the Accreditation of Counseling and Related Educational Programs (CACREP), an independent organization founded by APGA.

The final characteristic of a profession suggested by Moore is *autonomy*. On that characteristic counselors must be ranked well below the traditional professions of law and medicine. Counselors are similar to social workers, whom Ruzek (1973) called "captive professionals." They are captive because they tend to be employees rather than independent practitioners.

Discussions of professions typically include the concept of professionalization, the process by which occupations become professions. The brief review presented above suggests that counselors have achieved much in their struggle to become professionals. We must, however, underscore Ritchie's (1978) conclusion that in three critical areas—legal recognition, training standards, and enforceable ethical codes—the process of professionalization is far from complete. Chapters 2 and 3 will address those areas of concern in more detail.

The Professionalization of Counselors

As occupational groups strive to become professional, they achieve a culture (Greenwood, 1966) and formalized organization (Moore, 1970). Those attributes of professional occupations are associated with membership in professional organizations. Counselors might belong to any of several relevant professional organizations, but the most likely choice is the American Personnel and Guidance Association (APGA).

THE CHOICE IS YOURS

You should know right from the start that your public, regardless of your projected work setting, will not receive you with open arms. The effectiveness of counselors has been challenged by mental-health agencies, human service agencies, business and industry, the clients of private practitioners, correctional institutions, the military, colleges, and schools. So you've got to be ready to take the lumps earned by all those others who came before you.

Of course, it wasn't your fault that they were ineffective! But it wasn't their fault, either. The fault was in the training they received and the training opportunities they never received. They were victims of professional preparation that ignored or underemphasized at least three areas of critical need: (1) career development (2) organization and supervision and (3) an adequate repertoire of ways to deliver counseling services.

The contemporary counselor needs to know how to help counselees learn practical methods and techniques for finding and landing jobs of their choice. Administering interest inventories and providing anxiety-reduction counseling won't put bread on your counselees' tables. Nor will their career choice and job problems be solved if you merely give them the address of the nearest job placement agency. No concern is common to more people in today's society than careers, and today's counselors are expected to help their counselees with this vital dimension of their lives. So you've got to learn how. Yesterday's counselors were taught almost nothing about programming, organizational management, and supervision. Many superb and dedicated counselors "died on the vine" because they were never taught how to create, refine, and enlarge their programs of services or how to use their interpersonal skills when interacting with the guardians of budgets. Today's counselors need to learn how to create effective working relationships with their noncounselor colleagues. They need to learn how to use their counseling skills in consulting activities yesterday's counselors never had a chance to learn. Professional counselors of the 1980s must be taught how to enlarge not merely their program of services but the numbers of people receiving their services. One-to-one counseling is a far too inefficient method for reaching the masses, and today's counselor must have opportunities to learn how to work with large as well as small groups, how to provide psychological education, and where to find and how to use the variety of instructional materials currently available.

As a last word, today's counselor must be taught that counseling is a process, not a bag of tricks. All the techniques in the world will not a counselor make. You need to be taught the steps in the process, when to take each one, and when to proceed to the next. Counseling is a systematic process within which many differing techniques can be used. You don't have any choice about the reputation you've inherited, but you do have a choice about changing it. Yesterday's counselors were crippled by their training. You don't have to be—but the choice is yours.

—A Yesterday's Counselor

Before examining the history and current structure of APGA, I will describe the potential contributions of professional organization membership to counselors.

Only through some formal organization can counselors have a means to speak as a profession. A collective voice is necessary for counselors because much of funding, and thus determination of the objectives for counseling programs, is provided by public appropriation. On both the local and national levels, professional organizations provide the means for counselors to speak on professional issues. In addition to representing their members on matters that are vital to members' welfare, professional organizations provide a voice for members to speak collectively on social issues. As providers of a service, counselors, in their concern to expand their programs could be viewed as self-serving, but that is true of all professional groups in their lobbying efforts.

Not all members agree on social issues, and some reject the position of the organization majority, as has happened, for example, regarding approval of the Equal Rights Amendment and convention sites. However, on such matters as professional codes of ethics, standards for service, and counselee advocacy, the professional organization position represents nearly all members. For professionals to have the potential for autonomy and self-regulation, which are attributes of a profession, counselors must have a professional voice. As issues of licensure, standards for training, and competence endorsement increase in importance, the necessity for counselors to have a means to influence decisions and speak collectively magnifies the importance of professional organizations.

The individual member also gains directly from affiliation with professional groups. Professional organizations publish the journals that are "the literature" of the profession and provide the vehicle for sharing research findings and new techniques as well as a forum for the exploration of professional issues. Another means by which professionals share is the operation of conventions. The conventions or professional association meetings can be state, regional, or national. Conventions typically offer training workshops to allow practicing counselors to develop and refine skills. Convention program sessions allow a format for presentation of research findings, demonstrations, and professional issues in a way that allows for presenter/audience interaction. Conventions also provide an exhibit section so that publishers and other organizations can display their "wares" and ideas. The exhibit section of a convention allows counselors to know of and examine the latest materials as well as interact with representatives of organizations that want to influence counselor thinking.

Professional associations typically produce monographs, books, films, and other materials, which are sold to members at reduced costs. Group-insurance purchase privileges for personal protection as well as professional liability coverage are other typical benefits of associations.

A final but important service of professional organizations to their members is job placement. Their newsletters have classified sections that list both positions available and persons seeking positions. A placement service is a feature of national conventions. The placement service provides a means for employers and job seekers to meet without either having the burden of travel time and expenses.

As indicated in the following section, not all counselors have similar work, work settings, or even job titles. For that reason counselors can affiliate with a number of professional organizations. A detailed presentation on the history, organization, purposes, and membership requirements of all these organizations is not possible here. The APGA is the organization professional counselors are most likely to choose. I shall describe it, as representative. Appendix A provides information about other professional organizations in which counselors might have an interest.

The American Personnel and Guidance Association

The development of the American Personnel and Guidance Association mirrors developments in the profession it represents. Counselors usually cite Frank Parsons and his 1909 organization, the Vocational Bureau of Boston, as a historic benchmark for counselors. Just as counselors have developed professionally from a vocational counseling base, so did APGA. The National Vocational Guidance Association (NVGA) was organized in 1913, and from this organization came much of the leadership and initiative to form councils and confederations of professional organizations and to investigate new structures. A new structure, the Personnel and Guidance Association of America, was formed in 1951, and it became the American Personnel and Guidance Association (APGA) in 1952 to avoid name confusion with the PGA (Professional Golfers Association). APGA began its organizational life with four charter divisions. The four original divisions were quickly joined by a fifth, so that the first five divisions in the list of APGA divisions are considered the pioneer divisions. The expansion of the divisional membership to include rehabilitation, public employment, public offender, and mental-health divisions reflects an expanding definition of the counselor's role from vocational and student-oriented to a comprehensive view of counseling. This trend continues to be reflected in current proposals for APGA to change its name to one emphasizing counseling as well as, or in addition to, personnel and guidance.

Each division of APGA (see Table 1-1) has a national organization with bylaws, officers, and a budget derived from member dues. However, membership in APGA is a prerequisite for divisional membership. State branches of APGA are chartered and organized in a way that mirrors the national structure. The state organizations, each designated by the state name followed by *Personnel and Guidance Association,* typically have some divisions that parallel the national divisions. State branches usually have local chapters, which are the "grass roots" organizations of counselors in a geographic area. State branches encourage APGA membership, but it is not mandatory.

TABLE 1-1 Divisions of American Personnel and Guidance Association

Name	Journal	Founded	Approximate membership
American College Personnel Association (ACPA)	Journal of College Student Personnel	1952	7500
Association for Counselor Education and Supervision (ACES)	Counselor Education and Supervision	1952	3100
National Vocational Guidance Association (NVGA)	The Vocational Guidance Quarterly	1952	6000
Association for Humanistic Education and Development (AHEAD)	The Humanist Educator	1952	1800
American School Counselor Association (ASCA)	The School Counselor	1953	9100
American Rehabilitation Counseling Association (ARCA)	Rehabilitation Counseling Bulletin	1958	2900
Association for Measurement & Evaluation in Guidance (AMEG)	Measurement & Evaluation in Guidance	1965	1600
National Employment Counselors Association (NECA)	Journal of Employment Counseling	1966	1400
Association for Non-White Concerns in Personnel and Guidance (ANWC)	Journal of Non-White Concerns in Personnel and Guidance	1972	1600
Association for Religious and Value Issues in Counseling (ARVIC)	Counseling and Values	1973	1900
Association for Specialists in Group Work (ASGW)	Journal of Specialists in Group Work	1973	3000
Public Offender Counselor Association (POCA)	Journal of Employment Counseling	1974	700
American Mental Health Counselors Association (AMHCA)	AMHCA Journal	1978	5700

APGA is governed by a board of directors, which includes national officers and representatives from divisions and regional branch assemblies, reflecting the organization of state branches into four regions. APGA also has a full-time executive vice-president and professional staff headquartered in Falls Church, Virginia, a suburb of Washington, D.C. APGA has approximately 40,000 members and publishes the *Personnel and Guidance Journal* and the *Guidepost,* a professional newspaper.

Related Occupations

Counselors are not the only people who have chosen an occupation whose objective is to help others deal with educational, vocational, social, and emotional problems. The list of professional organizations in Appendix A demonstrates the breadth of our possible focus. This brief overview of some other helping professions that have goals similar or related to those of counseling is included because students enter counselor education programs from a variety of undergraduate and experience backgrounds. A consideration of other occupations may seem dissonant, but as the chapters in Part 2 will show, counselors share many methods and techniques with other professions.

Although the systematic theory on which counseling is based is not unique to counseling, to be a counselor is to have a distinct occupation. However, we recognize that many students in counselor education programs will secure entry-level jobs which are not positions for counselors *per se*. Occupations that share some of the theory base, methods, and techniques of counseling are listed in the DOT under the occupational groups Occupations in Medicine and Health; Occupations in College and University Education; Occupations in Secondary Education, Personnel Administrative Occupations; and Occupations in Social and Welfare Work. Those occupational groups are in addition to Occupations in Psychology, the occupational group that includes "counselor."

The greatest potential for confusion exists between counseling and psychology. That *counselor* is defined under the DOT group Occupations in Psychology shows the close relationship of counselors to the occupations in that group that have the title *psychology*. Psychology includes occupations with diverse practices and purposes. The distinction between counselors and developmental, engineering, experimental, educational, industrial, and social psychologists is not difficult. Counselors have the greatest degree of shared theoretical base and purpose, and therefore the greatest potential for confusion about role, with the psychologists who provide services to individuals and groups—clinical, counseling, and school psychologists.

Before considering the distinctions among the goals of these occupations, some technical distinctions are in order. Use of the title *psychologist* is now regulated in all states. The regulation typically provides for licensure of doctoral-level psychologists. The *Occupational Outlook Handbook* states "A doctoral degree almost always is the minimum requirement for employment as a psychologist" (1979, p. 529). As indicated in Appendix A, membership in the professional organization of psychologists, the American Psychological Association (APA), is limited to holders of doctoral degrees.

There are distinctions in goals and clients that go beyond the structural distinctions between counselors and the psychologists who work with clients individually and in groups. The clinical psychologist deals with persons who have mental and emotional disorders, whereas the clients of counselors are not considered to have disorders, but rather to have problems or concerns of living. The school psychologist typically deals with assessment and planning unique programs for students identified as having special needs, whereas school counselors develop programs for all students. Individual and group counseling by school counselors is focused on issues and concerns typical for the age group of their students.

Many of the pioneer counselors are identified with the field of counseling psychology, and the DOT definition of *counseling psychologist* is remarkably similar to that of *counselor*. The only simple distinction between counselors trained at the doctoral level and counseling psychologists is that counseling psychologists are licensed as psychologists. This is due to the close relationship between counseling and psychology and the fact that counselors in many states have been forced to become licensed as psychologists in order to practice their profession. With the exception of counseling psychology, there are distinctions between the training and professional objectives of psychologists and counselors, even though a great overlap exists between the theoretical bases of the two groups.

Psychiatrists are medical doctors who have elected a medical specialty in the area of mental, emotional, and behavioral disorders. The psychiatrist achieves the specialty by completing a three-year residency after medical school and internship. After the residency and successful experience for two years, the candidate must pass an examination administered by the American Board of Psychiatry and Neurology to be certified as a psychiatrist. Some physicians practice as psychiatrists without completing the certification process.

The population served by the psychiatrist is similar to that served by the clinical psychologist, but the medical qualification of psychiatrists is a critical distinction. As seeking help with personal problems has become acceptable in our society, psychiatrists now have some patients with problems of living that might be dealt with by counselors. It is common to find psychiatrists treating many of these outpatients with the same methods and techniques that counselors would use.

Psychiatrists are usually considered a group apart from other medical doctors, as evidenced by the DOT introduction to the group Physicians and Surgeons, which states "Includes practitioners of medicine, psychiatry, and ophthalmology" (p. 52). Unlike members of other medical specialties, psychiatrists are seldom viewed simply as "doctors." Further potential for confusion exists because many equate psychiatry, and to a lesser degree all fields that offer assistance with social and emotional problems, with psychoanalysis. Gross (1978) has estimated that only one of seven psychiatrists is a psychoanalyst. The vast majority of psychoanalysts are physicians who have specialized training based on Sigmund Freud's theory of human behavior.

There are a few nonmedical psychiatrists who are called "lay analysts." The American Psychoanalytic Association has rigid requirements for the training of those who want to become members, including an extensive period of analysis for the trainee.

An occupational group which is dissimilar to the medical group in most ways but which also includes occupations in which counseling techniques are used is Personnel Administration Occupations. Included in this group are personnel manager, director of placement, and employment interviewer/recruiter. In the occupations of this group, many of the interviewing and counseling techniques used would be difficult to distinguish from those of the counselor. Many college and university placement directors have been placement counselors and consider counseling to be a vital aspect of their work.

College career-planning and placement counselor is one of four counseling specialties covered in the *Occupational Outlook Handbook*. A recent trend has been for placement officers to add the term *career planning* or *career development* to their names to indicate that they do more than just arrange placement interviews. Likewise, many interviewers in public employment offices consider themselves counselors because they have some duties like those of counselors.

Listed under the DOT occupational group Occupations in Social and Welfare Work are occupations in which counseling skills are vital. Social workers proper, sometimes called "caseworkers," have a well-defined professional structure. The social worker usually has an M.S.W., a two-year master's degree. The social worker takes more direct action than a counselor to alleviate or eliminate the client's problem because social workers tend to view the source of the problem as external to the client more often than do counselors. Despite recent trends for counselors to focus more on social and community factors, and for social workers to work more on developing the individual client's resources, the professions are different. The distinctions are heightened by regulations that reserve certain positions for those credentialed as social workers and others for counselors. Also part of the same occupational group are probation and parole officers and military human relations and drug and alcohol counselors. Persons trained as counselors hold many of these positions, and counselors hold positions in a variety of community human service agencies.

Many student personnel workers in higher education have graduate training in counseling. Occupations in college and university education that are closely related to counseling are foreign-student adviser, dean of students, financial aid officer, director of admissions, director of student affairs, and registrar. Those occupations, added to that of dean of students (assistant principal), listed under secondary education, demonstrate the numerous avenues open to the counselor education student who wants to work in an educational setting.

This brief discussion of occupations employing the same skills and techniques that a counselor uses, or similar ones, is not intended to be an adequate review of those occupations. It is an attempt to demonstrate the sometimes confusing fact that the use of similar techniques does not eliminate the occupational distinctions and to demonstrate, further, that a legitimate basis exists for maintaining that counseling is a separate and distinct occupation from the many to which it is related by virtue of shared goals and activities.

Diversities, Commonalities, and Opportunities

Some counselor education graduates gain initial employment in positions titled "counselor"; others enter related positions. Some of these related positions may require as much use of the skills of the counselor as other positions that are labeled "counselor," or even more. The distinction may be merely one of the title given the particular job.

It's Not Where We Do It

Some students gain initial positions that are not labeled "counselor" because they are not, in fact, counseling positions. One reason is the reality of a labor market in which seekers of counseling positions outnumber vacancies. An additional reason is that many people enter counselor preparation programs with the goal of entering related career fields in which counseling skills and techniques are useful, if not vital, to satisfactory performance.

It is not unusual to find students who want to be college student personnel workers of various types, students who want to work in a variety of community-based helping programs, and students who want to be school counselors in the same graduate department. In fact, most counselor education programs not only accept students with diverse goals but actively encourage diversity in students. The authors of this text are among those who believe counseling skills and techniques can be effectively used in a variety of work settings and applaud variety among counselor education students. We hope that many students who do not plan to, and who will not, enter positions labeled "counselor" will nevertheless come to view the philosophical basis, professional ethics, methods, techniques, and outlook of counselors as their own.

It's the Way We Do It

Counselors believe the primary purpose of their services is developmental, as opposed to therapeutic or remedial. I believe that this single and relatively simple notion is the basis for distinguishing counseling as a profession from the many other occupational groups that offer assistance to individuals. The remaining chapters in Part 1 will explore the legal status of counseling as a profession and its ethics; additional sections will deal with some of the methods and techniques used by counselors and with the counselees we serve. All the following presentations are based on the idea that counselors are unique helping professionals and that counselor uniqueness is based on a developmental view of the helping services we offer.

Just what is a developmental view? Simply put, a developmental view is that all individuals are faced with certain tasks, challenges, or issues to be resolved as they progress through the life span. These challenges were called developmental tasks by Robert Havighurst (1972), who defined a developmental task as

> a task which arises at or about a certain period in the life of the individual, successful achievement of which leads to his happiness and to success with later tasks while failure leads to unhappiness in the individual, disapproval by the society, and difficulty with later tasks [p. 2].

The counselor does not view the need for assistance in mastering these developmental tasks as a disorder to be treated or cured. The counselor recognizes that individuals will differ in which, if any, of the developmental tasks or challenges will prove difficult but rejects the notion that seeking to learn the skills necessary to master the task is a sign of disorder.

To put the concept in even simpler terms, counselors do not believe there is anything fundamentally wrong with their counselees that the counselor will put right. Although it is true that the goals and objectives of an elementary school counselor will differ from those of a rehabilitation counselor, both are concerned about enabling their counselees to use their present resources and to develop new resources to live more productively and effectively in their environment.

The governing board of the American School Counselors Association (1979, p. 11) has approved a definition of *developmental guidance* that I believe could be used as a definition of *developmental counseling*.

> Developmental guidance is that component of all guidance efforts which fosters planned intervention within educational and other human services programs at all points in the human life cycle to vigorously stimulate and actively facilitate the total development of individuals in all areas, i.e. personal, social, emotional, career, moral-ethical, cognitive, and aesthetic; and to promote the integration of the several components into an individual life style.

If the term *counseling* is substituted for the term *guidance* in the ASCA definition, we see that developmental counseling requires the counselor to take a broad view of individuals and to be concerned about all aspects of their lives, not just education or career. Likewise, the concept of programs suggests that the developmental counselor—and the authors of this text believe that professional counselors are developmental counselors—does more than just sit and wait for those who are experiencing difficulty coping with life to ask for assistance. Counselors must be active in determining the needs of the client population they serve and developing programs to meet those needs. We further recognize that one of our tasks may be to encourage our potential counselees to take advantage of the programs and services we offer.

Starting from a developmental perspective means that although the counselor is not a specialist in disorder or deviance, counselors know the challenges typical of the life stage of their counselees. While we recognize that instances exist in which counselors' work is difficult to distinguish from that of their professional colleagues who focus more on disorder than development, we believe the distinction between perspectives to be a critical starting point.

In addition to having a developmental perspective, counselors focus on the counselee as the primary recipient of their services. The authors of this text recognize that counselors are members of a society that has many ills, and we further recognize that counselors are in a unique position to see the results of poverty, deprivation, and discrimination in all its ugly forms. We believe that the individuals we serve have the first claim on our professional time and energy.

As concerned citizens with a unique professional obligation, we should work for the removal of any obstacle to human development, but we must be committed to our counselees. The counselor will often face the dilemma of whether to invest time on causes or results, and no simple answer can be offered. However, we suggest the counselees to be served as an organizing point for the professional counselor's activities. This point of view will mean that the counselor views the counselee as a responsible person and that although conditions and circumstances may present barriers and obstacles, the counselor believes counselees have the potential for productive behavior to reduce the limiting effect of those barriers.

The developmental perspective means that counselors view education—education in its best and broadest sense, learning living skills—as a vital part of counseling. Counselors have for too long been apologetic about the connection of many counselor training programs with schools and/or departments of education. While we recognize that schools are only one setting in which counseling occurs, we suggest that counselee education and reeducation is a vital part of the counseling endeavor regardless of the setting.

We need only survey the literature of professional associations of counselors to see how often the terms *education* and *training* are mentioned. Assertiveness training, training groups, career education, values education, and relaxation training are some prominent examples. Developmental counselors recognize that education is a vital part of their enterprise and work to develop the skills necessary to teach their counselees skills to live more effectively.

The importance of career or occupation in the lives of counselees is another concept endorsed by counselors. Despite the heritage of counseling, with its historical ties to the vocational guidance movement, not all counselors consider themselves career counselors. However, from the elementary school counselor who assists elementary school teachers to enhance children's career awareness to the rehabilitation counselor who recognizes that vocational restoration may be more important to the self-concept of the disabled than physical treatment, counselors recognize that the concept of productive work is a vital part of their counselees' lives.

Last in this brief consideration of the attributes of the professional counselor is the concept of an eclectic approach to methods and techniques. Abraham Maslow is given credit for the observation "If the only tool you have is a hammer, you tend to see every problem as a nail." Because counselors are dedicated to seeing their counselees as unique individuals, they cannot be limited to one approach or technique.

In the chapter on counseling research, you will learn that one function of counseling research is to determine what counseling methods and techniques work best for different counselees. As Robert Carkhuff (1966) established in his proposal for a systematic eclectic stance, to be eclectic does not mean to have no system or to attempt to help others by a trial-and-error approach; rather, it means not to define counselee concerns in terms of one way of viewing problems. Likewise, Blocher (1974) has proposed a systematic eclectic model of developmental counseling. The professional counselor systematically chooses helping techniques on the basis of counselees' resolution of the problems they face.

Who Needs Us

To determine where counselors work and the employment outlook for counselors, you are encouraged to review the most recent material available, because changes in social priorities and the labor market can make our material misleading although it is not chronologically obsolete. Because you will be encouraged to undertake some personally relevant research in a following section, detailed statistics related to the employment of counselors are not included here.

Two cautions must be noted about the statistics on the current employment of counselors. First, as I have tried to show throughout the previous section, not all counselors have jobs that carry the title *counselor,* and to view career opportunities as being limited to those jobs and even to those mentioned would be a narrow perspective. Second, you should remember that opportunities for employment come both from expansion of the career field and from replacement positions. Replacement positions are those that become available owing to death, disability, retirement, promotion, and the other reasons that can cause an existing position to become vacant. Despite well-publicized data on the impact of the stabilizing and declining birth rate on schools and the employment outlook in schools, there are opportunities. To determine opportunities, one must study the characteristics of persons who have existing positions as well as the potential for new positions.

The information in the *Occupational Outlook Handbook,* coupled with estimates by Shertzer and Stone (1981), provides a basis for the following capsule of where counselors work. Most counselors work in educational settings. Approximately 54,000 counselors are employed in schools K–12. Of those, over 35,000 are in secondary schools, with middle and elementary schools combined having about half the number of counselors as secondary schools. Another 6000 counselors are in counseling centers of two- and four-year colleges and universities. Rehabilitation counselors number 19,000 and are the second largest group in occupations titled counselor. A closely related occupational field, that of corrections, which many consider to be a specialized type of rehabilitation, is estimated by Shertzer and Stone to have 15,000 counselors. Employment services, both publicly supported employment offices and private agencies, have about 6000 counselors.

These data represent the easily visible part of the counseling iceberg; whether the easily visible part is the tip or some larger part is a matter of perspective. Counseling job opportunities exist in community agencies of various kinds, but we have no clear picture of how many such jobs exist, and we know uniform hiring regulations do not exist.

Private practice is another career option for counselors. The number of counselors currently in private practice as a primary source of income is difficult to estimate, since it is a relatively new and rapidly growing trend. An increasing number of counselors are extending their formal training beyond the master's degree program for the express purpose of entering private practice. A variety of factors has contributed to this movement. The most prominent among them may be the changes that have occurred in state professional licensure laws regulating private practice by counselors. The recent enactment of such laws reflects higher standards of quality in professional preparation provided by programs of counselor education. Further, recent changes in state regulations allow payment for certain counseling services by third parties—insurance companies and health plans. However, the issue of what types of psychological helping services, if any, may be provided by persons other than physicians is a current subject of legal and insurance regulatory agency dispute in most states.

Similarly, we can make no good estimate of the number of professional counselors whose counseling careers are being sought in business and industry. However, we know that a growing number of students are identifying business and industry as career goals, either directly in that work setting or as members of consulting firms that handle the employee assistance programs for business and industry.

Another major source of employment opportunity for professional counselors is in college student personnel. For example, the *Occupational Outlook Handbook* does indicate that 3800 people are employed as career planning and placement counselors. The number of deans, registrars, activities directors, housing directors, foreign-student advisers, financial aid officers, and admissions recruiters is many times that number.

People do work as counselors in a variety of settings and with a variety of job titles. Many who do not have the title *counselor* will in fact see themselves as, and be, counselors because they subscribe to the ethical and philosophical bases of counseling in addition to using the methods and techniques of counselors.

Perspectives for the '80s

To this point we have explored the current status of counseling. We have considered how counselors are defined, their professional status, related professions, where counselors now work, and what they do. One way to view the 1980s would be to examine changes that might occur in each of these areas. Many of those specific projections for the profession are included in the "perspectives" section of the following chapters. What is attempted here is a perspective on the context in which counselors will work during the next decade. We will face issues of professional status, licensure, and program funding, but those issues and others will be faced in a decade of social change.

The focus of the role and functions of the counselor in the 1980s will remain unchanged. It will continue to be *the assistance of individuals* in accomplishing those developmental tasks appropriate to their life stages so that they can become concerned, mature, and contributing members of society. How effectively we provide this assistance in the '80s will be determined by our responsiveness to societal change.

Responsiveness to change always has required, and always will require, open-mindedness. A prerequisite to prognostications about the future is a critical analysis of the status quo. Unless we are willing to take a long, hard look at the way things really are instead of how we would like them to be, we will never abandon our old, familiar ways of doing things and adopt new, creatively effective interpretations of our functions. Rather, we must be able to understand, and willing to accept, the signs of the times.

Societal change is rooted in economic, legal, technological, and philosophical concerns. These influences are all prominent in the attempt to critically analyze today's status quo and are reflected in the recommendations made by the writers of the chapters that follow for the counselor of the 1980s.

For example, a realistic assessment of the status quo requires an acknowledgment that the present generation of young people is the first in our history who will have less than their parents had. Our position as a world power has diminished, and our economic future has been placed in jeopardy by spiraling inflation and continuing recession. The earliest public reaction to these circumstances was to look out for one's own self and to let everyone else do the same. Quite clearly, this response did not solve the problem.

Now, there is a heightened awareness of the need to give up the self-absorption that characterized the "me" generation and become instead a "we" generation. With the realization of restricted economic opportunity came an increased desire to control the forces that shape our lives. We are beginning to realize that we cannot shape our own lives unless we can control the forces that shape them. We have developed a sense of urgency to work collectively for the common good. We are learning that "looking out for Number One won't work" but that "we can make a difference" (Terry, 1980a).

Evidence for these observations can be found in almost all segments of society. Educators no longer dictate what the schools shall do or how they shall do it. School boards have been forced by taxpayer groups to reduce their budgets. Members of Congress have not been returned to their seats in the House and the Senate because they did not respond to well-organized lobbying efforts of their constituencies. The passage of Proposition 13 in California reverberated all the way to Capitol Hill.

Students no longer hold demonstrations and carry placards on campuses; they are conducting organized lobbies on both the state and federal levels for budget cutting, nuclear power, ecology, solar energy, and almost all other issues associated with the quality of life. There is a growing concern with society and how it relates directly to all its members (Terry, 1980a). The "me first" movement has been expanded, and the question has become "How does this affect me, my neighbor, the world we live in, and the future we face?" (Terry, 1980b).

These observations of the status quo seem too imply that our counselees of the '80s will have an evolving set of needs. Counselors of the '80s will need, not a different repertoire of skills, but a different interpretation of their skill repertoire. For example:

> If our counselees are concerned with the quality of life and how it relates to all members of society, then the concerns they bring to us will be a need to learn how to understand *others* and how to relate more effectively *to others*.

Put another way, their primary concern will be a concern not only with self-exploration but also of self in relation to others.

> If our counselees are concerned to control *the forces* that shape their lives, then counselors of the '80s will need to provide not only individual counseling services but also group opportunities for their clients to learn how to organize and manage groups and how to become effective change agents.

Implied here is the need for us to "give our skills away." We must educate others about group dynamics and group leadership.

CHAPTER 1 PROFESSIONAL IDENTITY: CRISIS OR CHALLENGE   23

If our counselees are concerned with their economic future, then counselors of the '80s will have to learn how to serve our counselees more "cost effectively" and how to "prove versus sell" the worth of our services.

We will discover new methods of delivering our services, and we will be delivering them from a variety of settings: schools, colleges and universities, community agencies, mental-health centers, private practice, business and industry. Our career options will be greater than ever before, and our presence in society will be more prominent than at any other period of our professional development, because we will be more competently trained. But regardless of the setting in which we choose to develop our career goal, our objectives will be the same, because a counselor is a counselor, not a setting.

It is the view of the writers of this text that the 1980s pose not only a challenge for society but a challenge for the professional counselor. When a society tightens its belt, not only the purse strings come closer together; the people do, too. And when people discover how to work cooperatively with one another, they usually find ways of excluding those who will not. After almost two decades of helping others understand and appreciate their own individuality, some counselors will find the decade of the '80s an impossible adjustment. But professionally committed, competent, and open-minded counselors of the '80s will be able to help their counselees learn how to express their sense of community and still retain their individuality.

Summary

Individuals and occupational groups that use the title *counselor* are not scarce. Students embarking on a graduate program to prepare for a career as a counselor will properly ask how the career they are preparing to enter is distinct from the many others that use the title *counselor*. A similar but perhaps more difficult question is how a counselor differs from the other helping professionals who use many similar methods and techniques. Counselors are recognized by the federal government as a distinct occupational group in the *Dictionary of Occupational Titles* and the *Occupational Outlook Handbook*. Counselors are certainly legitimately called professionals when they are evaluated on the basis of characteristics attributed to professions. The term *professional counselor* has a legitimate meaning, and professional counselors are those engaged in the full-time occupation of counseling, who have completed a graduate training program in counseling, and who follow the ethical codes of counseling. Likewise, professional counselors can be distinguished from other helping professionals by their adherence to a developmental approach to helping.

The developmental approach, together with counselor focus on the counselee, recognition of counselee learning, recognition of the importance of work, and an eclectic approach to methods, provides a further basis for that distinction. Many students in counselor preparation programs do not plan to enter positions that have the title *counselor*. Of those who seek counseling positions, some will find initial jobs in closely related occupations in which all or part of their work may be counseling but which have other occupational titles.

Now It's Your Turn

The following activities are suggested as means for the counselor education student to begin the process of developing a professional identity.

1. What job do you hope to get after finishing your counselor preparation program? Find that job in the *Dictionary of Occupational Titles* (DOT) and *Occupational Outlook Handbook* (OOH). Any surprises?
2. Review as many counseling-related jobs in the DOT and OOH as you can find. Do any of them have more appeal to you than the one you selected as your top choice?
3. What are your chances of getting the job you want? What will you need to do to have a reasonable chance to find the job you want? If you don't get your first choice, what are your alternatives?
4. Have you spent some time with and observed the daily activities of a person with a job similar to that you are seeking? If not, ask your instructor to help you arrange such an experience.
5. Make the best one-page case you can for the idea that a counselor is a professional.
6. Can you distinguish among counseling, psychology, and social work? If not, review the DOT and OOH.
7. One of your friends says "I think you are trying to psychoanalyze me; I don't need my head shrunk." What would you want your response to communicate to that friend?
8. How would the following define or describe a counselor?
   a. A psychologist
   b. A social worker
   c. A counselee
   d. An agency or school board member
   e. A person on the street

References

American School Counselor Association. Position statement on developmental guidance. Approved by American School Counselor Association (ASCA) governing board December 1978. Published in ASCA *Newsletter,* April 1, 1979.

Blocher, D. H. *Developmental counseling* (2nd ed.). New York: Ronald Press, 1974.

Carkhuff, R. R. Counseling research, theory and practice—1965. *Journal of Counseling Psychology,* 1966, *13,* 467–479.

Dunlop, R. Counseling as a profession: Toward occupational maturity. *Focus on Guidance,* 1969, *2*(1), 1–10.

Greenwood, E. The elements of professionalization. In H. M. Vollmer & D. L. Mills (Eds.), *Professionalization.* Englewood Cliffs, N. J.: Prentice-Hall, 1966.

Gross, M. L. *The psychological society.* New York: Random House, 1978.

Havighurst, R. J. *Developmental tasks and education* (3rd ed.). New York: McKay, 1972.

McCully, C. H. The school counselor strategy for professionalization. *Personnel and Guidance Journal,* 1962, *40,* 681–689.

Moore, W. E. *The professions: Roles and rules.* New York: Russell Sage Foundation, 1970.

Ritchie, M. H. The professional status of counseling. Unpublished doctoral dissertation, University of Virginia, 1978.

Ruzek, S. Making social work accountable. In E. Freidson (Ed.), *The professions and their prospects.* Beverly Hills, Calif.: Sage Publications, 1973.

Shevlin, M. The "professionalization" of guidance counselor. In R. Dunlop (Ed.), *Professional problems in school counseling practice.* Scranton, Pa.: International Textbook, 1968.

Shertzer, B., & Stone, S. *Fundamentals of guidance* (4th ed.). Boston: Houghton Mifflin, 1981.

Terry, S. Did activism graduate with '60s? *The Christian Science Monitor,* January 15, 1980, p. 1.(a)

Terry, S. The new student activism from marches to memos. *The Christian Science Monitor,* January 16, 1980, p. 13.(b)

U.S. Bureau of Labor Statistics. *Occupational Outlook Handbook* (1978–79 Edition). Washington, D.C.: U.S. Government Printing Office, 1978.

U.S. Department of Labor. *Dictionary of Occupational Titles* (4th ed.). Washington, D.C.: U.S. Government Printing Office, 1977.

CHAPTER **2**

The Law and the Counselor

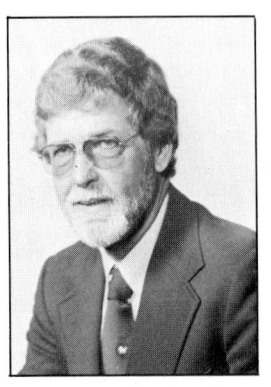

Carl D. Swanson

Carl Swanson is professor of psychology and coordinator of the counselor education program at James Madison University. He is an attorney and a member of the Virginia Board of Professional Counselors and the Virginia Behavioral Science Board. Dr. Swanson was the leading force in securing counselor licensure in Virginia and is a nationally recognized authority on legal matters affecting counselors.

The profession of counseling has developed from humble beginnings in vocational guidance to a multidisciplined profession having a generic body of knowledge and skills and many subspecialties. The need for unique services not offered by other professions has resulted in movement to fields such as rehabilitation, substance abuse, marriage and family counseling, and mental-health counseling.

The struggle for legal recognition and status has been waged in the courts and legislatures, resulting in a legal definition of counseling, privileged communication statutes for counselors, and professional licensing. With increased identity, recognition, and status, responsibilities to both clients and the public have also increased. Counselors are no longer "mere teachers" (as one court described them) with few professional responsibilities but are now professionals who are expected to exercise a high degree of care and provide competent, professional service.

The following sections show the development of the profession from the standpoint of emerging ethical standards and their relation to federal and state statutory, administrative, and case law. Statutory laws are those acts (codes) passed by a legislative body (U. S. Congress or a state legislature) and duly signed into law by the chief executive (U. S. president or a state governor). Administrative law is that body of regulations promulgated by agencies duly constituted and empowered by federal and state statute. Case law consists of all cases decided by the courts (U. S. or state), constituting a body of law that gives precedents for future cases.

No longer are counselors immune from ethical standards, statutes, or administrative and case law once thought applicable only to psychiatrists, attorneys, psychologists, or other professions of long standing. In fact, a recent computer (LEXIS) search, by the author, for a five-year period (covering only federal courts) found counselors involved in 298 lawsuits.

Standards have changed for counselors, and the prudent professional will become aware of statutory, administrative, and case law and professional ethical standards. The counselor is under an obligation to protect the public and deliver consistently high-quality services.

An Emerging Profession

Counseling is often described as a rapidly emerging profession but one having identity problems both legally and with the public. Great strides have been made from the early seventies to the present. One aspect of this professionalization has been the advent of certifying and licensing boards, such as the National Academy of Certified Clinical Mental Health Counselors ("American Mental Health Counselors Association . . .," 1979), Commission on Rehabilitation Counselor Certification (McAlees & Schumacher, 1975), Virginia Board of Professional Counselors (*Code of Virginia,* 1976), the Arkansas Counselor Licensing Board ("Arkansas to License Counselors," 1979), Alabama Counselor Licensing Board ("Alabama Licensing Approved," 1979), and certifying agencies within state departments of education (Woellner, 1981).

There are many forms of professional credentialing and regulation. School counselors are either certified or licensed by the state's department of education for practice only within the school systems. National certification by professional associations only recognizes an individual's qualifications and does not entitle the person so certified to practice. Examples are the Certified Clinical Mental Health Counselor and the Certified Rehabilitation Counselor. The states (*Code of Virginia,* 1979) themselves regulate or credential professionals, usually by means of one of the following:

1. *Inspection,* the lowest form of regulation. A state agency periodically examines the activities of a profession's practitioners to ascertain whether they are practicing the profession in a fashion consistent with the public safety, health, and welfare.
2. *Registration.* A practitioner of a profession may be required to submit information concerning the nature, location, and operation of his or her practice.
3. *Certification.* A state board or department issues a certificate to a person certifying that he or she has minimum skills to properly engage in his or her profession and that it knows of no character defect that would interfere with professional practice.
4. *Licensure,* the highest form of credentialing, includes the provisions of (3) and also means that the practice of the profession is unlawful without the issuance of a license. This is also known as "title protection."

Counseling as a profession was not always recognized as an entity on its own, as seen in an early court case. A college counselor was sued for "wrongful death" of a client who committed suicide. The judge, in ruling for the defendant, described counselors, here one with a doctoral degree (Ed.D.), as "mere teachers" who received training in education departments (*Bogust v. Iverson,* 1960). As a result, the same professional standards could not be applied to the counselor as would be applied to psychiatrists. Even within schools it was obvious that counselors did not have the same professional status or identity as school psychologists, nurses, or physicians. (Counselors took lunchroom, hall, recess, and even bathroom duty along with teachers.)

For legal status and professional recognition and identity, counseling needed to be defined. By 1977 counseling "had moved from the relative security (and to some, obscurity) of vocational and educational information giving and student record keeping to personal counseling, individually and in groups" (Swanson & Van Hoose, 1977) in a wide variety of areas ranging from rehabilitation (McAlees & Schumacher, 1975) to marriage and family counseling (Nichols, 1974).

Beginning in 1971, a new, emerging role was foreseen for counselors. An *Iowa Law Review Note* saw the counselor's function expanded and redefined from that of educational/vocational counseling to personal-problem counseling. The "Note" pointed out the importance of counselors (in schools) as "sources of aid for students with personal problems." This article, which argued for privileged communication for school counselors, thrust the profession into the 1970s.

Counseling received further definition in 1974 from another legal source. In *Weldon v. Virginia State Board of Psychologists Examiners* it was held that counseling constituted a separate and distinct profession. The Board of Psychologists Examiners sought an injunction against John Weldon to prohibit his continued practice as a counselor. He had attempted to become licensed as a psychologist but was rejected on the grounds that he was a counselor. The board held, and the judge affirmed, that he needed such a license, as he used the "tools of psychology." He was therefore enjoined from further practice, creating quite a dilemma for other counselors who wished to practice privately. Judge Smith's opinion, however, further stated: "The profession of personnel and guidance counseling is a separate profession [from psychology] and should be so recognized."

The United States House of Representatives was the next legal entity to further define and recognize counseling as a profession. H. R. 3270 (94th Congress, 1976) held counseling to be "the process through which a trained counselor assists an individual or group to make satisfactory and responsible decisions concerning personal, educational, and career development." In establishing a licensing board for professional counselors, the *Code of Virginia* (1976) defined counseling as "assisting an individual through the counseling relationship, to develop understanding of personal problems, to define goals, and to plan action reflecting his [client's] interest, abilities, aptitudes, and needs as these are related to educational progress, occupations and careers, and personal-social concerns." The act further provided for counselors to engage in appraisal activities, which "means selecting, administering, scoring, and interpreting instruments designed to assess an individual's aptitudes, attitudes, abilities, achievements and interests." Finally, the Virginia act (1976) saw counseling as a generic profession, having included within the generic body of knowledge and skills subspecialties requiring additional and/or specialized training. The specialty areas set forth included, but were not limited to, the following: marriage and family counselor, career counselor, pastoral counselor, substance-abuse (alcohol and drug) counselor, research counselor, and rehabilitation counselor. This gave additional breadth and depth to the profession. Alabama, Florida, Arkansas, Texas, and California, as well as Virginia, provide for the licensure of counselors. In addition, at least seven states license marriage and family counselors.

Another step in professionalization and the defining of counseling (with increasing legal responsibility and higher standards of care) has been the adoption of ethical standards or codes of ethics. The American Personnel and Guidance Association, the American School Counselors Association, the National Academy of Certified Clinical Mental Health Counselors, and the Virginia Board of Professional Counselors (1976) have all adopted these professional ethical guidelines. The legal implications will be seen in the following section.

A final step in the identity and professionalization of counselors came with the adoption and implementation of minimal standards of preparation for professional counselors. Representative of these are the "Standards for the Preparation of Counselors" (1977), Qualifications for Licensure of Professional Counselors (Virginia Board of Professional Counselors, 1976), and Standards for Providers of Counseling Psychological Services (American Psychological Association, 1978). As an example, the Virginia

(1976) and AMHCA regulations provide for a graduate degree in counseling from an accredited university with at least 60 semester hours of completed study. Virginia also requires two years of postgraduate, full-time supervised experience under a supervisor deemed satisfactory by the board. The APA's standards for the counseling psychologist (American Psychological Association, 1978) require a doctoral degree from a program that is primarily psychological in nature and at least two years of appropriate professional experience.

Professional associations have also set national standards for the certification of counselors. Both the American Rehabilitation Counseling Association (McAlees & Schumacher, 1975) and the American Mental Health Counselors Association ("American Mental Health Counselors Association . . .," 1979) have set such standards. A national registry of clinical mental-health counselors has been released by the National Academy of Certified Clinical Mental Health Counselors ("NACCMHC News," 1979). APGA has now established a National Board for Certified Counselors (NBCC). The standards for certification thereunder will be comparable to existing standards.

It appears that a minimum graduate program for professional counselors is moving to the 60-hour credit level plus supervised experience. This is quite a dramatic shift from some guidance programs of the 60s which required only nine credit hours in counseling. As early as 1976 the Counseling Students Association (1976) urged the New York State Board of Regents to "expand all existing graduate programs throughout the state in guidance and counseling to sixty credit hours . . . leading to the Master of Education degree." It would also appear that at least 60 graduate credit hours in counseling are needed to fully meet the "Standards for the Preparation of Counselors" (1977). To further strengthen the profession, greater uniformity in training throughout the nation is needed, which, it is hoped, will result from NBCC standards.

In spite of gains made toward professionalization of counselors and other mental-health service providers, even a long-established profession —psychology—runs into serious challenges in the area of professional training and identity. A federal judge in the *Berger* (1975) case ruled in favor of a plaintiff (who had a degree in accounting!), ordering the Board of Psychologists Examiners to administer an examination. The judge felt that the plaintiff might well be as qualified as one with a psychology degree and that he should be given the opportunity for an examination by the board. The language used by the judge was most significant: "But the very reason psychology has not been regulated before [in the District of Columbia] is that it has been and remains an amorphous, inexact, and even mysterious discipline. Possession of a graduate degree in psychology does not signify the absorption of a corpus of knowledge as does a medical, engineering or law degree. . . ."

In light of the *Berger* case it appears that graduate credit hours alone are insufficient. Accordingly, supervised postgraduate experience and the further development of competency-based examinations (American Institutes for Research, 1979) are rapidly becoming a part of the professionalization and training of counselors.

Because counseling is still looked on by some as only a segment of the guidance function, further efforts in professionalization are required. Identity problems still exist throughout the profession, as an article in the *APA Monitor* (Asher & Asher, 1978) illustrates. Therein a counseling psychologist parodied (tongue-in-cheek?) some stereotypes, claiming counseling psychology wanted to be neither "*fish* (fish are clinical psychologists; they are cold fish who believe in the medical model . . .) nor *foul* (foul are counselor educators or guidance and counseling graduates; they stink. They are not too bright and were ill-trained in ridiculously easy education departments where they took such rinky-dink courses as Pupil Personnel III: The Counselor's Bulletin Board. They try to pass as counseling psychologists . . .)."

Work is still ahead in the professionalization process as long as such images exist. However, on the other side of the coin, counselors (four subspecialties thereof) were recognized as "other allied health professionals" in the report of the President's Commission on Mental Health ("Mental Health Commission . . . ," 1979).

The Counselor and the Law: Ethical Standards

The development of ethical standards by and for a group is needed for professional status, as explained in Chapter 3. It gives the members a standard of professional conduct while further defining the profession. This is another step in obtaining legal status and sanction.

Standards or codes of ethics are designed to protect the public and also to give guidelines to the practitioner so that difficulty with the law may be avoided by the person who follows the profession's code (Swanson & Van Hoose, 1977).

Some professional organizations have procedures for handling violations of their ethical codes, such as state bar associations and the American Psychological Association. So far the American Personnel and Guidance Association (APGA) and other professional counselors' associations have not established procedures for implementing their codes. The Virginia Counselors Association (a branch of APGA) is an exception, as seen in Appendix C.

The courts have recognized for the past 35 years that there is not a complete body of law that explicitly applies to all actions of professional practitioners. Therefore, in legal actions the profession's own code of ethics *may* be introduced to aid the court in coming to a decision in a particular case. The professional standards, though not incorporated into the law, at least serve as quasi-legal guidelines governing professional services or conduct (*Cherry v. Board of Regents*, 1942). This use of professional groups' codes of ethics increases the level of responsibility and standard of care for the professional, together with the large body of statutory and common law. The professional counselor is faced with a grave responsibility in offering mental-health services to clients.

Statutory Law—Acts of the Legislature

The body of statutory law will be examined in the following sections. Owing to the breadth of the field, representative examples will be given. Further study is recommended not only because today's law is complex, but also because many cases are arising. For example, the Virginia Board of Behavioral Science (1979) reviewed more than 35 ethical charges brought during 1978 against psychologists, social workers, and counselors in the Commonwealth of Virginia alone.

Privileged Communication Statutes

The counselee's civil liberties and the counselor's obligation to keep confidences arising out of the counselor-client relationship go hand in hand. Confidentiality, under the law, demands that information resulting from that relationship be kept in confidence. Even in court the duty still exists to exhaust all avenues short of contempt, under the rules of evidence, in maintaining the confidence.

"The major threats to a counselee's civil liberties are most likely to arise when a counselor works both for his client and for an organization . . . too often counselors are really tools for administrators" (Ladd, 1971, pp. 262–263). "Counselors have an ethical obligation to help their clients understand the legal constraints under which they, the counselors, work and the limits of the confidential relationship that exists between them" (Stude & McKelvey, 1979, p. 455).

As such importance has been put on the confidential nature of the counseling relationship as a means of protecting civil liberties and enhancing the therapeutic effects of that relationship, at least 14 states have enacted privileged communication statutes for school and some college counselors. Virginia legislation (1982) grants privilege of communication to "licensed professional counselors, clinical social workers and psychologists." It is surely the intent of the client sharing problems with the counselor that the communication remain confidential.

The case for statutes providing privileged communication for counselors was well stated by a law-review article (1971): "In order for counselors to fully realize their potential for benefitting students with personal problems, there must be a free flow of communications between the student and counselor . . . A testimonial privilege in this situation may substantially diminish [these] inhibitions by prohibiting disclosure of personal, privileged communications in court." The privilege statute also strengthens the confidential nature of the counselor/counselee relationship. Privileged communication statutes have been passed because of the value to society of "full and complete disclosure by the client, penitent, patient . . . if the client knows that what he says will be kept secret, it is expected that he will speak more freely. The professional is then able to render better assistance following full disclosure by the client, and as a result, it is argued, society benefits" (Comment, 1974).

A statute typical of those 14 states' acts giving privileged communication to school counselors is the South Dakota law (*South Dakota Laws, 1972*):

> No counselor certificated in accordance with the certification regulations of the state board of education and regularly employed as a counselor for a private or public elementary or secondary school or school system in the State of South Dakota, may divulge to any other person, or be examined concerning any information or communication given to him in his official capacity by a student, unless: (1) This privilege is waived in writing by the student; or (2) The information or communication was made to the counselor for the express purpose of being communicated or of being made public.

The 1974 amendments to this act provided for another exception: "(3) If a counselor has reason to suspect, as a result of that information or communication, that the student has been subjected to child abuse or that the student's physical or mental health may be in jeopardy." This is an excellent statute, as it protects the client in prohibiting the counselor from divulging any information received from the client, subject to the exceptions. It further protects the counselor from having to testify in court but, at the same time, protects the public from such ills as drug use or child abuse.

It may be noted that rehabilitation and/or marriage and family counselors have the privilege in 5 states, whereas 35 states give this privilege to psychologists (Nichols, 1974). (For further discussion see 23 *Maine L. Rev.* 443, 450, and 56 *Iowa L. Rev.* 1344, 1351.) Where obtained, privileged communication statutes raise the professional and legal status of counselors.

Other Statutes

Most states have other laws that directly affect a counselor's practice. They were passed to protect the public or some significant segment thereof. Counselors must be aware of their legal responsibilities under rights of minors acts, freedom of information acts, and privacy protection acts, which are part of the codes of most states. Of course, there are also numerous federal laws the counselor must adhere to, such as the "Buckley

IT'S MY AX AND I'LL GRIND IT

A few years ago I wouldn't have been as honest about my master's degree program, but now I can tell you straight out. One year isn't enough! It doesn't train counselors for the jobs they go after. As a result our profession is the subject of more "badmouthing" than almost any other. What's the cure? More training!

Now, I'm not making a pitch for doctoral programs. I'm saying that counselor educators had better start providing two years of professional preparation in their master's program or you counselors-in-training had better start requiring it of yourselves. If you don't, then you will graduate, like all the rest of us, with the mistaken idea that you are capable of more than you really are. And you, along with our profession, will go farther down the drain.

And another thing, how did everybody get brainwashed into believing that doing therapy, getting licensed, and helping sick people is the only really important work for counselors? That isn't the top of the heap. It's more like the pits. First of all, professional counselors are trained for, and dedicated to prevention and development. *The ultimate goal of our profession is to wipe out the need for clinical services.*

Maybe we won't ever reach our goal—100%—but what's wrong with reaching for it? It's better than pretending to be able to do things we were never trained to do. So stand tall and take pride in your career goals as a developmental counselor, because you will be doing work your training prepared you to do. And remember, if you hang in there, you'll put the clinicians out of business.

Where do I get off taking all these potshots? I'm the product of a couple of counselor education departments and two degree preference programs. As a professional practitioner, my practice preference is prevention and development. My experience includes schools, colleges, agencies, government, and private-sector personnel establishments. I think I'm dry behind the ears, and so maybe I've earned the right to bend yours.

There's an enormous need for your services but too little funding to support you. Because your product is too invisible or confidentiality-bound to earn you much appreciation, you've got to learn to accept such occupational hazards gracefully. Complaining will only increase your frustration. It's counterproductive, so use your program of services, design accountability methods and procedures, and increase your own education and professional skills.

Your job won't be an easy one, but I'll bet you never know a more gratifying one.

—A Concerned Counselor

Amendment," the Developmental Disabilities Assistance and Bill of Rights Act of 1978, the Education for All Handicapped Children Act, known as P.L. 94–142, and the Federal Privacy Protection Act.

An example demonstrating the need for counselors to be aware of laws that may affect the conduct of their practice is a rights of minors act (*Code of Virginia,* 1977). This act (statutory law), typical of most, reads:

> A minor shall be deemed an adult for the purpose of consenting to:
> a. Medical or health services needed to determine the presence of or to treat venereal disease or any infections or contagious disease which the State Board of Health requires to be reported.
> b. Medical or health services required in case of birth control, pregnancy or family planning. . . .
> c. Medical or health services needed in the case of outpatient care, treatment or rehabilitation for substance abuse. . . .
> d. Medical or health services needed in the case of outpatient care, treatment or rehabilitation for mental or emotional illness.

It is obvious that counselors hereunder have a duty to keep information in these areas confidential, including withholding such knowledge from parents, which changes the old dictum of informing parents and obtaining their consent (Gottesman, 1975).

Rights of privacy acts are for the purpose of protecting the individual and maintaining the sanctity and accuracy of records. Probably the best known of these statutes is the Family Educational Rights and Privacy Act of 1974, known as the "Buckley Amendment." This act gives parents the right to inspect and review all official records, files, and data directly related to their children and, probably more important, gives parents

> an opportunity for a hearing to challenge the content of their child's school records, to insure that the records are not inaccurate, misleading or otherwise in violation of the privacy or other rights of students, and to provide an opportunity for the correction or deletion of any such inaccurate, misleading, or otherwise inappropriate data contained therein.

Other state and federal privacy protection and freedom of information acts do much the same, extending these rights to records of other government agencies in addition to the schools.

Recordkeeping is now under close scrutiny. The professional is well advised to enter only necessary data and put all comments in behavioral terminology. Moreover, it is clear that material arising from a counseling relationship should be released only with the express consent of the counselee. The contents of records may be challenged as well as inspected, imposing a duty to avoid any statements that may be defamatory (*Lopez v. Williams,* 1973).

Special acts dealing with specific populations must also be considered in the practice of counseling. An example is the Education for All Handicapped Children Act of 1975 (P.L. 94-142). An excellent, thorough publication discussing this legislation is entitled "The Public Law Supporting Mainstreaming" (1977). P.L. 94-142 has broad implications

(Humes, 1978) for school counselors, based on the act's major provisions, which include the following:

1. *Free, appropriate public education* is required for all children.
2. To the maximum degree possible, handicapped children are to be placed in the *least restrictive environment.*
3. An *individual education plan* (IEP) must be developed for each handicapped child and reviewed annually.
4. *Due-process procedures* are required, giving parents the right to challenge decisions made by the school team.
5. *Identification and recordkeeping* for the handicapped child are required.

Several authors, including Humes (1978), Henchert and Krouse (1979), Kameen and Parker (1979), and Noble and Kampwirth (1979), seem to agree that counselors could play a major role in the implementation of P.L. 94–142. Most agree that counselors should participate in team meetings, development of the IEP, monitoring progress, parental counseling, extracurricular planning, classroom consulting, in-service training, and recordkeeping. The resulting challenge seems to be twofold: (1) assuming extra duties under P.L. 94–142 while still handling the other responsibilities inherent to the counselor's office, and (2) securing additional funds for more counselors; here there will be plenty of competition for a limited number of dollars by school psychologists, special-education professionals, and other specialists. For a complete discussion of counseling handicapped persons see the December, 1979 *Personnel and Guidance Journal.*

Child-abuse laws and reporting statutes have developed across the nation to protect children. First, criminal and neglect statutes developed that made it illegal to "inflict cruelty on children" or to "contribute to the neglect of children." Both kinds of statutes were hard to enforce because few persons wanted to report criminal activity of their neighbors and because the neglect statutes were vague. Second, reporting statutes have arisen to supplement the criminal and neglect laws. The objective of these statutes is to identify the abused child and make reporting mandatory. Most require teachers (or counselors), social workers, and doctors to file reports of suspected child abuse. Counselors should check the statutes of the state in which they practice to determine their coverage and extent of responsibility. An excellent discussion of children's legal rights is contained in Gottesman (1975).

The Common Case Law

It is clearly established in law that the counselor is expected to maintain the confidential nature of the counseling relationship. This is equally true for written and spoken material.

Confidentiality and Recordkeeping

Liability on the part of the counselor can arise when this confidentiality is broken, especially if any of the material happens to be defamatory. *Guidelines for the Collection, Maintenance, Dissemination, and Security of Student Records* (North Carolina, 1975) is available through most state education departments. For persons in private or agency settings, guidelines are found in ethical codes and regulations accompanying various rights of privacy acts.

A confidential relationship is not limited to the formal office setting but has been held to arise when one "occupies toward another such a position of advisor or counselor as reasonably to inspire confidence that he will act in good faith for the other's interest" (*Kahan v. Greenfield,* 1949). In order for confidentiality to arise, the relation need not be legal; it may be moral, social, domestic, or merely personal. Release of material deemed confidential can amount to invasion of privacy and a right by the client to sue for damages and, if defamatory as well, a right also to sue under libel and slander laws.

Exceptions to these rules are seen in the "qualified privilege" defense. Hereunder a counselor may be excused because of the social importance of the client's statements. Instances of this privilege may arise when a client is likely to do harm to self or another (*Tarasoff v. Regents,* 1976). The ethical standards for counselors also provide for this. Testimony given in courts is protected from libel and slander charges through the qualified privilege, unless negligence or intent to harm can be shown (Pedersen, 1974).

A counselor must make every reasonable attempt to safeguard the confidential relationship before releasing any information. Even if subpoenaed, the counselor must exhaust all arguments (short of being held in contempt and jailed) before testifying in court. An argument can be made that testimony is hearsay, that the worth of the testimony as proof would be minimal, and that it is in the interest of the public to protect confidential communication. It is clear that the societal reason for breaching the privacy right must be persuasive. A New Jersey court (*In re State,* 1972) held that "children are entitled to constitutional rights... The right of privacy must be preserved against the unmitigated zeal and 'insolence' of government officers at all levels."

The Good Faith Doctrine

"Good faith in the law means being faithful to one's duties or obligations consistent with the generally accepted sense of professional responsibility of one's profession" (*Good Faith Doctrine,* 1974). Good faith has been further defined (Elliott, 1978) as acting with good motives and intent, honestly, without fraud, deceit, or collusion while being faithful to one's professional duty. Counselors act in good faith, for example, when they notify parents of minor children whom they believe to be seriously ill even though this could normally breach the confidential relationship. Further, counselors should in no way take advantage of a client—for example, socially, sexually, or financially.

A trend today under the good faith doctrine is to require counselors to recognize their limitations as well as their skills. Walz and Benjamin (1977) urge counselors to provide professional service only within their competencies and to make referrals when a situation requires knowledge or skills that they do not have.

Malpractice has been seen as the opposite of acting in good faith. It has been defined as the failure to render proper service through ignorance or negligence, resulting in injury or loss to the client. What was acceptable practice in the 1960s may well be flagrant malpractice in the 1980s. Recent cases have held counselors liable for damages when bad advice was given. If a client relies on the advice of an "expert" and suffers damage as a result, recovery may be had in a civil action. The professional must not succumb to the temptation to be all things to all persons. A higher level of care is demanded as professional standards, training, and legal recognition develop. The counselor must look to tomorrow for standards of professional conduct. In all matters the counselor must act skillfully, avoid misleading a client, give only accurate information, and adhere to high personal and ethical standards to avoid being held negligent. Any person holding himself or herself out to the public as capable of rendering a service based on special training, expertise, or skill may be responsible in tort for failure to do so, even without having been negligent (Pedersen, 1974). The counselor is responsible today for acting skillfully and with due care in dealing with the public. This is a far cry from the *Bogust v. Iverson* (1960) case previously cited.

Constitutional Rights

Rights guaranteed by the First, Fourth, Fifth, and Fourteenth Amendments to the U. S. Constitution have been extended to students. In *Tinker v. Des Moines School District* (1969) the Supreme Court held: "It can hardly be argued that either students or teachers shed their constitutional rights to freedom of speech or expression at the schoolhouse gate."

It appears that minors and college students do not give up their right to due process and their safeguard against unreasonable search and seizure. However, the courts have been prone in this area to balance the common welfare with an individual's rights. One court held that the privacy rights of public school students must give way to an "overriding governmental interest in investigating a reasonable suspicion of illegal drug use" by students. The court, while permitting an incursion into a constitutionally protected area, however, added: "Rights . . . are no less precious because they are possessed by juveniles" (*In re State,* 1972). It is clear that the societal reason for breaching the privacy rights of a student must be persuasive.

The school or college is no longer an enclave outside the constitution. A 1972 federal case (*Lopez v. Williams,* 1973) affirmed the extension of constitutional rights to university students in stating: "Although university administrators once had an almost unrestricted power to deal with students under the theory of *in loco parentis,* it is now clear that constitutional restraints on authority apply on campuses of state supported educational institutions with fully as much sanction as on public streets and in public parks."

School and college administrators must now safeguard all rights of the individual. As an example, a student accused of cheating has full rights to due process of law within the school. The accused has the right to confront the witnesses, to counsel, to an open and fair hearing, and to appeal. This is a far cry from the days of *in loco parentis,* when the school or college was deemed to stand in the shoes of the parent. Counselors must be in the forefront of protecting the rights of students, as advocates if necessary.

Perspectives for the '80s

The issues of the legal status and professional recognition of counselors are being raised in the areas of ethics and of statutory licensing and certification and by the courts. The *Tarasoff* (1976) decision is the latest in a series of cases raising professional standards in the mental-health field. The court held:

> When a psychotherapist determines, or pursuant to the standards of his profession should determine, that his patient presents a serious danger of violence to another he incurs an obligation to use reasonable care to protect the intended victim against such danger, that discharge of such duty may require the therapist to take one or more of various steps.

In *Tarasoff* it is seen that the professional should have known what his client would do and that he then did not go far enough in his efforts to protect the victim. In this instance the psychologist had only informed the campus police. The court made it clear that the obligation to protect a patient's confidences must yield when a therapist determines, or should determine, that a patient presents a serious danger of violence to another person. This case clearly expands the professional mental-health practitioner's (including the counselor's) duty.

Even though there is controversy over professional credentialing, it is generally thought that professional licensing and national certification have raised the legal status of counselors. It appears that there is broad support for licensure among professional counselors (Sweeney & Witmer,

1977; Cottingham & Warner, 1978; Swanson, 1976). The American Mental Health Counselors Association is in the process of certifying clinical mental-health counselors ("American Mental Health Counselors Association...," 1979). These movements will have a tremendous impact on the training of counselors. Performance/competency-based training, increased supervision, and expanded counselor education programs should result (Stripling, 1978; Cottingham & Swanson, 1976). With an increasing emphasis on credentialing brought about by state mental-health regulation and Health, Education and Welfare proposals for national credentialing, the trainee must be more aware than ever before of various legal and professional requirements (Bradley, 1978; Swanson, 1979; Vogel, 1978). In fact, in October 1981 licensed professional counselors were recognized by Blue Cross/Blue Shield of Virginia as health service providers. It appears that standards are rising and that counselor education programs will no longer be referred to as "ridiculously easy... rinky-dink" (Asher & Asher, 1978).

As all these standards rise, counselors will have to be better informed about what is taking place in the legal field. It appears that professional responsibility will entail carrying liability insurance. Continued training for counselors after they are in the field appears to be coming rapidly. Many state bar associations already require such postgraduate training for members to renew their licenses.

The counselor is now a full-fledged professional but will still have to face identity problems and strive for greater legal recognition in many states, as in the securing of privileged communication statutes. Counselors will also have to reach out and include all types of counselors in their professional organizations. Strength will be found in this unity. The road ahead is bright, but there are still many rough spots that need smoothing.

Summary

This chapter examined the relationship between the counselor and the law. It was observed that changes in the counselor's professional preparation were accompanied by changes in the counselor's rights and responsibilities. The discussion of these changes included examples of legal judgments of court record relative to counselor behavior and liability. Various categories of professional credentialing were defined and the historical development of counseling professionalism was selectively reviewed.

Ethical standards as they influence the counselor's legal status were reviewed with reference to differing legal statutes operative on both state and federal levels. The discussion of common (case) law included observations about confidentiality, record keeping, and malpractice. Finally, constitutional amendments pertaining to counseling were identified and certain contemporary court decisions were cited as influential for the 1980s.

Now It's Your Turn

Questions

1. Licensure is title protection as well as "definition." What may the counselor call himself or herself? How is practice defined? Who may use what titles? What are the limitations in your state? (Check your state's department of professional regulation.)
2. Counselor/teachers have specific ethical responsibilities. What are these? Where are the ethical standards for counselors found?
3. How does the practice of counseling (generic, career, and so on) differ from that of the clinical social worker, school psychologist, and clinical psychologist? How does it differ from the work of a certified alcoholism or drug counselor?
4. What does professional responsibility and competence mean today? What are the liabilities arising thereunder?
5. Explain confidentiality. What are some limitations on confidentiality? How does confidentiality differ from privileged communication?
6. The old common-law good faith standard is covered in the Counselors' Ethical Standards (American Personnel and Guidance Association, 1974). What does this standard mean to the professional counselor? What is "good faith"?
7. What is the issue raised by the (new) doctrine of "informed choice"? What are the responsibilities thereunder?
8. What are the responsibilities of counselors to their employing agencies or institutions? Can these responsibilities be in conflict with federal and state statutory, administrative, and case law?

Cases

1. You are a professional counselor working in a public school. You have just received a printed brochure in the mail that advertises the following:

OFFERING THREE ONGOING GROUPS

An Introduction to Transactional Analysis
Personal Growth Awareness Learning Group
Human Relations—Personal Growth Marathon

TO GET YOU STARTED JOIN

The Free Personal Growth Session, February 1st

! NO FEE !

"Everything you have wanted to learn about groups and never dared ask!"

Fill out the attached form and mail to:

_____,
Marriage Counselor, Group Facilitator, Personal
Growth Counselor, and Human Relations Trainer.

Questions occur to you as a professional counselor. Now that you have read the ad, what are your responsibilities?

What do you need to investigate?

What, if anything, is "improper"?

What would be your responsibilities if you were in private practice rather than employed by a public school system?

2. You are a professional counselor working in a private counseling center. You read the following ad in the paper:

FIND A WAY OUT OF YOUR PROBLEMS!
YOU CAN BE HELPED!

Intensive Care, Personal Counseling, Crisis Confrontation

We help with different life-event stresses, including drunkenness, abortion consequences, depression, aging, demon and occult possession, marital infidelity, sexual difficulties, guilt and fears, and many others!

We help with problems of people who for years have consulted with psychiatrists or other counselors but with nothing ever really accomplished. Our remedial therapy is distinctively biblical. Don't wait any longer to make your life easier and happier. Find a way out of your problems by calling:

_____, R.S.W.
(phone and address given)
Qualified Counselor and Therapist

Nominal Expense

What points of the above advertisement would you question as a professional counselor?

What steps should you now take?

In what ways does this differ from case number 1?

3. You are a professional counselor working in a middle school. You have contact with many parents as well as students, as they know they can come to you about their children's problems. From time to time you have been able to refer parents to a person in your community with a fine reputation as a "family counselor."

Now, from various people in the community, you hear that the family counselor's wife has become his secretary. You also hear that his wife has access to the counselor's personal records, and the evidence tends

CHAPTER 2   THE LAW AND THE COUNSELOR   43

to show she is spreading stories around town that could have been known only if she either listened to the counseling sessions or was reading the personal records.

What is your analysis of the facts?

What is your responsibility?

What is the meaning of "personal records" in the eyes of the law, and how do they differ from "official" office or agency records?

What is required in keeping personal records and in keeping agency records?

What is your duty in making referrals?

How would you answer the above questions if you were a counselor in a community agency or in private practice rather than working in a school setting?

4. You are a professional counselor whose best friend is in a "growth group" being led by another counselor. This friend shares with you the names of the persons in the group. At the same time, the friend points out that there was no screening and that two persons in the group have been seeing a psychiatrist for several years.

   As a result of the group experience, one person under the care of the psychiatrist has become badly disturbed. (Only your friend knows that the two members are under the care of a psychiatrist.) Your friend believes the disturbed person may commit suicide and is also afraid he might actually kill his mother-in-law.

   What are your responsibilities?

   How would they differ if the group leader were a licensed psychologist?

   What are the primary legal obligations and responsibilities of counselors doing group work?

   What obligations do the members of the group have to the group?

5. You, a professional counselor, have had three male clients during the past six months who were former patients of a prominent local psychiatrist. They all tell you similar stories about their previous experiences in therapy. The psychiatrist had told each one that he was probably homosexual, but had neglected to substantiate his perception with any evidence.

   As a part of their therapy they each had been asked to strip during the sessions and would remain without clothes with the therapist for an hour or more. They also were required to watch a series of slides showing nude males. The psychiatrist had told them that this was a desensitizing process that was very important for their progress in therapy.

   After several such sessions all three left therapy. This was brought about when the therapist told them the next step was for him to massage them, again as a part of treatment, to see "how you are progressing." The clients are now venting their anger at this approach to therapy, which they do not feel was justified. They feel they have wasted their money and have been used.

What action might you take?

What implications result from the fact that the other professional was licensed by the medical board?

What procedure might you follow?

What are some of the ethical problems involved in this case?

6. You are director of counseling in a community college. A former student, Betsy, comes to you stating she was advised by John, a counselor working in your center. She tells you that John filled out her complete two-year program of study and assured her that Eastern State University would accept all 60 semester hours. She has now learned that Eastern State will accept only 30 hours. She feels she has been wronged, as John's advice will cost her over $3500 and an additional year in order to get her bachelor's degree.

What are your professional responsibilities as director of counseling?

What is John's professional liability?

What will you advise Betsy?

What difference (if any) would there be in this case if the counseling had taken place in a private counseling center and had been done for a fee?

References

Alabama licensing approved. *Guidepost,* August 16, 1979, p. 1.

American Institutes for Research. *A manual of models for integrating competency-based resources in the certification, training, and differentiated staffing of career guidance personnel* (Draft). Palo Alto, Calif.: American Institutes for Research.

American Mental Health Counselors Association credentialing of professional counselors. *AMHCA News,* February 1979, p. 2.

American Personnel and Guidance Association. *Ethical standards.* Washington, D. C.: American Personnel and Guidance Association, 1974.

American Psychological Association. *Standards for providers of psychological services.* Washington, D. C.: American Psychological Association, 1974.

American Psychological Association. *Standards for providers of counseling psychological services, draft IV.* Washington, D. C.: American Psychological Association, 1978.

Arkansas to license counselors. *Guidepost,* June 14, 1979, p. 1.

Asher, J., & Asher, J. Setting psychology's house in order. *APA Monitor,* 1978, 9 (9, 10), 8, 44.

Berger v. Board of Psychologists Examiners, 521 F. Supp. 1056 (District Court, D. C., 1975).
Bogust v. Iverson, 10 Wis. 2d 129, 102 N. W. 2d 228 (1960).
Bradley, M. K. Counseling past and present: Is there a future? *Personnel and Guidance Journal,* 1978, 57, 42-45.
Cherry v. Board of Regents of the State of New York, 44 N. W. 2d 405 (1942).
Code of Virginia 54-932 (1950, as amended 1976).
Code of Virginia 32-137 (1950, as amended 1977).
Code of Virginia 54-1.18 (1950, as amended 1979).
Comment, *An analysis of the 1972 South Dakota Counselor-Student Privilege Statute.* 19 S. Dak. L. Rev. 378, 380, 1974.
Confidentiality, 15-A C.J.S. 355 (1967).
Cottingham, H. F., & Swanson, C. D. Recent licensure developments: Implications for counselor education. *Counselor Education and Supervision,* 1976, *16,* 84-97.
Cottingham, H. F., & Warner, R. W. APGA and counselor licensure: A status report. *Personnel and Guidance Journal,* 1978, 56, 593-598.
Counseling Students Association. *Resolution.* Presented to New York State Board of Regents, September 1976.
Elliott, K. P. Legal considerations for the South Carolina counselor. *Carolina Counselor,* University of South Carolina, 1978.
Family Educational Rights and Privacy Act. *32 Congressional Quarterly* 3477, December 28, 1974.
Good Faith Doctrine, 76 C.J.S. 133 (Supp., 1974).
Gottesman, R. *Children's legal rights in counseling.* Washington, D. C.: Community Mental Health Institute, 1975.
Henchert, C. M., & Krouse, J. P. L. 94-142: Implications for the school counselor. *Virginia Personnel and Guidance Journal,* Fall 1979, 7, 2.
H. R. 3270, *Congressional Record,* 94th Congress, Washington, D. C., 1976.
Humes, C. W., II. School counselors and P. L. 94-142. *School Counselor,* January 1978, 25, 3.
In re State, 121 N. J. Super. 108, 296 A. 2d 102 (1972).
Kahan v. Greenfield, 165 Pa. Super. 148, 67 A. 2d 567 (1949).
Kameen, M. C., & Parker, L. G. The counselor's role in developing the individualized educational program. *Elementary School Guidance and Counseling,* February 1979, *13,* 3.
Ladd, E. T. Counselors, confidences, and the civil liberties of clients. *Personnel and Guidance Journal,* 1971, *50,* 261-268.
Lopez v. Williams, 372 F. Supp. 1279 (So. Dist. Ohio, 1973).
McAlees, D., & Schumacher, D. Toward a new professionalism: Certification and accreditation. *Rehabilitation Counseling Bulletin,* 1975, *18,* 160-165.
Mental Health Commission labels counselors "other allied" profession. *Continuing Education Units Clearinghouse,* Spring 1979, pp. 3, 12.
NACCMHC news. *AMHCA News,* December 1979, p. 3.
New Virginia Regulations. *AMHCA News,* April 1978, p. 1.
Nichols, W. C., Jr. *Marriage and family counseling: a legislative handbook.* Palo Alto, Calif.: American Association of Marriage and Family Counselors, 1974.
Noble, V. N., and Kampwirth, T. J. P. L. 94-142 and counselor activities. *Elementary School Guidance and Counseling,* February 1979, p. 3.
North Carolina. *Guidelines for the collection, maintenance, dissemination, and*

security of student records. Raleigh, N. C.: State Department of Public Instruction, 1975.

Note, *Testimonial Privileges and the Student Relationship in Secondary Schools,* 56 Iowa L. Rev. 1323-1326 (1971).

Parks, A. L., & Roussea, M. K. *The public law supporting mainstreaming.* Austin, Texas: Learning Concepts Press, 1977.

Pedersen. *Federal-State Privilege Proposals Compared,* 53 Neb. L. Rev. 373 (1974).

South Dakota Laws, SDCL. 19-2-5.1, Supp. 1972.

Standards for the preparation of counselors and other personnel services specialists. *Personnel and Guidance Journal,* 1977, 55, 595-601.

Stripling, R. O. Standards and accreditation in counselor education: A proposal. *Personnel and Guidance Journal,* 1978, 56, 608-611.

Stude, E. W., & McKelvey, J. Ethics and the law: Friend or foe? *Personnel and Guidance Journal,* 1979, 57, 455.

Swanson, C. D. A case supporting licensure. *APGA Guidepost,* August 19, 1976, p. 5.

Swanson, C. D. Counselor certification for private practice now a reality. *Valley Educator,* Summer 1975, p. 2.

Swanson, C. D. I need a license? *Virginia Personnel and Guidance Journal,* 1979 7, 9-11.

Swanson, C. D., & Van Hoose, W. H. *Legal and ethical aspects of school counseling.* Atlanta, Ga.: Pioneer CESA Guidance Project, 1977.

Sweeney, T. J., & Witmer, J. M. Who says you're a counselor? *Personnel and Guidance Journal,* 1977, 55, 589-594.

Tarasoff v. *The Regents of the University of California,* 17 Cal. 3d 425, 131 Cal. Rep. 14 (1976).

Tinker v. *Des Moines School District,* 393 U. S. 503, 506 (1969).

Virginia Board of Behavioral Science. *Minutes.* Richmond: Virginia Department of Commerce, January 23, 1979.

Virginia Board of Professional Counselors. *Regulations.* Richmond: Virginia Department of Commerce, 1976.

Vogel, F. J. Counselor certification trends and predictions. *Journal of Counseling Services,* 1978, 2, 14-20.

Walz. G. R., & Benjamin, L. *Legal concerns for counselors.* Washington, D. C.: American School Counselor Association, 1977.

Weldon v. *Virginia State Board of Psychologists Examiners,* Corp. Ct., City of Newport News, Va. (Oct., 1974, Unrep.).

Woellner, E. H. *Requirements for certification.* 1981-1982. Chicago: University of Chicago, 1981.

CHAPTER *3*

Ethics and the Counselor

Carl D. Swanson*

Neither client nor counselor can remain free of the ethical imperatives of life. Effective counseling involves dealing with ethical understanding, legal responsibilities, and moral realities of living. This chapter will identify and discuss issues facing the counselor, the impact of ethical conduct on counseling procedures and outcomes, and some steps in ethical decision making. The role and responsibility of professional associations in developing and implementing ethical standards will also be examined.

The relationship between a counselor and a client is much more complex than what is said or done in a given session. Counseling is affected by numerous additional factors, including attitudes, beliefs, personal behavior, and views about right and wrong acts. Techniques and information are important to the counseling process, but the manner and conditions in which they are used are critical. The counseling profession is not lacking in techniques, approaches, or theories of helping, and there is certainly no shortage of "experts" or "leaders" purporting to represent these approaches. What the profession seems to lack, however, is comprehension of, adherence to, and enforcement of clear professional ethical standards. The professional counselor, in order to be effective, cannot ignore the ethical dimension of human behavior on the part of clients or self. Counseling occurs not in a fantasy world but in a world of reality where people are required to make ethical choices and decisions as they live their lives and play their roles in society. Adherence to professional ethical standards protects both the public and the counselor (see Hoffman, 1979).

A climate of doubt and mistrust, which appears to surround

---

*The author wishes to acknowledge the contributions of William H. Van Hoose to this chapter.

government institutions and public officials, has now engulfed members of other professions. Consequently, the public has lost much of the respect once freely given to several of the learned professions. In the negative attitudes toward the leading professions, it is obvious that the problem is more specific than a sense of impatience with the establishment. Public distrust seems specifically related to unethical conduct.

Although counseling, unlike medicine and law, has not been attacked by a president or a chief justice, it has not escaped public scrutiny and criticism. There is considerable evidence that the behavioral science professions are becoming more vulnerable, as attested to by the rising number of cases in Virginia brought to the State Board of Behavioral Science (1980). Psychiatry, always viewed by some as an offspring of witchcraft, magic, and palm reading, has been particularly hard hit during the past decade. Practitioners of this craft have been buffeted with malpractice suits and charged with and convicted of fraud, incompetence, and of having improper relationships with clients. Their colleagues in clinical psychology have fared little better. Parallel grievances about this group include incompetence, improper treatment, deception, and mutual protection through professional associations. Counselors, too, have had their problems with disaffection, mistrust, and public criticism. Counselors are also being charged with malpractice actions, including incompetence and unethical behavior (State Board, 1980).

Over its first six years the Virginia State Board of Behavioral Science (1976-1980) has handled numerous cases brought against practitioners in psychology, social work, and counseling. These cases include improper sexual relations with clients, false or misleading advertising, improper financial involvement with clients, double billing, gross overcharging, breaches of confidentiality, practicing in areas without competence to do so, and abuse of alcohol or other drugs by the practitioner.

This era has been described as an "age of psychiatry." Persons suffering from emotional handicaps or seeking optimum development of their personal resources turn to psychiatrists, counselors, and other therapists because they believe that their services are beneficial. There is evidence that counseling does help people with emotional problems, as well as ordinary people who desire assistance with personal planning and decision making (Van Hoose & Kottler, 1977).

Counseling has proliferated during the past four decades and during that period has become a significant force in Western society. This growth and public acceptance is a result of substantial achievements in treating people with mental-health problems and in assisting people in dealing with developmental issues in living. It is therefore unfortunate that the counseling profession has not dealt with some issues that now threaten public acceptance of counseling functions and perhaps the existence of the profession. These issues are discussed below.

Counseling has failed to clearly define its goals, scope of services, and relations to the larger society. Although there is ample evidence that counseling meets most of the criteria for a profession, this evidence is known mainly to members of the profession. An equally serious and related problem is the failure of counseling to control entry into the profession and to monitor the professional behavior of counseling practitioners. Finally, the counseling profession seems little aware of, and even less concerned about, the ethical dimensions of counseling activities.

The upshot is that laypeople, other professionals, and—judging by their actions—even some counselors are quite confused about who gets counseled, by whom, and for what. Counselors are variously viewed as "shrinks," guidance workers, vocational advisers, spiritual healers, and assorted "do-gooders" who smile a lot and say "Uh-huh." Those who try to emulate psychiatrists or clinical psychologists, while wishing they were, contribute further to identity confusion for counseling. Lack of professional or legal controls has led to numerous abuses and unethical practices. One writer (Szasz, 1978) has noted that sex, nudity, dance, divorce, painting, poetry, and pets have all been described as "therapy" by doctors and other experts on mental health. Quacks, "healers," and charlatans call themselves counselors and get away with it. The professional associations have been strangely silent and inactive in such matters.

Incompetent and Unethical Behavior

In this author's opinion, most members of the counseling profession are competent, ethical, and dedicated. They have a sense of duty to clients, to society, and to the profession. Unfortunately, however, there are persons in the profession who are either unaware of or unconcerned about the ethical standards of professions and who follow no professional guidelines except their own. They feel no responsibility to anyone, appear to be motivated primarily by personal recognition and financial gain, and seemingly have no moral conscience.

Incompetent Behavior

Incompetent professional behavior, though closely linked to unethical practice, is somewhat different. Incompetence is generally defined as inadequate knowledge and absence of skills necessary for professional performance (Van Hoose & Kottler, 1977). Pietrofesa and Vriend (1971) suggest that one test of a counselor's competence is his or her own objective assessment of whether he or she is qualified to provide counseling to a given client. If not, the counselor is ethically obligated to acquire the skill or refer the client to someone who is prepared. This view is consistent with a point made earlier in this discussion: counselors are first of all personally responsible for monitoring their own behavior and for judging the appropriateness of their own acts.

There are also persons calling themselves counselors who have little training for the job and who may be unaware of their own unethical/incompetent practices and oblivious to the damage they are doing to clients. Some of these persons are protected by professional counselors who are reluctant to admit that the profession has its share of charlatans and incompetents or are reluctant to deal with such issues for fear their own practices may be suspect. Professional associations tend to ignore these issues for similar reasons. To date, legal regulation of such activities is almost nonexistent.

Unethical Behavior

Counselors are often confronted with possible ethical conflicts, although some counselors are not always aware of these conflicts. Such issues as privacy and confidentiality are frequently used as examples of ethical problems in counseling, and these are, in fact, major concerns in practice.

Unethical counselors are those who lack the integrity, moral commitment, and sound professional judgment to adhere to acceptable standards of right and wrong actions in professional practice. They may be unaware of ethical codes and ignorant of or unconcerned about the rights of others or the possible negative consequences of their unethical acts. Wrong professional actions, whether they result from ignorance, inadequate training, self-interest, or faulty judgment, are still unethical. Some of these will be summarized in the following paragraphs.

Violating confidences. Confidentiality is both an ethical and a legal problem in counseling. Professional counselors believe they have a right and, in fact, a duty to safeguard information presented in a counseling interview. Clients, too, have a right to expect that information revealed to a counselor will be held in strict confidence. These views often conflict with legal demands and with the views of some administrators who may believe that the public's or the institution's right to know transcends client privacy rights.

The legal aspects of confidentiality are discussed in Chapter 2 of this text. Here we are concerned with the ethical side of confidentiality. However, it is appropriate to mention that the counselor/client relationship is protected by statute or court ruling in 14 states (Swanson & Van Hoose, 1977). This means that in those states a school or college counselor cannot be required to divulge information provided in counseling.

The ethical code of the American Personnel and Guidance Association (APGA) specifies that information resulting from the counseling relationship is confidential except when the client's behavior appears destructive to self or others or when the counselor may have to work with others in an effort to assist the client. In such cases the client must be informed of circumstances limiting confidentiality.

Intentional breaches of confidentiality constitute one of the most critical ethical violations in counseling. Yet, they are common (in spite of the Buckley Amendment), particularly in schools where administrators, teachers, and even many parents insist on knowing "everything that is going on." The pressure on counselors to inform others about client problems often exceeds the counselor's commitment to clients and to his or her code of ethics. There are several other reasons that confidentiality is often breached: to meet the counselor's own needs, to protect the client, or to protect others who may be endangered by the client's actions. In addition, a counselor can often make an honest mistake and inadvertently break confidences. Although it is important to examine and understand the counselor's intentions and motivations in breaching confidentiality, nothing alters the fact that a moral contract has been broken.

Exceeding professional competency level. Counselors often find themselves facing problems outside their area of knowledge and expertise. To some extent every client is different and requires specialized treatment.

Each time counselors are confronted with a problem for which they are ill prepared, untrained, or inexperienced, they are faced with the ethical dilemma of whether to try to help the client or to refer the person to someone with special or different skills. Van Hoose and Kottler (1977) write that counselors must recognize their strengths and limitations in order to serve their clients in the most competent manner. When a particular area of weakness is discovered, the counselor has an ethical obligation to become educated in this area or to refer clients with particular problems to other experts.

Claiming expertise not possessed. This is an age of specialization, and that fact has not gone unnoticed among members of the helping crafts. Thus, one finds various descriptors used with the term *counselor*. "Marriage counselor," "vocational counselor," "sex counselor," "loan counselor," "credit counselor," "counseling psychologist," "qualified reality therapist," and "rational-emotive therapist" are a few illustrative examples. The titles, perhaps self-awarded, supposedly indicate an area of expertise not possessed by other helpers. A study of how this expertise was acquired may be revealing. Training in one specialty, including doctoral-level preparation, does not necessarily qualify a person for practice in other specialties. For example, graduate-level preparation in vocational counseling does not qualify a person for sex counseling, and a Ph.D. in clinical or counseling psychology does not by itself produce a marriage counselor. Similarly, a one-day workshop in rational-emotive therapy, regardless of how many signatures appear on the attendance certificate, does not necessarily mean that one is a qualified practitioner in the Ellis school of counseling.

The American Association of Marriage and Family Therapy (AAMFT) carefully monitors and approves counselors for that specialization, but practitioners in some of the other specialties mentioned above are not regulated, and one suspects many are untrained or at least not skilled in their area of practice. The ethical problems inherent in these conditions are obvious. The ethical standards of the APGA state that counselors should not claim qualifications not possessed, but that is as far as they go. There is little evidence that the APGA is able to deal with problems of misrepresentation among its own members, and this association is not yet ready to tackle the problem of dishonesty in the marketplace.

Beyond-the-couch relationships. Becoming personally involved with clients beyond appropriate limits is an ethical conflict that counselors sometimes encounter. Dependency, sexual relations, and social interactions with clients are issues that frequently arise.

The belief that it is unethical and perhaps counterproductive to engage in sexual relations or to have a romantic affair with a client is not universal. The American Psychiatric Association specifically prohibits such relationships, but the American Personnel and Guidance Association code of ethics is silent on this issue. Generally the courts have taken a dim view of sexual activities between clients and therapists, and some psychiatrists have discovered that having intercourse with clients to "speed their recovery" is an expensive technique—for the therapist.

Nevertheless, some well-known writers are convinced that sexual relations between clients and counselors are not only fun but quite healthy. Ellis (1958), for example, has been an exponent of such relations for over 20 years. In his book *Sex without Guilt* he attacks old taboos, such as homosexuality, adultery, and premarital sex. Martin Shepherd, M.D. (1972), also uses sex as a counseling technique. In *A Psychiatrist's Head* he describes an approach to therapy that includes group-therapy orgies, regular sex with both male and female clients, and LSD trips.

To say that intercourse between consenting adults not hampered by traditional mores is wrong is a moral judgment that we are not presently prepared to make. But when sex is invoked as a therapeutic technique, the counselor is most certainly treading on sensitive moral ground, with probable negative psychological consequences to the client. Moreover, there is little or no scientific validation for sex as a counseling technique. It is our judgment that the counselor who engages in sex with persons who are his or her clients not only is on thin ice ethically but is taking serious legal risks as well.

Other unethical behavior. Other examples of unethical counselor behavior include, but are not limited to, the following:

1. Imposing one's own values on clients. A positive responsibility of the counselor is to become totally aware of his or her values and their impact on others.
2. Creating dependency on the part of clients to meet the counselor's own needs.
3. Improper advertising, especially advertising that holds the counselor out to have skills or competencies and/or credentials that he or she

does not actually possess. A weekend workshop in a new theory or approach does not create a skilled or experienced group leader!
4. Charging fees for private counseling for persons who are entitled to free services through the counselor's employing institution and/or using one's job to recruit clients for private practice.
5. Involvement in fee splitting or false or double billing.
6. Other examples of unethical behavior are identified in the APGA *Ethical Standards* (Appendix B) and in the Virginia Board of Professional Counselors Regulations (Appendix D).

There is no suggestion here that counselors can always be ethically correct in all their professional actions. Counselors are human, after all, and errors of judgment and of interpretation are to be expected. Counselors, too, have values, and although they can try to prevent values from interfering with counseling, personal values often creep in.

Basically, most counselors are competent, ethical, and socially conscious professionals. Unfortunately, just as in other professions, counseling has its share of misguided individuals, as well as quacks and conscious rogues who are deceiving their clients and the general public. Sooner or later, the profession must deal with the actions of these persons; otherwise we may all suffer the consequences of acts by the irresponsible.

Ethical Codes

Ethical codes or standards of professional societies, such as the American Personnel and Guidance Association (Appendix B), are designed to provide some guidelines for the professional behavior of members. The codes or standards formulated by professional associations represent a consensus of members' beliefs and concerns about ethical behavior. These guidelines are quite useful to counselors and other mental-health practitioners, but they do not always provide specific directions when ethical decisions are necessary. Ethical actions reflect the practitioner's values, experiences, competency, and prejudices, and although codes can provide some useful directions, only the individual can make ethical choices.

Ethical codes serve several purposes. First, they protect members of the profession from practices that may result in public condemnation. Second, they provide some measure of self-regulation for the profession, thus giving the professional group some freedom and autonomy. Third, they may provide clients some degree of protection from charlatans and incompetents. Finally, ethical codes help protect counselors or psychotherapists from the public. If counselors adhere to the code, they have some protection if they are sued for malpractice.

Ethical standards may also help a group achieve professional status and identity. Counselors and psychotherapists sell a service rather than a

NOBODY EVER PROMISED . . .

First you plow the ground. Then you nurture the seedlings, and finally you harvest the crop. Sounds simple, doesn't it? Well, it isn't. It means long hours—9 to 9 during the peak season. Boredom and frustration during the off season. And disappointments during the midseason.

Oh, there are plenty of lighthearted moments when you and all your competitors hit the road in the fall and try to outsell one another at each stop along the high school circuit. There is a sense of camaraderie because you're traveling together and visiting the schools as a group. The competition among you is good-natured and helps to sharpen your wits. The night sessions are your real test. In the day sessions you're talking to students, but at night you've got to answer to their parents. It's not easy. You've got to know your business and how to explain it—truthfully and competently. On your second go-round, from December to spring, you're traveling alone, and so are all your competitors. The travel schedule you planned was tailored to your institution's follow-up needs. Being on the road is lonely, but it's not the only demoralizing experience for this season of the year. Getting kids into your institution of higher learning is not the primary goal of high school counselors, and so no red-carpet reception is in store for you. You'll be neglected and ignored. Even the number of kids who are interested in listening to you is fewer. The big, enthusiastic crowd you addressed in the fall was big because it was a general assembly. And the students were enthusiastic because their classes had been canceled. Now, you have to really beat the bushes to find those kids who, first, really want to go to college and, second, might want to go to your college.

So you get back to your college to find your desk piled high with applications and folders that must be searched and analyzed and a phone that doesn't stop ringing. Naturally, the questions that must be answered have no answers—at least no easy answers. And if you happen to work in a small college, you can't make any of the big decisions anyway. The director makes all those from the reports you must prepare.

What's in it for me? A lot of things. It feels good to stand up in front of people and share information with them. There's a lot of satisfaction in learning all you can about the college you work for and in being able to tell someone else about it. Most of all, it's hard to match the sense of well-being that comes from helping all those kids and their parents make a very critical decision in their lives. Then, too, the director just might get promoted someday.

—*Assistant Director of Admissions*

---

product. When anyone performs a specialized service which is not easily evaluated and which is intangible, he or she incurs an obligation that is ethical in nature. In this sense the professional is distinguished from amateurs, who are not paid, and also from merchants, who sell a product that can be weighed, measured, and touched. In these circumstances therapists have a serious obligation to provide a useful and appropriate service even though they may at times fail to do so without being caught at it.

Some professional groups have established specific procedures to be followed when their ethical code is violated. The American Psychological Association (APA), as an example, has a published code and casebook and a committee that rules on charges of unethical conduct and often expels members who are found guilty. To date, the American Personnel and Guidance Association (APGA) has no specific procedures for dealing with violations of its ethical code. Some state branches of the APGA, however, have developed guidelines for dealing with unethical behavior of members. The Virginia Counselors Association, for example, has a detailed set of procedures for dealing with ethical abuses in counseling (Appendix C).

As noted earlier, ethical codes such as those mentioned here do not provide clear answers to ethical questions. They can, however, provide some useful directional guidelines and may in fact provide some legal support for some professional actions of counselors.

The Counselor's Ethical Orientation

Research on ethical behavior and the ethical orientation of counselors is quite minimal, considering the magnitude of this topic. Much of the research is descriptive, dealing with ethical issues such as confidentiality, use of tests, and release of records. If answers to some important questions are to be found, more theoretically based research on the counselor's ethical behavior will be necessary. For example, it could be theorized that counselors do impose their values on clients. (Is it possible for a counselor not to model a set of values?) This question could be researched through the use of taped sessions with clients, much in the same manner as currently practiced in counselor education training programs. In the same vein, it could be theorized that counselors do create and/or encourage dependency in clients, and this, too, could be tested through the judging of actual tapes. As the counselor progresses through the ethical hierarchy, it could be theorized that unethical behaviors such as the above would become less frequent, if they occurred at all.

Several steps in this direction have been taken within recent years. Van Hoose and Paradise (1979) conceptualized the ethical behavior of counselors along a developmental continuum. They proposed that the ethical orientation of counselors—that is, the rationale underlying ethical decision making—could be viewed from a model of five qualitatively different stages of ethical reasoning:

- Stage I. Punishment orientation: Counselor decisions, suggestions, and courses of action are based on a strict adherence to prevailing rules and

standards; that is, one must be punished for bad behavior and rewarded for good behavior. The primary concern is strict attention to the physical consequences of the decision.
- Stage II. Institutional orientation: Counselor decisions, suggestions, and courses of action are based on a strict adherence to the rules and policies of the institution or agency. The correct posture is based on the expectations of higher authorities.
- Stage III. Societal orientation: The maintenance of standards, approval of others, and the laws of society and the general public characterize this stage of ethical behavior. Concern is for duty and societal welfare.
- Stage IV. Individual orientation: The primary concern of the counselor is for the needs of the individual while avoiding the violation of laws and the rights of others. Concern for law and societal welfare is recognized but is secondary to the needs of the individual.
- Stage V. Principle or conscience orientation: Concern for the individual is primary, with little regard for the legal, professional, or societal consequences. What is right, in accord with self-chosen principles of conscience and internal ethical formulations, determines counselor behavior.[1]

It can be seen that at Stage I the ethical orientation is exclusively dependent on external rationale. Counselor functioning at this stage is governed by the sanctions and physical consequences of the behavior involved. When the counselor is faced with an ethical dilemma, reasoning becomes restricted and absolute. At Stage II, the rules and policies of the institution or agency with which one is associated provide the ethical decision-making rationale. There is little room for conflict with the expectations of higher authorities. One follows orders or "goes by the book."

At Stage III reasoning is based on general societal welfare. Judgment is derived from the norms and laws set by society. When the individual and society are in conflict, the individual is secondary to society.

Stage IV reflects judgment based primarily on what is best for the individual, though the needs of society are not overlooked. The counselor functioning at this stage considers the individual his or her primary concern and the societal context secondary. At this stage, the reasoning underlying ethical judgments is internally oriented, in contrast to the preceding stages, where guidelines and expectations were external in origin.

Stage V is the highest level of ethical orientation. It is here that the individual is primary, with little concern for legal and societal consequences. Right is defined by individual decisions of conscience and justice consistent with one's own defined internal ethical code. The counselor

---

[1] Reprinted by permission of the Carroll Press. Cranston, RI from Van Hoose & Paradise: *Ethics in Counseling and Psychotherapy.* Copyright 1979, page 38.

operating under this orientation reflects on his or her principles of ethics and morality without regard to external pressures, consequences, or situational factors.

Within this theoretical framework, Van Hoose and Paradise (1979) proposed the following formulations:

1. Most counselors do not function solely at one given stage, variations being a function of situation, training, and related variables.
2. The proposed ethical orientations not only describe qualitatively discrete stages but reflect an underlying continuum of ethical reasoning that forms the basis for ethical judgments. Thus, the conclusion that certain ethical judgments are more adequate, appropriate, or correct appears to be a safe assumption.
3. The basis for the counselor's judgment, when faced with an ethical dilemma, is characterized in terms of the counselor's dominant stage of ethical orientation.
4. The stages of ethical orientation are continuous and overlapping, suggestive of movement toward higher levels of ethical reasoning (Paradise, 1978).
5. Movement in ethical judgment, the reasoning process underlying ethical decision making, is forward and irreversible, whereas ethical action, the overt behavior associated with an ethical dilemma, need not be forward and is reversible. That is, one may reason at a high level, but one's behavior may reflect a much lower level.

Ethical Decision Making

As stated earlier, counselors operate from their own personal style of ethics. Generally, this is sufficient for the most part. It is only when one is faced with a dilemma for which there is no apparent good or best solution that problems arise. It is for this reason that counselors need to understand and develop their own process for ethical decision making. The universal or absolute models of ethical conduct suggested by the theorists, the law, society, or the professional organizations may not always be totally compatible with the counselor's own system of morality.

Development of a process for ethical decision making is a personal and individual responsibility of each counselor. Self-examination, a vital aspect of this process, raises four questions: First, what am I now doing in sessions with clients? What do I hear on my tapes? An honest awareness of where we are is the starting point. Second, what are my ethical beliefs (values) now? How have these been formulated? Third, what steps do I take in coming to ethical decisions? Do I use an organized approach (such as the one that follows) in my self-examination? Finally, what tools do I need in order to grow ethically? Additional reading, group discussions of ethical issues, consultation with another professional, and seeking feedback on professional work are all tools we might use to develop our ethical decision-making process.

For the counselor, nearly every intervention—indeed, almost everything said and done—has potential ethical ramifications. Therefore, an appropriate rationale for all counselor actions is always important. The reasoning underlying counselor judgments related to ethical dilemmas may be attributed to five qualitatively different ethical orientations, restated here for the reader's convenience.

- Stage I. Absolute dogmatic beliefs of right and wrong, good and bad.
- Stage II. Right and wrong as defined by higher authorities.
- Stage III. Right and wrong as defined by societal or legal expectation.
- Stage IV. Right and wrong as defined by what is best for the client, considering the societal and legal ramifications.
- Stage V. Right and wrong as defined by general principles of conscience regardless of legal and societal consequences.

This framework is presented as model from which the individual should explore his or her own rationale for the particular moral and ethical judgments that have been made or need to be made. Using this approach can serve as the first step in synthesizing a personal system of moral and ethical behavior.

Whatever the approach to analyzing one's ethical decision making, it should consider the following elements:

1. *Identify the problem or dilemma.* What is the source of conflict? Is it between the client and society, the client and the institution, the institution and society, or something else? The ethical orientations presented earlier can help to accurately identify where the conflict lies.
2. *Do any rules or guiding principles exist to help resolve the dilemma?* When there are expectations or rules, whether from the institution, society, or the standards of the profession, the individual's agreement with these guidelines must be examined. Perhaps guidelines exist that are in conflict with the counselor's own personal expectations.
3. *Generate possible and probable courses of action.* List the courses of action that are possible and probable so that each can be examined from the perspective of its underlying rationale. Here the rationale for the stages of ethical orientation may be of help.
4. *Consider potential consequences for each course of action.* What are the implications and ramifications of each course of action? How likely is each consequence to occur? Another important issue to consider in this element of the process is where and to whom your responsibilities lie—to the individual, to society, to the institution, to your supervisor, and so on. Are you serving your needs or someone else's?
5. *Select the best course of action.* Once decided, it is your decision to live with. As Browne (1973) warns, "If you are wrong, you will suffer for it. If you're right, you will find happiness" (p. 59). This is precisely why one must be ready to justify actions in an appropriate and meaningful way.

The counselor or psychotherapist is *probably* acting in an ethically responsible way concerning a client if (1) he or she has maintained personal and professional honesty, coupled with (2) the best interests of the client, (3) without malice or personal gain, and (4) can justify his or her actions as the best judgment of what should be done based upon the current state of the profession. Whenever these four components are present, ethically responsible behavior is likely to be demonstrated.

Perspectives for the '80s

The relationship between effective counseling and ethics and the law is a key issue within the profession. Society today provides fewer guidelines for personal conduct, and many traditional institutions have lost their influence in guiding human behavior. Ethical codes have been developed by professional counseling associations to provide guidance. The impact of these codes is limited, however, as appropriate procedures for dealing with unethical acts have not been developed. The law has had to step in to fill this void, as witnessed by the rise in litigation involving counselors.

Where counselors are licensed, disciplinary standards have been established and become part of administrative law. An example of this governmental action is seen in the Regulations for the Virginia Board of Behavioral Sciences (Appendix E). It may be noted that, in addition to the usual reasons for disciplinary action, such as commission of a felony, fraud, or misuse of alcohol or other drugs, the following are also grounds for revocation of the professional counselor's, social worker's, or psychologist's license:

- Negligence in conduct of their profession or nonconformance with the code of ethics.
- Performing functions outside the board-certified area of their competency.
- Being mentally, emotionally, or physically incompetent to practice their profession.

As the profession continues to develop and gain identity and credibility, a greater degree of policing from both within and without the profession will occur. Upgraded counselor training programs are at the base of this trend. Professional associations will be exercising an increased role in policing the profession. Finally, the states will be moving more into this area as licensure for counselors becomes more widespread.

Summary

This chapter included a discussion of certain ethical standards that should guide professional conduct. Various kinds of counselor behavior that militates against rather than facilitates the resolution of a client's problem were examined, and such behaviors were identified as incompetent and unethical. Ethical codes and the purpose they serve were discussed with particular reference to a counselor's ethical orientation, and a developmental continuum conceptualizing ethical behavior was offered. Finally, the dilemmas inherent in ethical decision making were examined and some perspectives for the 1980s were proposed.

Now It's Your Turn

Mark true or false and explain.

T F   1. The client is referred for evaluation and report by the school system; as a result, the client is not entitled to the protections of the ethical code, since your relationship and responsibility is to the school.

T F   2. A 10-year-old comes to you with bruises and a mark on her upper arm that looks as though fingers have squeezed her hard. You suspect abuse but should be careful to collect more evidence before you report your suspicions to the welfare department.

T F   3. John, age 12, was tested (here at the clinic) at the request of his parents because they thought he was gifted. His teacher would like to see the results so she can plan a curriculum for him. You will have to gain a release from the parents before the teacher can see the record even though John will probably benefit.

T F   4. You don't want Jenny's (age 8) parents to know her IQ score because, as laypeople, they don't know how to interpret the number and might label her. You have a right, as a professional, to refuse to show the score to the parents.

T F   5. Anything you write in a record of your client is confidential and cannot be subpoenaed by a court.

T F   6. You have heard of the Rorschach inkblot test and would like to use it to see what interesting responses your client might produce. You believe this might help you to help your client, but you have not had a course in its use. If you study the test on your own, could you use it? (true = yes; false = no)

T F   7. The court has referred Ted for a clinical impression and report regarding his ability to stand trial. You should tell him at the beginning of the interview that you will have to report everything he says that may be of use to the court.

T F   8. Your best friend is convinced that you are the only person who can counsel her because you know her so well. You should, nevertheless, refer her.

T F   9. Gail is 14 and pregnant. Her parents don't know yet and are against any form of sex education outside the home. Gail wants the phone number of Planned Parenthood. You have it, but you can't give it to her.

T F 10. A client comes to you stating that he is seeing another counselor but wishes to begin counseling with you instead. You should not agree to see the client.

T F 11. Jake, a 10-year-old child, was just administered an IQ test by a school psychologist and obtained an extremely low score. On the basis of this test, he can now be placed in a special-education program.

T F 12. Janet has a mild learning disability, and she is recommended to be "mainstreamed." This means that she will be in a special class for the entire day.

T F 13. Sally has a speech impairment. According to P.L. 94–142, she is entitled to special-education services.

T F 14. Fred was deemed eligible for placement in a program for the seriously emotionally disturbed, but his parents objected strongly. Fred must remain in his regular classroom, because his parents refused permission for special placement.

T F 15. Linda is in a class for the seriously emotionally disturbed. Her IEP lists "staying on task for at least 20 minutes" as a long-term goal. This goal will be evaluated for the first time at the end of her second year in the program.

T F 16. Ray is a 16-year-old learning-disabled student. His IEP lists "career counseling" as a related service. Since Ray is in a special-education program, a guidance counselor would definitely not provide this service.

T F 17. You know that a colleague of yours has violated ethical standards. You discuss your concern with him, and he replies "Oh, everyone does it," and so your ethical responsibility has been satisfied.

T F 18. A 12-year-old child was determined eligible to be placed in a program for the emotionally disturbed. The IEP committee recommended placement in a residential program as being the "least restrictive environment." However, the school budget was recently cut. This means the placement is legally permitted to be indefinitely delayed.

Questions for Discussion

1. Were ethical standards devised to restrain you or aid in your professional development?
2. Have you accepted the standards because they have always been present or because you have personally determined that they are in consonance with your own value system?
3. What would you be willing to do for money? For example, would you continue a client relationship when you are aware you can no longer be of any meaningful help?
4. On what are the rewards and payoffs that you obtain from your work as a counselor based?
5. Under what circumstances would you lie to a client?

6. To what extent would you attempt to provide services for which you are not properly trained or experienced?
7. When would you find it necessary to divulge confidential information?
8. How tolerant are you of the unethical practices of your colleagues? Under what circumstances would you take action against an unethical act?
9. How often do you use the counselor/client relationship to satisfy your own needs?
10. By what method do you evaluate your effectiveness?
11. How would you handle situations of transference and countertransference with clients of the other sex?
12. To what extent do your own personal problems interfere with your work as a counselor?

References

American Personnel and Guidance Association. *Ethical standards.* Washington, D.C.: American Personnel and Guidance Association, 1981.

Browne, H. *How I found freedom in an unfree world.* New York: Avon, 1973.

Ellis, A. *Sex without guilt.* New York: Lyle Stuart, 1958.

Hoffman, J. C. *Ethical confrontation in counseling.* Chicago: University of Chicago Press, 1979.

Paradise, L. V. What price ethics? *Counseling and Values,* 1978, 23(1), 2–9.

Pietrofesa, J. J., & Vriend, J. *The school counselor as a professional.* Itasca, Ill.: F. E. Peacock, 1971.

Shepherd, M. *A psychiatrist's head.* New York: Dell, 1972.

State Board of Behavioral Science. *Minutes.* Richmond: Virginia Department of Commerce, 1976–1980.

Swanson, C. D., & Van Hoose, W. H. *Legal and ethical concerns.* Atlanta, Ga.: Pioneer CESA Guidance Project, 1977.

Szasz, T. S. *The myth of psychotherapy.* Garden City, N.Y.: Anchor Press/Doubleday, 1978.

Van Hoose, W. H., & Kottler, J. A. *Ethical and legal issues in counseling and psychotherapy.* San Francisco: Jossey-Bass, 1977.

Van Hoose, W. H., & Paradise, L. V. *Ethics in counseling and psychotherapy.* Cranston, R.I.: Carroll Press, 1979.

Virginia Board of Professional Counselors. *Regulations.* Richmond: Virginia Department of Commerce, 1981.

PART 2

The Work of the Counselor

The work of the professional counselor is, of course, counseling. Nevertheless, as you will learn from the chapters in this section, counseling comes in many sizes and assumes many forms. You will discover that a substantial number of your counseling services are provided under labels that seemingly dissociate them from your unique professional heritage and identity. But do not be misled. The various labels resulted only from a need to classify the multiple functions included in the comprehensive role described for professional counselors.

For example, the skills, attitudes, resourcefulness, and creativity needed for your counseling relationships are precisely those needed for effectively performing the other services described by your professional role. If any difference exists, it is only in the degree to which these competencies must be internalized so that they may be generalized. Your counseling skills must be sharpened to the highest level in order to effectively perform group counseling, consulting, programming, and research and evaluation activities. Professional counselors who have achieved this level of understanding of the counseling process have the insight and versatility to apply it in all other dimensions of their work. The interpretations and the applications may *seem* different from counseling, but regardless of the activity to be performed, effective counselors will use the counseling process to perform it.

And it isn't easy. Only those with skill and knowledge have the confidence and courage to perform in public. The visibility inherent in these activities differs greatly from the privacy experienced in one-to-one counseling relationships. Many inept practitioners have retreated from the multiple services expected of them because they have failed to understand the unlimited possibilities of their counseling skills and/or they feared exposure of their limitations. However one explains our reluctance to become involved in the full range of our professional responsibilities, it cannot be excused in professional counselors of the '80s.

The most familiar aspect of the counselor's work is individual counseling, and it is also the most critical. We believe the acid test of a professional counselor's competence is the ability to work effectively in a one-to-one facilitative relationship.

John D. Boyd, in Chapter 4, provides his readers with a definitive discussion of individual counseling. Certain skills are essential prerequisites for establishing helping relationships without assuming responsibility for counselees' lives. But a helping relationship requires more than merely establishing a good relationship. John explains that the essential element, regardless of the counseling approach, is the provision of learning opportunities. Counselees must be given opportunities to learn new ways to view themselves and others, and themselves in relation to others. They must be helped to learn new ways to interpret the events of daily living and new skills for coping with the world. He also defines the counselor's responsibilities to include more than discovering the source of a counselee's dissatisfaction. Counselors must help their counselees learn how their ways of dealing with the world contribute to their expressed dissatisfaction. More important, professional counselors must help their counselees learn alternative and more satisfying ways of behaving. John Boyd describes the professional counselor, unlike a teacher armed with a syllabus that indicates what is to be taught, as someone who must help counselees develop and implement their own syllabuses.

Chapter 5, by Gerald Corey, is your introduction to the group counseling process: why it is useful, what it includes, and how it is performed. The term *group counseling* has been used to describe a wide range of activities that extend from what other observers would label "teaching" or "preaching" to exotic involvements that many critics are unable to accept. The common thread running through all group work is intimately related to the essential principles of the counseling process. Counseling, whether performed individually or in groups, requires a respect for, and a complete understanding of, the process as systematically organized. It is *not* a collection of gimmicks or a bag of tricks. The author's discussion of the skills and knowledge critical to group leadership is a strong argument for competent group counselors.

Chapter 6, by Jeannette A. Brown, gives you an opportunity to examine for yourself the versatility of your counseling skills.

Counseling competence has a wide range of applicability, and it is far too valuable to be reserved for special occasions and special populations. Jeannette examines consulting from this perspective and suggests that when professional counselors learn how to give their skills away, they will not only have increased their own stature and that of their profession, but they will also have made a valuable contribution to society. Through examples, Jeannette Brown offers you a vicarious experience in how consulting could be performed.

The assessment and information-giving functions of the counselor are discussed in Chapter 7 by Robert H. Pate, Jr. The chapter combines assessment and information giving because the related functions present similar problems and opportunities in the work of the counselor. Pate discusses the contribution that information and assessment can make to the work of the counselor and presents a survey of what professional counselors should know about assessment devices and informational materials. The social, legal, and ethical issues surrounding counselors' use of information and test results are reviewed. The chapter also includes suggestions appropriate for counselors' use of informational materials and the results of assessments.

Chapter 8, by N. Kenneth LaFleur, examines our need, as professional counselors, to clearly demonstrate the worth of our services. Evaluation and research are discussed from a practical rather than an academic perspective. Ken identifies our primary research and evaluation obligations to be a concern to know how well we do what we do. We must evaluate the effectiveness of our services and determine whether they meet the needs of those we serve. Implied here is that research and evaluation are not merely the responsibility of researchers; they are a professional expectation for all counselors. Ken LaFleur's discussion of research and evaluation approaches is practical, and his examination of our accountability problems is unequivocal. If we cannot provide society with evidence of our contributions, then society cannot continue to provide us with its contributions.

The chapters in this section are designed to inform you of the full range of the professional expectations held for you. The work of the counselor includes more than counseling, but none of this work can be competently performed without a thorough knowledge and intense appreciation of the counseling process and its versatility and adaptability. Once learned, it will become the framework for the performance of your individual and group counseling, your consulting, programming, and managing, and even your research and evaluation services.

CHAPTER *4*

Individual Counseling

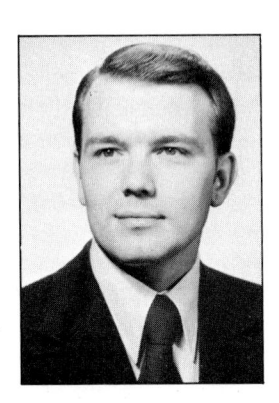

John D. Boyd
John D. Boyd is an associate professor in the Institute of Clinical Psychology, University of Virginia, and a practicing clinical psychologist. His clinical interests span a variety of topics and activities, including cognitive-behavioral psychotherapy, hypnotherapy, and other experiential techniques as well as the supervision of counselors and clinicians. Dr. Boyd has authored Counselor Supervision, *coauthored* Rational-Emotive Therapy: A Skills-Based Approach, *and published numerous articles on counseling skills and techniques.*

During the last three decades, the role and function of the professional counselor have broadened and the counselor's work settings have multiplied. During the formative years of the guidance and counseling profession (1940–1955), vocational matters received most of the counselor's attention, and guidance was delivered in private or government-sponsored placement/employment centers and in a few public schools. The late 1950s and particularly the '60s saw school counselors gain a permanent place in American education with the assistance of federal funding. They maintained their historical responsibility for promoting career development, and they took on the additional task of facilitating the social, educational, and self-development of school-age youngsters. Counselors in postsecondary education likewise established themselves as facilitators of psychological development.

Continuing through the 1970s and into the '80s, the counselor's work and settings have continued to expand, the prominent feature being an increase in the number of counselors preparing for and entering nonschool sites where various kinds of human services are delivered (Austin, Skelding, & Smith, 1977). Professional counselors are now establishing themselves in any setting where people seek help for the problems they encounter in life. They are adapting their skills to the contemporary needs of the human population—for example, through abortion services, retirement planning, geriatric and hospice counseling, crisis counseling, consumer advocacy services, health care counseling, guidance for minority issues and problems, parenthood training, and drug abuse services.

Throughout the expansion and evolution of the professional counselor's role and function, from the 1940s to the present day, one thing has remained unchanged: *counseling is a generic activity*. Regardless of the counselor's work site and his or her specific job description, counseling is a primary service. Role statements from professional organizations such as the American Personnel and Guidance Association have always placed counseling at the center of the counselor's activities, and over the years the lay public has developed a strong association between counselors and counseling. Ask the average person "What do counselors do?" and the usual response is "They counsel." Stated simply, counselors are expected to help others by means of their counseling interactions.

Another reason for counseling to be called a generic activity of the counselor is that it consists of *foundational helping skills*. The skills used in counseling are prerequisites to many other helpgiving modalities, and if a person does not possess counseling skills, it is unlikely that he or she will be competent in other counselor functions.

Because counseling is generic to counselors, it is an appropriate activity with which to begin this section on the work of the counselor. It is also appropriate to devote an entire chapter to the counseling of individuals and another one to group counseling. Although individual and group counseling overlap in terms of their skills and process, there is enough difference to justify separate treatment. The remainder of this chapter, then, will focus exclusively on answering the question "Individual counseling—what's it all about?"

Conversation, Counseling, and Psychotherapy

A first step toward discovering what individual counseling is all about is to differentiate it from two other forms of helpful dyadic (two-person) interaction—conversation and psychotherapy. When an individual enters counseling, something special is expected to happen, something different from the experience of talking to a friend. Further, counseling is usually considered by the public and by helping professionals to be different from psychotherapy. What goes on in therapy somehow differs from the operations of counseling. Very few people would argue that conversation, counseling, and psychotherapy are the same, but *how* do they differ— that's a tough question to answer. What criteria can we use to distinguish among the three interactions?

Conversation and Counseling

There are numerous differences between conversation and counseling that are not apparent to the untrained observer, and *interpersonal focus* is one of these. In conversation the focus is directed at both parties, and participants often talk about themselves. Counseling, however, places the focus on one participant—the counselee. Counselors rarely talk about themselves at length; instead, they keep the interaction focused predominantly on the counselee.

During the counselee-focused interaction, counseling promotes *exploration*—that is, the exploration of a problem, a stage or task of psychological development, or whatever topic the client wants to discuss. Conversation does not foster exploration and often inhibits it because participants vie for topics of interest to themselves.

The exploratory interchange of counseling, as opposed to the nonproductive discourse of conversation, is *empathic* and is directed at factors instrumental to the counselee's concerns and psychological development. Counselors communicate an empathic understanding of counselees' experiencing—their thoughts, feelings, impulses, and so on— and through this kind of communication counselees gain self-awareness. The counselor also guides the interaction toward an exploration of *psychologically important topics* such as personal goals, self-esteem, emotions, attitudes and beliefs, plans, and social relationships.Conversation does little of this; conversationalists may politely listen but then respond in a way that indicates they didn't hear the core of what the counselee was saying. When psychologically important factors are raised, conversation brings about premature closure rather than exploration.

Another difference between counseling and conversation involves *goals*. The general goals of conversation are polite discussion, an exchange of information, making or continuing a friendship or acquaintance, and sometimes offering supportive listening and perhaps advice to a distressed friend. These goals are valuable, for as personality theorists have stressed, the social interest and interpersonal stimulation spawned through conversation are necessary for successful living. Conversation does not always reach its goals, for it can breed interpersonal conflict, and when a person seeks counsel for a difficulty through conversation, frustration and discouragement often result. Nevertheless, pleasant conversation does have a beneficial role to play in society.

The goals of counseling are certainly compatible with the ultimate social objectives of conversation, but the goals of counseling are more professionally than socially based. Counselors are committed to fostering the counselee's welfare in general and psychological development in particular. This fostering of welfare is called "helpgiving"; counseling is designed to offer professional help. When a conversationalist tries to offer help, it is out of personal concern, an altruistic act with no professional responsibility. Counselors, however, have the responsibility to offer accountable helpgiving services. They too have altruistic motives, but their actions are also guided by professional intent and training.

Counseling also has immediate and explicit objectives that conversation does not have. During the counseling process, usually after the exploration and increased understanding of a topic or concern, the counselor and counselee set a mutually acceptable goal to work toward. Such goals are concrete, specifically stated, and observable. Here are examples of goals, which could be made more specific when counseling with a particular counselee.

1. Choose two or three career alternatives that can be explored further in the next year.
2. Overcome speaker's anxiety and make a presentation to a group of people.
3. Improve study habits.
4. Learn how to be assertive with bossy people.
5. Make friends.
6. Decide whether to change jobs.
7. Learn how to look for a job.
8. Stop angry outbursts.
9. Improve communication with a spouse.
10. Learn how to discipline a disruptive child.
11. Resolve an interpersonal conflict.
12. Find out why I am doing poorly in school.

Literally, any constructive step furthering the welfare and psychological development of the counselee can be an immediate objective for counseling. The counselee is helped to explore a concern, to understand it and clarify it into one or more goals. Then the counselor employs a strategy to help the counselee take the necessary action to attain the goals.

Strategies, composed of techniques and methods based on the principles of developmental psychology, learning theory, and therapeutic behavior change, are the last point of differentiation between conversation and counseling. Laypersons in conversation do not use strategies to help others better their welfare. They may offer advice, dictate solutions, or merely listen, but they do not have the professional knowledge and skills to use approved counseling strategies.

Counselors use strategies that are designed to help counselees mobilize and utilize their resources. Although counselors may offer direct assistance, as through brief skill training, testing, attitudinal restructuring, or information giving, these techniques give counselors additional tools with which to activate and use blocked or dormant resources. For example, the strategy for helping a counselee identify several potential careers might involve (1) assessing and examining abilities, interests, and personality characteristics, (2) finding and digesting career information, (3) exploring personal issues related to career choice, such as values, expectancies, ideals, and fears, and (4) observing and talking with people in certain careers. Each of these four steps requires counselee effort and responsibility, and by following them the counselee learns how to make informed career choices in the future.

To summarize the distinction between conversation and counseling: Conversation is social discourse, which can be an enjoyable and valuable part of everyday living. It is a necessary form of communication in civilized society for practical and psychological reasons. Counseling is not a natural social entity but, rather, is a professional helpgiving activity consisting of specific counseling skills to promote counselee welfare and psychological development. The skills of counseling are communicatory in nature but go beyond simple communication to include the use of technical psychological knowledge and methods.

Psychotherapy and Counseling

The distinction between psychotherapy and counseling is not nearly as clear as that between counseling and conversation. There are so many similarities between the two that many authors treat them synonymously. Both counseling and psychotherapy are helpgiving processes devoted to the welfare of helpees; they use many of the same techniques and methods, and the major approaches to psychotherapy have been adapted to counselors' work. Thus, we see titles such as "client-centered counseling" and "client-centered psychotherapy," "behavior therapy" and "behavioral counseling," and "rational-emotive therapy" and "rational-emotive counseling."

Some past attempts to differentiate psychotherapy and counseling have been shown to have weak logic, and these are vanishing. The old notion that psychotherapy can be performed only by a Ph.D. psychologist or an M.D. psychiatrist has been dispelled. We also know that therapy can be performed in settings other than hospitals and psychiatric clinics. And research (Bergin & Garfield, 1971; Carkhuff, 1969b) has shown that many of the core ingredients of effective psychotherapy can be offered by counselors, paraprofessionals, and other therapeutic agents. Thus, it is fairly well accepted that counseling can promote constructive and "therapeutic" changes in counselees—that is, alterations in the emotional, cognitive, and behavioral realms. Yet, there are significant distinctions between psychotherapy and counseling. Although there is overlap, counseling and psychotherapy have somewhat different *purposes and methods,* and they deal with different *helper concerns.*

Counseling has the aforementioned purpose of promoting individuals' welfare and their psychological development. People are viewed as being in a constant process of development and change—meeting and grappling with the stages and tasks of life. Counseling attempts to help them successfully deal with their developmental process and reach ever-increasing heights of happiness, contentment, and actualization. Counseling is a facilitative and promotional endeavor, nurturing the individual's capabilities and encouraging independence and self-direction. It is "growth oriented" rather than "problem oriented."

The purpose of psychotherapy is narrower than the general objective of counseling. Psychotherapy exists for the amelioration of psychopathology. It is problem oriented, and clients present difficulties that are aberrations of normal psychological development. These problems are debilitating, they prohibit successful living, and they require more than the individual's resources for resolution. Neurotic disorders, functional psychoses, personality and character disorders—these are the province of psychotherapy.

Such problems are treated in psychotherapy with remedial and interventionistic procedures. The therapist assumes major responsibility for changing the person, though this is done at the client's request and with the client's cooperation and effort. A standard first step in psychotherapy is to conduct a psychological assessment—that is, gather information about the client's personality and problem through tests and an interview. The information is examined and a psychodiagnosis is established, consisting of a thorough description of the client and problem and the selection of a nosological (classificatory) label identifying the client's condition as a particular kind of psychopathological disorder (for example, anxiety neurosis, paranoid schizophrenia, sociopathic character disorder).

In the past, the traditional assessment and diagnosis steps of psychotherapy have contrasted with the exploration stage of counseling. Therapy clients tended to passively receive the psychotherapist's diagnosis and treatment, whereas in counseling the counselee has historically been an active participant, with expanded self-awareness as a goal. As contemporary psychotherapists have become aware of assessment-diagnosis limitations and the value of client involvement in the initial phase of therapy, practice has changed. Unnecessary assessments and psychopathological labels are avoided by many therapists, and client motivation and insight are encouraged.

Following assessment and diagnosis, psychotherapeutic treatment is applied to the client with the intention of resolving the psychological disorder. More specifically, this means changes in long-standing patterns of emotion, cognition, and behavior. Individual therapy sessions are held once or twice weekly, and after a few months of intensive treatment, appointments may be reduced in frequency. Problem severity and the rate of client progress determine how often therapy sessions are held. It is not unusual for psychotherapy to last a year or more, and for clients with chronic disorders, mental-health treatment can become a way of life.

Within the psychotherapy session, the therapist's behavior may differ slightly or greatly from counseling, depending on the approach being used. Client-centered therapy is virtually identical to the empathic, reflective styles of counselors who espouse a nondirective approach. However, behavior therapy for psychological disorders can differ markedly from behavioral counseling with developmental concerns. Generally speaking, psychotherapy strategies tend to be more forceful and directive than those in counseling, and the therapist's behavior is intended to have a strong impact on the client. Some therapy techniques are confrontive and evocative, and clients may have strong emotional experiences during sessions. Lately psychotherapy treatment has grown to include techniques and methods that rely on and strengthen the client's resources, such as self-management procedures (Thoresen & Mahoney, 1974) and biofeedback (Karlins & Andrews, 1972). This trend has brought the "treatment philosophies" of counseling and psychotherapy closer together.

Homework assignments are frequently part of psychotherapy treatments, although counselors also find them useful (Shelton & Ackerman, 1974). Through psychotherapy homework, clients work on making difficult changes in themselves; they apply their energies toward the resolution of emotional/behavioral disturbances. Counseling homework is more proactive and less remedial. Counselees implement plans for accomplishing such things as coping with transient adjustment difficulties, improving interpersonal relations, making decisions, or developing skills for effective living.

In summary, counseling and psychotherapy have many similarities, but they do differ in purpose, method, and clientele. Overlap and perhaps some confusion regarding the two will always exist, but this does not prevent the professional counselor from establishing a firm identity. Knowing who and what you are as a professional helper is the best defense against intraprofessional role conflict.

Three Categories of Individual Counseling

An understanding of the differences and similarities between counseling and other helpful interactions enables us to take a closer look at individual counseling, and three descriptive categories are offered to further our inquiry of what counseling is all about. These three categories are based on the premise that counselors try to match their helpgiving efforts to the needs of the counselee and that three broad types of counseling emerge: *developmental counseling, career counseling,* and *personal adjustment counseling.* The lessons to be learned from these categories are that the counselee's concern dictates, to a great extent, what will be done in

DON'T TELL ME, SHOW ME!

How polished are your interviewing skills? Do you know how to ask questions that help people tell you about themselves? Do you know how to listen to their answers and discriminate between fact and emotion, drives and skills, wishful thinking and tenacity? And then would you know what to do about it? If you've got all these things going for you, then business and industry will be going after you.

Your well-trained perceptive mind, coupled with a receptive and pragmatic attitude, will make you a natural for employment and placement sections of employee relations departments. And this setting is also a perfect match for your professional goals, because you will be helping people practically as well as personally. To help your company increase production, you must help it decrease employee absenteeism. But to reduce employee absenteeism, you've got to discover employees' reasons for staying away from work. When you help them solve their personal problems, you aren't just helping them lead more satisfying lives: you are helping them, and your company, operate more productively.

A lot of companies may not have a high level of appreciation for this kind of solution. Their only concern is production efficiency, and so they don't want to hear about anything else. This means that you've got to have first-rate interpersonal skills for working with company managers. You've got to get the results they want without arguing for or defending your methods. Your results are your only defense.

Getting results sometimes will mean spotting someone who is able to assume more responsibilities than those in his or her present job and then recommending this high-potential employee for advanced training. Sometimes it means providing preretirement or job termination counseling. At other times it may mean finding outside help for alcoholics, deserted spouses, battered wives, one-parent homes that need child care or teenager supervision. Whatever it means, if you can get it, then you have got the real meaning for living back into a lot of lives—including the corporate life of the company you work for.

—*A Business and Industry Counselor*

---

counseling and that there are at least three broad types of individual counseling.

Developmental Counseling

All counseling could be called "developmental" because, regardless of the counselee's specific topic of discussion, the counselor is generally trying to foster healthy psychological development (Blocher, 1966, 1980). And isn't everything in one's life an aspect of one's developmental process? Even a psychopathological disorder, though considered aberrant in terms of group norms, is part of the individual's developmental process.

But aside from the general nature of counseling as being developmental, there is a specific category of the counselor's work with individuals that can be labeled "developmental counseling." This category encompasses counseling interviews and multiple-interview counseling processes in which discussion centers on one or more tasks or stages that are part of normal psychological development. Ordinarily these tasks and stages do not cause undue emotional distress, although the individual may be genuinely concerned about them. When acute emotional distress does surround a developmental issue, the helpgiving process becomes "personal adjustment counseling," described later.

Developmental counseling rests on the proposition, underscored by the research and writing of Robert Carkhuff (Carkhuff, 1969b; Carkhuff & Berenson, 1976) that an interpersonal contact may have a facilitative or inhibitory effect on the development and well-being of the participants. Particularly when one party is deemed the "helper," his or her influence on the helpee may be for better or worse. This interpersonal potential for influence is often overlooked by "problem-centered" clinicians, but counselors view every professional contact as an opportunity to be a constructive influence on the helpee.

Examples of developmental counseling abound, and leading the way are school counselors, who have a continual flow of helping contact with youngsters. During the first hours of a typical school day, the counselor might orient a transfer student, help two youngsters settle an argument, help a disruptive student become aware of her responsibilities, and initiate counseling with a discouraged student who is having academic difficulties. The majority of helping encounters between a school counselor and individual students are in the developmental counseling category, some being brief contacts and others full-fledged counseling processes having goals and strategies.

College counseling centers perform a similar function with late adolescents. Developmental counseling is directed at stages and tasks such as establishing independence from parents, resolving roommate conflicts, planning an educational major, choosing a career, forming an identity, and building intimacy.

Developmental counseling in nonschool settings has been limited in the past, but presently the human services movement and a growing recognition of "adult counseling" offer optimism for the future. Professional counselors are infiltrating those agencies and service delivery sites where developmental counseling can be offered to adults in the early, middle, and later stages of their lives. Given public endorsement and reliable sources of funding, developmental counseling for adults could grow and become a widespread form of human service.

Such a picture is very tentative, though, because developmental counseling is an overlooked service—overlooked by the public, by clinical helpers, and by counselors who exclusively practice career or personal adjustment counseling. Counselees seek help for the stress of personal adjustment problems and for the societally valued tasks of choosing and changing careers. Only on occasion do they request counseling sessions for the purpose of facilitating their psychological development. For this reason the future of individual counseling with nonstressful developmental concerns seems brightest in educational settings, where close contact with counselees and their strivings is built into the counselor's position. Helpgiving methods other than individual counseling, such as *psychological education* (Ivey & Alschuler, 1973), may prove more practical for facilitating adult development.

Career Counseling

A second category of individual counseling—career counseling—has its roots in the historic beginnings of the guidance and counseling profession. Vocational guidance services in the early 1900s were the first systematic helping efforts to be recorded (Borow, 1964), and career counseling has been a mainstay of counselors ever since. Public appreciation for career counseling is perhaps greater than for any other type of counseling, and funding from the federal government for vocationally based guidance services has expressed this value.

The category of career counseling is defined in this chapter as individual contacts with counselees in which the counselor's main purpose is to facilitate the counselee's career development process. This definition and category would encompass counseling situations such as these:

- Helping an elementary school student become aware of the many occupations available for exploration.
- Helping a middle-school youngster think over learning from a career education unit.
- Interpreting an occupational interest inventory to a high school student.
- Assisting a teenager in deciding what to do after high school.
- Helping a student apply to a vocational-technical school or college.
- Role-playing a job interview with a counselee in preparation for the real thing.
- Counseling with a middle-aged man who is bored with his job.
- Helping a woman enter or reenter a career after 15 years as a homemaker.
- Counseling aimed at retirement planning.
- Promoting adjustment to retirement.

Career development begins when children first notice that people have careers and wonder about their place in the world of work, and it continues throughout life, being one of the most fulfilling aspects of living. Essentially, a fruitful career consists of purposeful and stimulating activity, an ingredient very important to one's psychological health. Inactivity or boring work can spawn depression and apathy, while productive and interesting activity usually leads to a sense of competence, mastery, and happiness.

Our sense of self-esteem is tied to our work, although the strength of this tie varies among people. A career promotion can buoy our confidence, and a demotion can shake our self-worth. Identity is likewise contingent on our work, and when we introduce ourselves, we usually mention our career position. Similarly, biographies detail the subject's career path.

Career development, then, is a major dimension in life and in our psychological development. It is not surprising that counselees find career counseling so valuable and that it consumes a large part of the professional counselor's time.

Career counseling practice demonstrates the three-stage process alluded to earlier. That is, the counselor assists the counselee to explore and understand a career concern, convert it to a tangible and concrete goal, and work toward the goal with a strategy. The principal methods within career counseling strategies are (1) assessment of interests, abilities, aptitudes, and personality, (2) gathering and assimilating information about careers, (3) gaining firsthand observations and experiences with prospective careers, (4) decision making, and (5) planning for future career development progress. These methods, and indeed the entire career counseling process, are tailored to the counselee's concern, which reflects his or her individual position in the career development process. To illustrate, the concern for a middle-school girl might be to explore scientific careers and find out whether there are "women scientists." Several years later this same girl might again assess the pros and cons of entering a science career and decide to pursue this direction by planning a "college preparatory" high school curriculum. In her third year of college, having nearly completed a biological science program of study, the young woman might possibly experience a growing dissatisfaction with this career direction. Through career counseling she might become aware of a shift in her values and interests and decide to alter her career direction toward becoming a medical doctor.

As illustrated in this case, career counseling follows and facilitates the individual's career development process throughout life. And although career development theories help the counselor recognize and understand some of the innumerable variables that affect career direction (Osipow, 1968; Whitely, 1976), each counselee has a unique path. The purpose of career counseling is to help the individual achieve career satisfaction by constructing and choosing a career path rather than helplessly accepting fate's offering.

Personal Adjustment Counseling

Complementing developmental and career counseling is the third category of counseling: personal adjustment counseling. This category forms a comprehensive triad with the other two because it contains counselee concerns that are disruptions and unusual stresses in the normal developmental process. The three categories together encompass many of the problems, stages, and tasks that fall under the normal developmental process.

Personal adjustment counseling deals with emotional distress and behavioral difficulties that arise when individuals must struggle to cope with developmental stages and tasks. Any facet of development can be turned into a personal adjustment problem, and it is inevitable that everyone will at some time encounter exceptional difficulty with an ordinary challenge of life. The examples in this list are representative.

- Anxiety over a career decision.
- Procrastination of an important but unwanted duty.
- Lingering anger over an interpersonal conflict.
- Insecurities about getting older.
- Depressive feelings when bored with work.
- Marital discord.
- Excessive guilt about a serious mistake.
- High stress due to child-rearing problems.
- A lack of assertion and confidence.
- Grief over the loss of a loved one.
- Disillusionment and loneliness after parents divorce.

Problems such as these are not psychological disorders, but they may become so if exacerbated and continued over a long period. At their usual level of magnitude they represent undue stress and behavioral difficulty with ordinary (though demanding) aspects of life. Counseling is the appropriate helping treatment for these personal adjustment problems, but if they surpass the counselee's coping ability, referral to psychotherapy would be the proper course of action.

Counseling for personal adjustment problems is intended to strengthen and enhance the counselee's coping ability. The innate resources of the individual are drawn out and utilized, changes in attitudes, emotions, and behavior are made, and new skills may be developed for more effective living. This type of counseling appears similar to psychotherapy, and it is. But discriminating features are that counselees, as opposed to therapy clients, are reacting to acute rather than chronic problems, they are struggling rather than having been overwhelmed and given up, and they evidence strong personality characteristics and resources (though perhaps dormant) rather than characterological deficits.

Categories and Counseling Practice

The three categories of developmental, career, and personal adjustment counseling are convenient descriptors for explaining what counseling is all about, and in the author's opinion they are valid categories. A large proportion of individual counseling cases can be placed neatly into the triadic framework. But there is a danger accompanying the framework. If counselors begin to structure their helping efforts according to categories and rigid frameworks, they risk the loss of their spontaneity and helping accuracy. They can inadvertently force counselees and their concerns into convenient descriptive guidelines rather than attending to unique and personal characteristics. Moreover, counseling becomes inflexible and prescriptive.

Experienced practitioners realize that counseling expertise involves attending to any and all counselee concerns by means of a smooth-flowing counseling process that sometimes violates categories and at other times merges categories. They use diagnostic categories and theoretical concepts to aid their deep understanding of the counselee, but they do not allow these mental sets to detract from the unique qualities of each counselee.

The following case example illustrates how counseling practice can encompass developmental, career, and personal adjustment counseling. Further, the case demonstrates an application of three *approaches* to counseling, which will be described later: *client-centered counseling*, the *rational-emotive approach*, and *behavioral counseling*.

Case Example

Jack is 27 years old and is employed as a carpenter. His wife, Karen, is a full-time homemaker with three youngsters to look after. When Jack and Karen were first married, they both maintained jobs, but for the last three years of their marriage Jack has provided the sole income. Rising inflation, increasing family expenses, and a wage rate that cannot be raised have placed Jack and Karen in financial difficulty. Worse yet is the strain on their marriage that has arisen from their practical problems. These concerns are related by Jack in a segment from an initial interview with a professional counselor.

Excerpt from First Session

Jack: The bills are just killing us; it seems as the kids get older, they need more and more. I don't know how other families do it!

Counselor: Yes, it is hard to see how others make ends meet when your paycheck doesn't go far enough.

Jack: I work harder than most people, and still there's not enough money to meet expenses. It just isn't fair. And now Karen is pushing me to enter a partnership with my father; he's a small contractor here in the city, but I don't want to leave carpentry. It's my work!

Counselor: You'd like to be able to work at carpentry, but it just doesn't seem to pay enough, and now you feel like maybe you're being pushed into something you don't want.

Jack: Yes . . . but if I don't get a better-paying job . . . [shakes head back and forth] I just don't know what to do.

Counselor: ... it seems like you can't win either way ...
Jack: Yeah [sigh].
Counselor: How does Karen react to the situation? You did say she was pushing you toward the partnership ...
Jack: Oh, she thinks the partnership would be a solution to all our problems, and my father wants it too.
Counselor: So they're both wanting you to take it ... but ... you'd have to give up something you love ... a kind of work that is a part of you.
Jack: I'm one of the best interior carpenters around here; lots of people say that!
Counselor: And you don't want to lose that skill, something which you do so well.
Jack: Yeah, and damn it, I shouldn't have to give it up. They don't understand!
Counselor: Karen and your father don't understand how much carpentry means to you; yet, you feel that they are pressuring you to give it up? Is that how it is?
Jack: Yes. My work, what I want to do, doesn't seem to matter.
Counselor: How have they told you or shown you they don't care about your interest in carpentry?
Jack: Well, I've been at the job for over five years; they ought to know by now how much I love it.
Counselor: They ought to know, but do they? Have you talked this over with Karen?
Jack: She wouldn't understand, anyway!
Counselor: You don't think she would understand your feelings.
Jack: I don't know, maybe ... but I hate to cry on her shoulder!
Counselor: That's what it would seem like to you?
Jack: And besides, I don't want to burden her.
Counselor: If she knew how you feel, she'd be burdened.
Jack: Yes, she'd worry.
Counselor: I think you're right—if she cares for you, she might be concerned about your unhappiness.

Jack's financial problems were not solved in the first counseling session. Indeed, the counselor chose to reflectively respond more to Jack's feelings and attitudes than to his practical problems. Not surprisingly, after the first session, Jack expressed his feelings to Karen, and a healthier line of communication was established. Jack related this experience to the counselor in the second session, and another aspect of Jack's financial problems was discovered.

Excerpt from Second Session

Counselor: Jack, it sounds like you and Karen had a really good talk about the situation, and she did understand!
Jack: Yes, and we discussed a number of things we could do to better our

financial situation. We ruled out Karen going back to work, at least for now while the kids are small. And we ruled out changing jobs; Karen wants me to stay with carpentry as long as it is what I want to do.

Counselor: Talking cleared the air, then, between the two of you.

Jack: Yes, but no easy solutions turned up. There was only one thing that made sense, but I want to think it over.

Counselor: What was that?

Jack: Well, Karen thought maybe I could get a foreman's job with my father's company, you know, overseeing the inside carpentry work for his projects. It would probably pay better than my present job, but . . . [sigh].

Counselor: I'm hearing a hesitancy in your voice . . . like you have reservations?

Jack: Well, Dad is bossy and perfectionistic, and I've never been able to please him. We've had conflicts.

Counselor: And you've really tried to please him.

Jack: All my life!

Counselor: And when you don't please him, you sometimes feel hurt? Later maybe angry? [Jack nods.] Then a conflict boils up.

Jack: You've got it! Is this a common thing? You sound as though you know about it.

Counselor: Yes, it's not unusual to have conflicts with a parent. In your case the conflict seems to be stopping you from considering business with your father.

Jack: You know, if I could get along with Dad, it would be a terrific opportunity, and I think he would like to have me as a partner. But getting along with him . . . and presenting the partnership idea to him . . . I just don't know.

Counselor: If you like, we could work on improving your interaction, and then you could decide if you want to pursue the idea with your father.

Jack: OK, but I'm warning you, I really get mad at him.

Counselor: Let's start right there. In what kind of situations do you get angry at him?

Jack: Like when I do something for him or do something I'm proud of, and he makes some kind of critical comment or else doesn't have even one good word to say.

Counselor: And you think he should say thanks, or be complimentary.

Jack: Well, at least a word or two!

Counselor: Jack, why *should* he give you that word or two?

Jack: Because any father would to that . . .

Counselor: . . . if he truly cared for his son? Is that how it seems?

Jack: [Silence, head nod, downcast eyes]

Counselor: So, when you look to your father for approval or a good word, and he doesn't give it, you say to yourself "He doesn't care for me, if he did he'd show it, he ought to give me compliments . . ."

Jack: Something like that.

Counselor: Jack, let's think that through. Does your father's lack of praise, and critical comments, show conclusively that he has not and never will care for you?
Jack: No, but . . . it would be nice just to have it sometimes.
Counselor: Right. It would be nice, but is it a necessity? *Must* you have good words from Dad to feel OK about yourself, to know you've done a good job, and so forth?
Jack: No. I guess not.
Counselor: Why isn't it necessary; how will you know you are a worthwhile person and son and that your work is of quality?
Jack: [Long silence] I guess . . . from other people . . . and . . . I can think for myself!
Counselor: Let's try out your independent thinking . . . suppose you are a foreman and have supervised and helped complete the interior work on a house . . . and you did a solid job, good work. But your father says to you "Why didn't you do it differently here and there, it doesn't look like the work my previous foreman did." How would you ordinarily feel and act?
Jack: Usually I would be a little tiffed; I'd feel like saying "Do it yourself!"
Counselor: You would feel angry, and what thoughts would be behind that anger?
Jack: Uh . . . why doesn't he let me do my work . . .
Counselor: Or perhaps "He *should* accept me and my work without comment; he *should* appreciate a good job, and since he doesn't, he's a louse of a father!"
Jack: [Laughing] Yeah, that's close!
Counselor: Those attitudes bring on anger and resentful behavior, but what could you think to keep your cool, to only feel irritated?
Jack: Uh . . . "That's just the way Dad is, a crank." And . . . "I think it's a good job even if he doesn't."
Counselor: Right! Does this crankiness mean he dislikes you?
Jack: No, I guess he can care for me and still be cranky . . . like we said before . . . there's no rule that he should be complimentary, even though it would be nice.
Counselor: How do you feel when thinking these new attitudes you are coming up with?
Jack: Gee, a lot better, still a little peeved, but OK.

In this second excerpt the counselor and client set the goal of improving Jack's relationship with his father. Specifically, this means decreasing Jack's hurt and angry feelings toward his father, thus freeing him to cope more effectively. The counselor's style has changed and is now more directive and confrontive. The counselor's responses force Jack to examine the thoughts and attitudes that underlie his anger and hurt. Other verbal leads ask Jack to logically examine his cognitions and dispute those that don't make sense (for example, father *should* give me approval; I'm not worthwhile unless Dad says so). In the last part of the segment Jack is helped to establish more accepting attitudes toward himself and his father. These new attitudes, and a lessening of emotional distress, prepare Jack to develop some specific assertive behaviors for interacting with his father.

Excerpt from Third Session

Jack: Our second session helped me see that I can handle a professional interaction with Dad, that I can control my anger, but it's not easy.
Counselor: Yes, it's difficult to change attitudes and feelings that have been a part of you for so long. This kind of change takes time and a lot of work. Can you hang in there and keep working at it?
Jack: Yeah, I'll keep working on it. But—this may sound silly—I am still unsure about how to present this partnership idea or what to say to him at those times when he is unfairly bossy.
Counselor: You're not accustomed to doing that, so it's not surprising that you are unsure. Would it help us to develop some basic assertive methods to get you started?
Jack: Yes, just some things I could say so I'm not lost for words.
Counselor: After this session I'll recommend some readings that will give you a lot of assertive techniques, but for now, what is one situation we could work on?
Jack: Asking Dad about entering the business as a foreman.
Counselor: OK, let's decide on what you want to say to him, and then we can practice through role playing. [Later in the session]
Counselor: Jack, I'll play you and you play your father. So, here we go. "Dad, I've been doing some thinking about my future in carpentry, and I'd like to explore an idea with you."
Jack: What kind of an idea?
Counselor: Well, I really enjoy interior carpentry, particularly finishing work, and I'd like to stay in it. But I'd also like more responsibility, such as a supervisor's job. I think I could handle a job like that . . .
Jack: Yes, yes, but what you really ought to do is go into building as an owner or partner. There's more future in that than being a supervisor.
Counselor: I can see why you say that—builders make more money than supervisors, and I suppose there's financial security in owning your own business—but I am darn good at interior carpentry and I want to stay with it—at least for now. I just don't enjoy the management and paperwork in being a contractor.
Jack: But don't you see how much better off you'd be?
Counselor: Financially better off but unhappy, and maybe not doing a good job at it. But I don't want to argue; what I want, Dad, is to ask if your company has a supervisory job I could apply for.
Jack: [Breaking the roleplay] I'll never remember to say those things.
Counselor: I wasn't outlining a speech for you, Jack, just expressing the motives and desires you've said you want to express. When we role-play

again, why don't you play yourself and try a few assertive statements? Just hang loose and be spontaneous, and gradually build up how to say what you want to say.
Jack: I see, I'm just not in the habit of saying what I want or how I see things. I need to work on this.

For the rest of this third counseling session, Jack continued to learn and practice some assertive techniques—the behaviors of standing up for his rights, expressing his desires, stating differences of opinion, making requests, resolving conflicts, and so on. As these new behaviors were developed, Jack also assessed his attitudes and emotions, working through any blocks to assertion. With readings in assertive techniques, practice, and effective counseling, Jack could reach his goal of bettering interactions with his father and securing a financially desirable job.

Three Approaches to Counseling

Thus far, in exploring what individual counseling is all about, this chapter has explained how counseling is distinct from conversation and psychotherapy, and three broad categories of counselee concerns have been described. But the most revealing piece of information about counseling has been saved for last, and this concerns the "hows." How do counselors counsel—what do they say, think, and do? And how do their actions influence the counselee?

The "hows" of counseling are contained in many *approaches*. As counseling and psychotherapy have developed and expanded over the last 80 years, an extensive list of approaches has arisen. Each approach is one (or more) helper's attempt to construct a set of procedures and methods, based on a personality theory or a set of hypotheses about human functioning, which is effective and somehow different from other, earlier approaches. Some of these approaches have survived, gained clinical support, and become prominent helping modalities. Others have not been strongly endorsed and remain peripheral, yet valuable because of their unique properties and techniques, which may sometimes be applicable in certain helping situations.

Three major counseling/psychotherapy approaches have been selected for presentation in order to illustrate and explain the "hows" of counseling. The client-centered, rational-emotive, and behavioral approaches will be briefly overviewed because they are major and prominent ones, because counselors have found them to be of significant value in individual counseling, and because the three seem to embody a large measure of the disparate elements and characteristics that separate other approaches. What follows is a brief overview of the three approaches and an explanation of how they were applied to the previous case example. Readers are encouraged to go beyond these three in their study of counseling approaches and to be aware that more thorough study and training in the three are necessary before practicing them can begin.

Client-Centered Counseling

The name of Carl Rogers is synonymous with client-centered counseling, for he is its founder and leader, having devoted his entire professional life to the practice, teaching, research, and refinement of the approach. Rogers's emerging ideas were first published in *Counseling and Psychotherapy* (1942), and two later books entitled *Client-Centered Therapy* (1959) and *On Becoming a Person* (1961) more fully explicated the client-centered approach and its underlying personality theory. Since its beginnings, a voluminous amount of literature has been amassed further refining and attesting to client-centered therapy, and it stands today as one of the most prominent approaches to counseling.

Counselors have found the client-centered approach to be particularly applicable to their work; many would argue that no other approach has so strongly influenced the field of counseling and guidance. A host of counselor educators and psychologists have embraced and extended Rogers's work, one of the most noteworthy contributions being that of Carkhuff and Truax (Carkhuff, 1969a, 1969b; Carkhuff and Berenson, 1967; Truax & Carkhuff, 1967).

Client-Centered Theory. Rogers's theory of personality development gives a rationale to the methodology of client-centered counseling. The crux of the theory is that humans have an inherent *self-actualizing tendency,* a movement toward developing one's capacities in ways that serve to maintain and enhance the individual. By following this innate drive and tuning in to one's organismic experiencing process, people can meet their needs, develop an accepting and valuing view of themselves, and interact in a socially beneficial manner. All this may not occur without natural distress or "growing pains," but theoretically, if humans can be attuned to and follow their inner experiencing and nature, they will move toward an actualized state of relative happiness, contentment, and general psychological adjustment (Patterson, 1980).

Problems in our personality development process arise when, inevitably, significant people in our lives (for example, parents, teachers, peers) place *conditions of worth* on us rather than unconditionally accepting us. They value us *if* we meet certain conditions and expectations. Because humans need regard from these others in order to create self-respect, we strive to meet the expectations of others, even though this often requires that we suppress or ignore our self-actualizing tendency and the opportunity to accept and value ourselves unconditionally. A phony self-image is created, based on meeting the conditions of worth, and we distort and deny reality in the quest to confirm our unrealistic self. Psychological maladjustment results.

The key to healthy personality development and the self-generated rehabilitation of psychological problems lies in the "necessary and sufficient conditions of personality change" (Rogers, 1957). These conditions consist in the counselor's expressing and the counselee's perceiving unconditional positive regard, empathic understanding, and congruence, or honesty. When counselees interact with counselors who behave in this manner, they begin to attend to their organismic experiencing, the self-actualization tendency is activated, they question and cast off conditions of worth, and they move toward unconditional acceptance and respect.

Application to the Case Example. Client-centered counseling attempts to enact Rogers's facilitative conditions. The counselor genuinely accepts the counselee, whatever the counselee's thoughts, feelings, and behavior. An unconditional respect is transmitted through the counselor's words and nonverbal behavior, and a deep empathic understanding is communicated to the counselee through *reflective responses*. In terms of skill or technique, the client-centered counselor is a master at hearing and reflecting the counselee's intrapersonal and experiential domain. On receiving such counseling, counselees deeply explore themselves and raise denied experiences, feelings, and attitudes into awareness and acceptance. A reorganization of the self takes place, and a more authentic person emerges, free of the previous defenses, disturbed emotions, and disordered behavior of before.

In the previous case example, an excerpt from the first counseling session demonstrated client-centered techniques. Most of the counselor's responses were reflective, attempting to mirror back the counselee's feelings and meanings to convey acceptance, respect, and honesty. From this feedback the counselee would gain self-awareness and self-acceptance, perhaps leading him to clarify the pressure and conflict he felt, to realize that he had not talked over his concerns with Karen and that she could not be expected to understand his innermost feelings unless he expressed them. It is also likely that the first session helped Jack own and accept his feelings, rather than feel guilty for not wanting to enter a partnership with his father.

Rational-Emotive Counseling

Rational-emotive therapy (RET) was founded by Albert Ellis, a clinical psychologist who has spent his lifetime practicing in New York City, most notably directing his Institute for Rational-Emotive Psychotherapy. Since its inception in 1955 RET has been a leader in the movement toward a cognitive-behavioral model of psychotherapy. And counselors are increasingly being influenced by RET, as evidenced by the outpouring of books and articles on rational-emotive counseling (Boyd & Ramer, 1980; Ellis, 1975; Protinsky, 1976; Schmidt, 1976; Tosi, 1974).

RET Theory. Underlying the practice of RET and its applications to counseling is a set of theoretical hypotheses about the emotional-behavioral functioning of humans and how it can be changed in psychotherapy (Ellis, 1977). At the center of these hypotheses is "the A-B-C paradigm"—an RET concept that states that *events* (A) do not force people to have *emotional-behavioral reactions* (C); rather, it is their *interpretation or thoughts* about events (B) that precipitate emotion and behavior. Therefore, the target for change in psychotherapy is "the B," those thoughts, attitudes, beliefs, and meanings that create emotional-behavioral disturbance.

Ellis theorizes that humans have the capacity to interpret reality in a clear, logical, and objective fashion, thus avoiding unnecessary emotional-behavioral upsets, but he also says that humans are predisposed to *irrational interpretations*. They are susceptible to crooked thinking, or drawing conclusions that are not logical, are not objective, and indeed are cognitive distortions of reality events. For example, following the A-B-C formula, an irrational interpretation occurs when (A) parents scold because of spilled milk; (B) the child concludes "I am a bad and inept person" and consequently (C) feels threatened and hurt and withdraws from the scene.

An irrational interpretation of reality such as the foregoing usually has two or three of these standard characteristics (Ellis, 1979): (1) it demands something unrealistic of the world, other people, or yourself, (2) it exaggerates the awfulness of something you dislike, (3) it concludes that you can't tolerate the thing you dislike, and (4) it condemns the world, other people, or yourself. These characteristics are expressed in a host of specific irrational ideas and beliefs, such as the following ten:

1. I must be loved or approved by everyone I consider significant.
2. I must be thoroughly competent and adequate in everything I do; I should not be satisfied unless I'm the best.
3. Some people are inherently and totally bad, wicked, and evil; they should be severely blamed and punished.
4. There's something that's not going my way or that I don't like, and it's awful! Catastrophic! I can't stand it!
5. My happiness is caused by events and other people; one's fate determines one's happiness; I have little ability to control my sorrow and disturbance.
6. There are dangers and calamities just around the corner, and I must constantly look for them and stay on guard in case they happen.
7. In my life there are difficulties and responsibilities that are best avoided because it would require so much discomfort and effort to deal with them.
8. It's best to do what others want, let them have their way, so that I can depend and lean on them to help me out.

9. Because of the earlier influences on my life, I am what I am, and I'll always be this way; I can't change.
10. There is a right and perfect solution to all problems, and I must find it in order to be happy and completely resolve my problems.

Case Example of Rational-Emotive Counseling. The process of rational-emotive counseling passes through four stages (Grieger & Boyd, 1979), the first being an exploration of the counselee's emotive-behavioral difficulties and an identification/*diagnosis* of those irrational interpretations that are precipitating the problems. Next the counselor helps the counselee gain *insight* into his or her irrational meanings and how they cause upset emotions and behavior. The irrationalities are then *challenged* and *restructured* to form more rational interpretations, and a *reeducative process* is followed so that counselees use their new rational thinking to establish adaptive life patterns of emotion and behavior.

In the excerpt from session two in the foregoing case example, the rational-emotive approach is evident. The counselor zeroes in on Jack's demand for his father's approval, helps him see how he bases his own self-worth on the father's praise, and then encourages him to dispute (think through) his irrational ideas. The counselor uses interpretative and confrontive techniques to foster insight and self-responsibility. Quickly Jack lessens his anger and hurt by thinking more rationally, and with further counseling and homework he could make these changes permanent.

Behavioral Counseling

A general definition of behavioral counseling is that it "consists of whatever ethical activities a counselor undertakes in an effort to help the client engage in those types of behavior which will lead to a resolution of the client's problems" (Krumboltz, 1965, p. 384). This definition is perhaps too general to fully portray the character and color of behavioral counseling, but it points out the two important facts that (1) there is no end to the variety of methods used in behavioral counseling, and (2) the goals of counseling—to resolve the client's problems—can be stated in behavioral terms. As will be explained, these two facts are interrelated.

The methods and procedures of behavioral counseling are based on social-learning theory—theories about how people learn and change their behavior. Forms of learning such as operant conditioning, classical conditioning, modeling, and cognitive processes are used to help counselees change unwanted behavior and/or develop new, productive behaviors. These forms of learning are translated into specific techniques, multiple-technique methods, and multiple-method strategies, which are used by the counselor and counselee to reach behavioral goals that they both agree on. A presentation of the many techniques and methods of behavioral counseling is not possible here, and readers are referred to sources such as the following for this material: Cormier and Cormier (1975); Krumboltz and Thoresen (1976); Mahoney and Thoresen (1974); Osipow and Walsh (1970). It is possible to say briefly that methods can be grouped into these categories:

- Changing and controlling the antecedents of behavior.
- Changing and controlling the reinforcers of behavior.
- Using models to recognize unwanted behavior and to learn desirable behaviors.
- Using imagery to extinguish and/or practice behaviors.
- Learning social skills.

Behavioral Counseling Process. The process of behavioral counseling flows through sequential stages. In the first stage, the counselor helps counselees to explore their concerns, and a behavioral analysis and assessment is conducted through questioning and perhaps a questionnaire or survey instrument. The counselor tries to analyze the counselee's concerns in terms of composite behaviors or deficits, and the extent of severity of these behaviors and deficits is assessed.

Next, the two parties set mutually acceptable goals, stated in behavioral terms. These goals are the targets for stage three—developing and implementing goal-oriented strategies based on learning-theory principles. As noted in Krumboltz's definition, quoted earlier, an accountable strategy is any set of ethical procedures that helps counselees to engage in behaviors that resolve their concerns. Accountability is reached in stage four of behavioral counseling, when counselee feedback indicates that the strategy was effective in promoting target behaviors and problem resolution.

Case Example of Behavioral Counseling. The excerpt from session three of the case example is an example of behavioral counseling. Jack wanted to improve his communication with his father; he wanted to express himself assuredly and not be "lost for words." Specifically, his behavioral goal was to ask his father for the type of job he desired.

The strategy for reaching this goal was *assertion training*—that is, learning to communicate assertively with the father. Role playing was the primary training method because it contains multiple learning modalities. The counselee can play the father's role and gain empathy for his position, observe and model the counselor's assertion techniques, critique the roleplay and make it realistic, perform assertive techniques in a lifelike situation, receive constructive feedback and reinforcement from the counselor, and practice assertive behaviors until they can be proficiently and comfortably performed.

FREE ROOM AND BOARD—AND A WHOLE LOT MORE

My job is a great one for a young person, but it can't be a career. I like it now, but part of my pay is an apartment and meal privileges when I'm on duty. How long can you live in a dorm? I don't make a lot of money, but I don't need much in my situation. The job has a lot of limiting features, but it's a good way to get a start, and that's what I wanted.

I'm responsible for setting up educational and recreational/social programs for people in my residence hall. It's as if I'm a speakers' bureau. I'm director, apartment manager, and social director all in one. But I do a lot of work through student committees. I'm just learning not to do it for them but to be a consultant and adviser. I'm a "doer," and I get frustrated by their inefficiency and "pokiness." I have to hold back a lot, but some of them are really good organizers.

I get to do a lot of counseling, and I like that. People come by my suite with all kinds of problems. I guess I'm safer than the counseling center. I get all kinds: money, roommates, sex, parents, majors—just whatever is on their minds. I really like it and am glad they trust me. Mainly I just listen— that's really what they want—but sometimes I get a chance to use counseling techniques as part of the process. I do a lot of practice confrontations with them; I think it was called role rehearsal in my courses. But most of the students just want to talk.

I have a lot of administrative stuff: maintenance, security, hall budget, and property damage. Twice already I've been contacted by parents who haven't heard from their daughters, and I would call and say they're OK. I can't think of it all; I do stay busy. What don't I like? I don't like trying to defend rules that don't make sense to me, like no smoking marijuana in students' rooms. They really put me on the spot. It's dead on break times. We get only a few days off, and I get bored just doing the paperwork and planning when students are not around.

This is a job for a young person; in a couple of years I'll be too old and will need to move out of the hall. It's a great way to get started. I was told there were residence jobs, and I had four interviews at NASPA and got this one. I guess it's not a popular job, but I like it.

—A Residence-Hall Counselor/Director

Perspectives for the '80s

What about the future? What will be the counseling perspective for the '80s? Will the *whats* and *hows* be different? As a believer in everyone's right to speculate about the future, I will not mince words; rather, I will offer a few speculations about individual counseling in the next decade.

First, concerning the problems counselees bring to individual counseling, there will be a continued trend toward personal/social or mental-health concerns. In the future counselors will see more emotional difficulties (for example, anxiety, depression, anger) arising from human confrontations with contemporary problems. This may come about because our current living conditions and world situation present us with more stress-producing factors and/or because we are becoming more aware and accepting of mental-health problems. Whatever the reason, statistics continually shock us with the apparent increase in divorce, child abuse, incest, violence, childhood and adolescent suicide, alcoholism, drug addiction, and the like. Articles in counseling journals suggest that counselors in the 1970s have seen more of the above-mentioned problems than the guidance pioneers of the '50s and '60s. Have we merely opened up our doors to such concerns, or are there more of them? Time will tell.

A second speculation, related to the first, concerns the counselor's area of expertise. Will counselors continue to move toward human services in nonschool settings, as they have during the late '70s? The author's best guess is yes, and furthermore, this expansion of the counselor's role (that is, dealing with personal/social problems) may influence school counselors to do likewise. They may also expand their role, in practice, to include service targets beyond the traditional vocational-educational helpgiving model of the 1950s and '60s. As mentioned in the first speculation, this expansion may already be happening in counseling as well as other guidance services.

The third and last speculation concerns interrelated changes in counselor training, counseling theory, and counselor practice. Counselor training has improved in the '70s and will continue to become stronger in the '80s. Accreditation standards set and administered by the Association for Counselor Educators and Supervisors will upgrade training, and a growing movement for state licensure of professional counselors will enhance the status of counseling. These two events will make counselors more skilled and confident at individual counseling. They will be better able to counsel with distressful concerns in addition to vocational and educational problems. In so doing they may use leading approaches and techniques of the '60s and '70s that heretofore they have been aware of but have not actually implemented. Client-centered and Carkhuff methods, plus behavioral techniques, could reach new heights in practice. Adler's "Individual Psychology" also has shown signs of proliferation in elementary and middle-school counseling (Allen, 1971). Additionally, applications of the presently emerging "cognitive therapy" (Beck, 1976; Mahoney, 1974; Meichenbaum, 1977) are likely to join RET in finding their way into individual (and group) counseling. The counselor's expertise is likely to increase, not just with personal/social problems but when counseling with any type of concern regarding human welfare.

The counseling perspective for the 1980s is positive. Professional counselors will become better prepared, strengthen their methodology, achieve an improved level of accountability and status, and grapple with a broader range of human problems than ever before. It's an exciting time to be entering the counseling profession.

Summary

What's individual counseling all about? It is certainly more than can be presented in this chapter! Yet, a few universal basics have been established. Though similar to helpful conversation and psychotherapy, counseling is distinctive enough to have its own identity. It helps individuals with developmental, career, and personal adjustment problems, and where there are no problems, counseling can foster healthy human development by increasing self-awareness and resourcefulness.

How is counseling done? Through many different approaches, methods, and techniques. The three approaches overviewed have focused on the affective domain (client-centered), the cognitive, or ideational, realm (RET), and counselee behavior (the behavioral approach). There are numerous other approaches and methods that influence these three realms of human functioning, and aspiring counselors have much to choose from. Ultimately, one's "how" in counseling consists of one's unique and idiosyncratic manner of helping others combined with the skill and knowledge acquired from approaches such as the three that have been reviewed.

Now It's Your Turn

A brief overview of three counseling approaches was presented, and each approach was illustrated by an excerpt from the counseling process. This material, ideally, gave the reader some initial understanding and awareness of how counseling is performed, but most important, it was intended to stimulate further reading, study, and thinking about counseling and its numerous approaches (for example, Gestalt, Adlerian methods, trait-factor, reality therapy, transactional analysis). Toward this end you are now asked to reexamine the three counseling approaches and their respective illustrations and examine the following set of questions. Read each question slowly, then stop, think about it and try to answer it, and then go on to the next.

1. Which counselor sounded like the type of counselor you want to be? Why? What did you value in that counselor's performance?
2. Which counselor would you choose to help you with a problem? What is there in that approach that you want when you have a problem?
3. What was the counselee's "real concern"?
4. What was the outcome of each approach? Which one was most effective?

5. How would an RET or behavioral counselor have handled the first session?
6. If client-centered or behavioral counseling had been used in the second session, what would have been the outcome?
7. Could the counselee have behaved assertively toward his father without assertion training? And did the first two counseling sessions prepare or help him toward assertion?
8. If you could reconstruct the three-session counseling process, using whatever approach, combination, or synthesis you wish, how would you handle the case?

Having entertained each of the foregoing questions, you may be experiencing some meaningful insights and conclusions about counseling, perhaps other questions have arisen in your mind, and/or you may have an uncomfortable feeling that the true answers have escaped you. Any, all, or even other reactions are a step in the right direction. Why? Because rather than a passive receipt of information, *reasoning* and deep *thoughtful involvement* are required if counselors are to examine, test, and choose those approaches and counseling methods that seem to fit their personalities and natural helpgiving talents. The foregoing questions can only begin this tough but exciting journey. The responsibility for completing it lies with the traveler.

References

Allen, J. W. The individual psychology of Alfred Adler: An item of history and a promise of a revolution. *Counseling Psychologist,* 1971, *3*(1), 3–24.

Austin, M. J., Skelding, A. H., & Smith, P. L. *Delivering human services.* New York: Harper & Row, 1977.

Beck, A. T. *Cognitive therapy and the emotional disorders.* New York: International Universities Press, 1976.

Bergin, A. E., & Garfield, S. L. *Psychotherapy and behavior change.* New York: Wiley, 1971.

Blocher, D. H. *Developmental counseling.* New York: Ronald Press, 1966.

Blocher, D. H. Some implications of recent research in social and developmental psychology for counseling practice. *Personnel and Guidance Journal,* 1980, *58*(5), 334–337.

Borow, H. *Career guidance for a new age.* Boston: Houghton-Mifflin, 1973.

Boyd, J., & Ramer, B. Teaching rational ideas. *National Middle School Journal,* 1980, *11*(2), 18–21.

Carkhuff, R. R. *Helping and human relations.* Vol. 1: *Selection and training.* New York: Holt, Rinehart & Winston, 1969. (a)

Carkhuff, R. R. *Helping and human relations.* Vol. 2: *Practice and research.* New York: Holt, Rinehart & Winston, 1969. (b)

Carkhuff, R. R., & Berenson, B. G. *Beyond counseling and therapy.* New York: Holt, Rinehart & Winston, 1967.

Carkhuff, R. R., & Berenson, B. G. *Teaching as treatment.* Amherst, Mass.: Human Resource Development Press, 1976.

Cormier, L. S., & Cormier, W. H. Operant procedures, self-management strategies, and recent innovations. *Behavioral Counseling.* Boston: Houghton Mifflin, 1975. (a)

Cormier, W. H., & Cormier, L. S. Initial procedures, individual and group strategies. *Behavioral counseling.* Boston: Houghton Mifflin, 1975. (b)

Ellis, A. Rational-emotive therapy and the school counselor. *School Counselor,* March 1975, pp. 236–242.

Ellis, A. Rational-emotive therapy: Research data that supports the clinical and personality hypotheses of RET and other modes of cognitive-behavior therapy. *Counseling Psychologist,* 1977, 7(1), 2–20.

Ellis, A. The clinical theory of RET. In R. Grieger & J. Boyd, *RET: A skills-based approach.* New York: Van Nostrand Reinhold, 1979.

Erickson, V. L. (Ed.). Developmental counseling psychology. *Counseling Psychologist,* 1977, 6(4), entire issue.

Grieger, R., & Boyd, J. *RET: A skills-based approach.* New York: Van Nostrand Reinhold, 1979.

Ivey, A. E., & Alschuler, A. S. (Eds.). Psychological education: A prime function of the counselor. *Personnel and Guidance Journal,* 1973, 51(9), special issue.

Karlins, M., & Andrews, L. M. *Biofeedback: Turning on the power of your mind.* New York: Warner Books, 1972.

Krumboltz, J. D. Behavioral counseling: Rationale and research. *Personnel and Guidance Journal,* 1965, 44, 383–387.

Krumboltz, J. D., & Thoresen, C. E. (Eds.). *Counseling methods.* New York: Holt, Rinehart & Winston, 1976.

Mahoney, M. J. *Cognitive and behavior modification.* Cambridge, Mass.: Ballinger, 1974.

Mahoney, M. J., & Thoresen, C. E. *Self-control: Power to the person.* Monterey, Calif.: Brooks/Cole, 1974.

Meichenbaum, D. *Cognitive behavior modification.* New York: Plenum, 1977.

Osipow, S. H. *Theories of career development.* New York: Appleton-Century-Crofts, 1968.

Osipow, S. H., & Walsh, W. B. *Behavior change in counseling.* New York: Appleton-Century-Crofts, 1970.

Patterson, C. H. *Theories of counseling and psychotherapy.* New York: Harper & Row, 1980.

Protinsky, H. Rational counseling with adolescents. *School Counselor,* March 1976, pp. 240–245.

Rogers, C. R. *Counseling and psychotherapy.* Boston: Houghton Mifflin, 1942.

Rogers, C. R. *Client-centered therapy.* Boston: Houghton Mifflin, 1951.

Rogers, C. R. The necessary and sufficient conditions of therapeutic personality change. *Journal of Consulting Psychology,* 1957, 21, 95–103.

Rogers, C. R. *On becoming a person.* Boston: Houghton Mifflin, 1961.

Schmidt, J. A. Cognitive restructuring: The art of talking to yourself. *Personnel and Guidance Journal,* October 1976, pp. 71–74.

Shelton, J. L., & Ackerman, J. M. *Homework in counseling and psychotherapy.* Springfield, Ill.: Charles C Thomas, 1974.

Thoresen, C. E., & Mahoney, M. J. *Behavioral self-control.* New York: Holt, Rinehart & Winston, 1974.

Tosi, D. J. *Youth: Toward personal growth.* Columbus, Ohio: Merrill, 1974.

Truax, C. B., & Carkhuff, R. R. *Toward effective counseling and psychotherapy: Training and practices.* Chicago: Aldine, 1967.

Whiteley, J. M. (Ed.). Career counseling. *Counseling Psychologist,* 1976, 6(3), entire issue.

CHAPTER **5**

Group Counseling

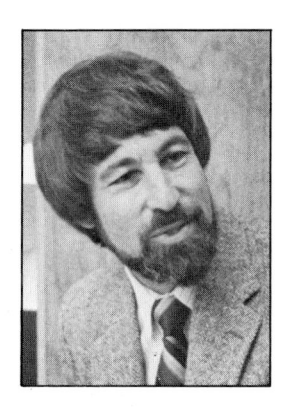

Gerald Corey

Gerald Corey is a professor of human services at California State University, Fullerton. He is a Diplomate in Counseling Psychology, American Board of Professional Psychology, and is a licensed psychologist. He is the author or coauthor of eleven books in the counseling field, and he has written several journal articles on group counseling. Dr. Corey is currently a member of the editorial board of the Journal of Specialists in Group Work, *and with his wife, Marianne, he serves as a cochairperson on the Professional Standards and Ethics Committee of the Association for Specialists in Group Work.*

If you are interested in pursuing the counseling profession, you are likely to discover that you will eventually need the skills to organize and conduct a counseling group. Many counseling centers, mental-health agencies, and rehabilitation institutions rely on group approaches as a way of reaching their clientele. Thus, if you are limited to competencies in individual counseling, you may be limiting your options as a mental-health worker or counselor. This chapter is in no way intended to give you the skills needed to lead a group, but it will, I hope, serve as a catalyst to get you to read more about groups and maybe even take a course or two in group counseling. If this chapter stimulates your interest in knowing more about how groups work and their possibilities, then its purpose will have been achieved.

Group Counseling for Special Populations

Groups offer particular advantages for working with a variety of populations, for groups can be designed to meet the needs of special populations such as children, adolescents, young adults, middle-aged persons, and the elderly. Special counseling groups with these and other populations are described in *Groups: Process and Practice* (Corey & Corey, 1983), which offers suggestions on how to set up such groups and on what techniques to use for dealing with the unique problems of each of these populations. What follows is a brief discussion of the value of group counseling for these special populations.

Children

In the school setting, group counseling is often suggested for children who display behaviors or attributes such as excessive fighting, chronic tiredness, violent outbursts, extreme withdrawal, inability to get along with peers, and neglected appearance. In small groups children have the opportunity to express their feelings about a wide range of personal problems. Children frequently experience learning difficulties in school as a result of inner turmoil. Some of these children suffer from anxiety over broken homes and disturbed family relationships. If the group is structured properly, these children can receive psychological assistance at an early age and will therefore stand a better chance of coping effectively with the tasks they will face later in life.

Adolescents

For most people, adolescence is a difficult period. It is a period characterized by paradoxes: they strive for closeness, and yet they often fear intimacy and often avoid it; they rebel against control, and yet they want direction and structure; while they push and test limits imposed on them, they see having some limits on them as a sign of caring; they are not treated as mature adults, and yet they are often expected to act as though they had gained complete autonomy; they are typically highly self-centered and preoccupied with their own worlds, and yet they are expected to cope with societal demands and go outside themselves by expanding their horizons; they are asked to face and accept reality, and at the same time many avenues of escape are available to them in the form of drugs and alcohol. With the adolescent years come some of these conflicts: dependence/independence struggles, acceptance/rejection conflicts, identity crises, the search for security, pressures to conform, and the need for approval. Because of the stresses of the adolescent period, these years can be extremely lonely, and it is not unusual for an adolescent to feel that there is no one there to help.

Group counseling can be very useful in dealing with these feelings of isolation because it gives adolescents a place to express conflicting feelings, explore self-doubts, and come to the realization that they share these concerns with their peers. A group allows adolescents to openly question their values and to talk freely about some of their deepest concerns. In the group, adolescents can learn to communicate with their peers, can benefit from the modeling provided by the leader, and can safely experiment with reality and test their limits. A unique value of a group situation is that it offers adolescents a chance to be instrumental in one another's growth and change. Because of the opportunities for interaction in groups, the members can express their concerns and be genuinely heard, and they can help one another on the road toward increased self-acceptance.

For those readers who are especially interested in a detailed treatment of working with children and adolescents in groups, I recommend *Developmental Groups for Children* (Duncan & Gumaer, 1980) and *Windows to Our Children* (Oaklander, 1978).

Adults

Special-interest groups of a wide variety can be developed for adults of all ages. For example, groups can be formed for couples, for single parents, for parents who want to explore problems they are having in relating to their children, for middle-aged people who are returning to college or changing careers, and for adults who want to explore developmental concerns such as the search for identity.

On the college campus, groups have become increasingly popular as a way of meeting the diverse needs of students who range from young adults to the elderly. Such groups can be designed for relatively healthy students who are experiencing some developmental crisis or for students who want to talk openly with others about concerns. The purpose of these groups is to offer the participants an opportunity to explore ways of changing certain aspects of their lives. In group situations, college students of all ages can deal with issues of career decisions, male/female relationships, the need for and fear of love, sex-role identity issues, educational plans, the meaning of life, challenging one's value system, the meaning of work, feelings of loneliness and isolation, learning to form intimate relationships, exploring marital conflicts, and other concerns related to becoming a self-directed adult. Through the college counseling center, students are likely to find a variety of groups designed for special concerns, including assertion training groups, women's groups, men's groups, groups for minorities, stress management groups, test-anxiety reduction groups, and personal-growth groups.

For readers interested in learning more about theme-oriented groups, I recommend *I Never Knew I Had a Choice* (Corey, 1983). This book deals with various personal issues facing adults, such as the search for autonomy, the body, sex roles, sexuality, love and intimate relationships, work, death and loss, loneliness and solitude, and the meaning of life. I have developed groups for adults by structuring them around these themes. The group becomes a place where people can discuss life choices at each period of adulthood; the group challenges members to take an honest inventory of how their past choices influence the person they are today and how they can make new decisions and change the present course of their lives.

The Elderly

As people grow older, they typically face feelings of isolation, and they may struggle with the problem of finding meaning in life. Some of these older persons may resign themselves to a useless life, for they see little excitement in their future. Like adolescents, the elderly often feel unproductive, unneeded, and unwanted by society. Another problem is that many older people have uncritically accepted myths about aging.

Themes that may be more prevalent with the elderly than other age groups include loneliness, social isolation, losses, poverty, feelings of rejection, the struggle to find meaning in life, dependency, feelings of uselessness, hopelessness and despair, fears of death and dying, grief over others' death, sadness over physical and mental deterioration, depression, and regrets over past events.

Older people have a great need to be listened to and to be deeply understood. Respect can be shown by accepting them through hearing their underlying messages and by not patronizing them. These individuals need support and encouragement, and they need the chance to talk openly about what they are feeling and about topics that concern them. A counseling group can do a lot to help the elderly challenge myths they may have bought that limit their lives; it can also help these people deal with the developmental tasks that they, like any other age group, must face in such a way that they can retain their self-respect. Groups can assist the elderly in breaking out of their isolation and encourage them to find new meaning in life.

Readers who would like to pursue the study of groups for the elderly would do well to consult the excellent book *Working with the Elderly: Group Processes and Techniques* (Burnside, 1978). This edited collection contains a wealth of practical information on subjects such as suggestions in working with older people, group-membership issues, responsibilities of group leaders, guidelines for leaders, and the future of group work with the aged.

Some General Goals and Purposes of Groups

All the special types of groups just described share some general purposes of the group experience. Group members decide for themselves the specific goals that give meaning and direction to the group they are in.

However, the following are a few of the general goals shared by most groups:

- To grow in self-acceptance and learn not to demand perfection.
- To learn how to trust oneself and others.
- To foster self-knowledge and the development of a unique self-identity.
- To lessen one's fears of intimacy and to learn to reach out to those one would like to be closer to.
- To move away from merely meeting others' expectations and decide for oneself the standards by which to live.
- To increase self-awareness and thereby increase the possibilities for choice and action.
- To become aware of one's choices and to make choices wisely.
- To become more sensitive to the needs and feelings of others.
- To clarify one's values and decide whether and how to modify them.
- To find ways of understanding and resolving personal problems.

Advantages of Group Counseling

Group counseling has advantages as a vehicle for assisting people to make changes in their attitudes, beliefs about themselves and others, feelings, and behaviors. One is that group members can learn more about the ways they relate to others and can improve certain social skills. By giving and getting feedback, members can come to understand how others perceive them.

Counseling groups provide a re-creation of the members' everyday world, especially if the group membership is diverse with respect to age, interest, background, socioeconomic status, and range of problems. This diversity helps to make a group a microcosm of society. The group process provides a sample of reality, for the struggles and conflicts that people experience in the group situation are much like those that they experience in their everyday lives.

Groups offer support and understanding, which foster the members' willingness to explore the problems they brought with them to the group. Participants are able to work toward achieving a sense of belonging, and through the sense of togetherness that develops, they learn ways of being intimate, caring, and challenging. In this supportive climate, participants can explore personal problems and experiment with new behaviors. They can practice these behaviors in the safety of the group itself, and they can learn ways of applying what they learn in the group to many situations that they face outside the group.

In setting up a group, I suggest that you begin by developing a written proposal to see the overall design. This proposal can be very useful if you have to "sell" your supervisor on the idea of doing a group. The issues that need to be thought through carefully are these: What type of group are you proposing? What population will it serve? What will be the leader's functions? What will be the main goals of the group? Where will the group be held? How long will it last? What topics will be explored? What will be the basis for including or excluding members? How will potential risks of group participation be dealt with? What kinds of ground rules and policies will govern the group? How much structure will there be? What are the ethical and legal considerations that need to be taken into account? What techniques and procedures will and will not be used? What are the qualifications and background of experience of the group leader (or leaders)? What kinds of evaluation procedures can be used to determine the level of effectiveness of the group? What kind of follow-up procedures will be used to help members integrate what they learn and evaluate this learning?

As a leader of a group, if you are not clear in your own mind about what you hope to accomplish, if you cannot demonstrate that you have the competencies to lead a group, and if you do not have a sound proposal, then you are likely to meet with rejection before you ever get your project off the ground. For this reason, I cannot overstate the value of the preparatory period in the formation of a group. Attention to basic pregroup concerns is crucial to the outcome of a group.

Evolution and Development of a Group

This section is designed as a road map of the stages that characterize the evolution of a group. It is a mistake to assume that the stages to be described flow in a neat and discrete way in the life of a real group. There is considerable overlap between the stages, and groups do not conform precisely to some preordained time sequence that theoretically separates one phase from the next. However, there does seem to be some generalized pattern in the evolution of a group, and it is to the stages that make up this pattern that the rest of this chapter addresses itself.

It is important for group leaders to have a general understanding and perspective of the stages involved in group process. By gaining such an understanding, group leaders also become aware of the factors that facilitate group process and of those that interfere with it. By learning about the problems and potential crises of each stage, leaders learn when and how to intervene. By getting a picture of the systematic evolution of groups, the leader becomes aware of the developmental tasks that must be successfully met if a group is to move forward.

Where to Begin: Formation of the Group

In forming a group, the place to begin is by clarifying the rationale for a particular group. It has been my experience that devoting considerable time to planning is well worth the investment, for if the planning is done poorly, and if members are not carefully selected and prepared, groups typically get stuck and much floundering occurs.

Announcing a Group and Recruiting Members

Assuming that you have been successful in getting a proposal accepted, the next step is to find a practical way to announce this group to prospective participants. How a group is announced influences the way it will be received by potential members as well as the kind of people who will join the group. I have found that personal contact with potential members is one of the best methods of recruiting membership. Through personal contact the leader can enthusiastically demonstrate that the group has potential value for a person.

In announcing a group and recruiting members, professional standards should prevail over a commercialized approach. In the recruitment process, potential clients have a right to know the goals of the group, the basic procedures to be used, what will be expected of them as participants, what they can expect from the leader, and any major risks as well as potential values of participating in the group.

The Association for Specialists in Group Work has developed *Ethical Guidelines for Group Leaders* (1980), which states that prospective members should have access to the following information, preferably in writing:

- A statement of purpose of the group and group goals.
- Qualifications of the leader.
- The types of techniques and procedures that may be used, especially any specialized or experimental activities in which members may be expected to participate.
- A statement of all fees and any services that can and cannot be provided within the particular group structure (including whether a follow-up meeting is covered in the fee).
- The personal risks involved in the group.
- Any recording of sessions.
- A statement concerning confidentiality and the limits of confidentiality.
- Statements concerning the division of responsibility of the leader and the participants.

Screening and Selecting Members

The ASGW's *Ethical Guidelines for Group Leaders* (1980) states:

> The group leader shall conduct a pre-group interview with each prospective member for purposes of screening, orientation, and, in so far as possible, shall select group members whose needs and goals are

compatible with the established goals of the group; who will not impede the group process; and whose well-being will not be jeopardized by the group experience [p. 1].

In keeping with the spirit of this guideline, after recruiting potential members, the next step is to determine who (if anyone) should be excluded. Elsewhere I discuss guidelines for screening (Corey, 1981), issues involved in screening and selection procedures (Corey & Corey, 1983), some basic techniques in screening and preparing members (Corey, Corey, Callanan, & Russell, 1982), and some ethical issues in the screening and orienting of members (Corey, Corey, & Callanan, 1979).

I consider screening a two-way process: as well as giving me the opportunity to judge the appropriateness of a given group for an individual, it includes the applicant interviewing me so that he or she can make an informed decision whether to join the group. The key question is: Is it appropriate for *this person* to become a participant in *this type* of group, with *this leader,* at *this particular time?* Some questions that can be productively explored in about a half-hour interview with each candidate are these:

- Why does this person want to join the group?
- How ready is the person to become actively involved in the process of self-examination that will be a part of the group?
- Does the candidate have a clear idea about the nature and purpose of the group? Does he or she have a view of what is expected?
- Are there any indications that the person might be counterproductive to the development of cohesion in the group? Might this group be counterproductive to the person?

In my view, screening and selection are not a process by which the "expert" makes an objective decision with a sense of certainty. My approach is merely a rough estimation of who might or might not profit from participating in a group, as well as giving candidates information about the group. If this screening and information-giving process is done well, my experience has been that many people will screen *themselves* out of the group if they come to see that the group is not for them. If I have reservations about admitting a person, I can discuss them with the candidate.

Some Practical Considerations in Group Formation

In selecting members for a given group, there are some basic factors to keep in mind:

1. *How large should the group be?* The ideal size of a group depends on the age of the members, your experience as a leader, the type and purpose of a group, and whether you have a coleader. For instance, a

group with elementary school children might be kept to four or five members, while a group of adolescents might have eight to ten. The group should be big enough to give ample opportunity for interaction and small enough for everyone to feel involved in the group.
2. *How often should a group meet, and for how long?* With children and adolescents, frequent short meetings may be better, to suit their attention span. If the group is taking place in a school setting, the meeting times can correspond to regularly scheduled class periods. For groups of well-functioning adults, a two-hour weekly session might be preferable. The frequency and duration of meetings should suit your style of leadership and the type of people in the group.
3. *Where should the group meet?* Physical arrangements and setting contribute to or detract from the climate of a group. Privacy and freedom from distractions are essential. Sometimes, for example, group leaders think that meeting outdoors is a good way to promote informality, but generally such a setting both lacks privacy and is a source of distraction.
4. *Will membership be voluntary or involuntary?* Although it is ideal to have a group composed only of those who want to be a part of the group, some groups consist of clients who are required to attend. According to Yalom (1975), in order to benefit from the group experience, especially group therapy, a person must be motivated to change. Attending a group because one has been "ordered" to go by someone else greatly curtails the chances for success. Yalom believes that people with a deeply entrenched unwillingness to enter a group should not be accepted. However, he thinks that many of the negative attitudes that involuntary candidates have about groups can be changed by adequately preparing members for a group. In my experience, many involuntary members are able to learn that a group counseling experience can help them make the changes they want to achieve. Since many agencies offer groups for an involuntary clientele, it is important to learn how to work within such a structure rather than clinging to the assumption that groups will be successful only with a voluntary population. Presenting to members the values of a group experience increases the chances that productive work will take place. The key to successful participation here lies in carefully orienting members and preparing them for being a part of the group, as well as in the leader's belief that group process has something to offer these prospective members.
5. *Should the group be open or closed?* An open group is one characterized by changing membership; a closed group adds no new members during the lifetime of the group. Closed groups have some distinct advantages, as trust can be developed and work accomplished. If the membership changes from week to week, as in some open groups, productive work as a group may be very difficult to accomplish.

HAVE YOU GOT YOUR ACT TOGETHER?

I like this work. I like working with and for people who are having trouble resolving a part of their lives, in need of support and help in reaching their potential for living fully. I like working as a member of a team—getting and giving support, getting feedback, helping solve problems. It's also great to receive heartfelt thanks from people who have overcome their adversities, reentered their homes, and years later send you cards still saying "thanks."

It is not enjoyable to rank below psychiatrists, psychologists, and social workers and to be discounted in some situations by some people. Neither is it fun to have people furious with you if you are unable to "cure" them or meet their every need in their distress. It's hard not to be distressed yourself. Why can't they realize that they must cure them, not me? And being responsible for helping to control acting-out or destructive patients means calls at all hours of the night—never mind the tons of paperwork, reports, and recommendations.

There is no typical day. Crises and other interruptions are standard procedures. But somewhere throughout the day the business of the agency has to get done. Staff meetings are held to report on the events of the previous evening and/or night, discuss problem patients, design treatment plans, air gripes, needs, and conflicts, and resolve the problems that come up when so many people live together in such limited space. There are some opportunities for individual counseling, like with someone who needs help because of something that happened in a group counseling session or maybe some vocational counseling. In group counseling you're a coleader, generally, because a psychiatrist is the leader and other staff members act as coleaders.

It is vital for counselors-in-training who are considering entering this setting to be able to deal with anxiety (yours and other people's) and stress and anger. You will also need to be able to leave your work at your job; otherwise you will never get any sleep or have any life of your own. You need to have your "act together," or you will never be able to give support, motivation, patience, etc., etc., etc. to others. Good luck!!

—A Mental-Health Counselor

Conducting a Pregroup Session

Once the members have been screened and the group formed, it is useful to conduct a preliminary, or pregroup, session with all the members who have been selected. The pregroup meeting can be an extension of the individual screening process, for it is an ideal way to present basic information, to help members get to know one another, and to help them decide whether to commit themselves to the group. Purposes of the preliminary meeting include introducing the leader and coleaders to the group, helping members get acquainted, clarifying personal goals and sharing reasons for wanting to be a part of the group, learning about how groups work and how to get the most from the experience, exploring any fears or reservations members might have about participating, discussing the possible dangers and risks involved in the group, clearing up common misconceptions about groups, talking about the importance of confidentiality and other ground rules and policies that are necessary for the effective functioning of a group, and beginning to develop the trust necessary for open exploration of personal issues. Depending on the nature of the group, certain ground rules will have to be established early in its history. For example, the following ground rules could be presented to most types of groups at the preliminary session in the form of a written contract that members can sign:

- Members are not to use drugs during a session and are not to come to a session under the influence of drugs, including alcohol.
- Members are expected to come to the sessions on time and be present at all the meetings, since absences do affect the entire group.
- Members must avoid sexual involvements with others in the group throughout its duration.
- Members may not smoke during the group sessions.
- Members must maintain the confidences of others in the group.
- Members are not to use physical violence in group sessions, nor are they to be physically or verbally abusive of others in the group.
- Members will be given a list of their rights and responsibilities so that they know what is expected of them before they join the group.
- For groups of children or adolescents, written consent must be given by the parents or guardians.
- If members decide to leave the group, they are expected to bring this up for exploration with the group before terminating; abrupt departures can be detrimental to the member leaving as well as the other members.

It is my bias that a group experience can be enhanced if the members are systematically prepared for becoming active participants; this includes teaching members how to get the most from the group, teaching them how groups work, discussing ways of getting personally involved during the sessions, and exploring the basics of group process. Of course, this can be done over several sessions and does not need to be completed in the preliminary session.

Stage 1—Initial Stage: A Time for Orientation and Exploration

Perhaps the most important period in the evolution of a group is the initial sessions, for they set the tone that will influence what occurs in later stages. Many groups do not get beyond the initial testing period, mainly because the pregroup issues that I've discussed were ignored or poorly handled.

Characteristics of the Initial Stage

During the early stage of a group, the central process involves orientation and exploration. At this time, members are getting acquainted, learning how the group functions, developing spoken and unspoken norms that will govern in-group behavior, exploring fears and hopes pertaining to the group, clarifying their expectations, identifying personal goals, and determining how safe this group might be for them.

At the initial session or two, it is common to see considerable tentativeness and a lack of clarity about what the participants hope to get from a group experience. Members tend to present aspects of themselves that they think others will accept, because of concern over such matters as acceptance versus rejection, being in the group versus being out of the group, being understood versus being misunderstood, being free to proceed at one's own pace versus being pushed to open up too quickly, being cared for versus being ignored or given conditional approval; and the issue of trust versus mistrust looms in the background. Whether or not members actually verbalize some of their thoughts and feelings, questions that are a part of their awareness early in the group's history include the following:

- Will I be accepted or rejected in here?
- Can I really say what I feel, or do I have to say what I think others expect?
- Am I like others in this group?
- Will I really get anything from this group?
- Will I feel pressured to perform and meet the expectations of others? If so, how will I handle this pressure?
- What kinds of risks will I take in here?
- Whom can I trust? Is there anyone I don't trust?
- Can I reveal the sides of myself that I generally keep hidden?
- What if I discover aspects of myself that I don't like?

Since most members are uncertain about the norms and expected behavior of the group situation, there are moments of silence and awkwardness. Some may be impatient to "get things moving" and at the same time be waiting for others to risk themselves first. If the leader provides very little structure, the level of anxiety is likely to be high because of the ambiguity of the situation. In this case, there is likely to be considerable milling around and requests from members for direction.

If someone does volunteer a topic for discussion, the chances are that some members will be oriented toward problem solving. Instead of allowing members to express a feeling and explore an issue, some members at this stage will offer "helpful advice." Soon the members will tire of ready-made solutions to every problem raised, and some participants will begin to express negative feelings about the superficial level of interaction.

Negative feelings might surface over a number of situations, a few of which are anger over the lack of direction given by the leader, impatience with those members who are quick to give others advice and tell them "how to live," boredom over the social chitchat and unwillingness of some to get to a deeper and more meaningful level, and resentment over the fact that some members remain quiet while others dominate the group sessions. Regardless of what is triggering any negative feelings, it is crucial that leaders be sensitive to these reactions and encourage members to express them openly. If leaders react defensively or cut off the exploration of negative feelings, then a norm is being established that only positive feelings are acceptable. Trust can be lost or gained by the way the leader handles the initial expression of any negative feelings. Members might say to themselves: "I'll risk myself by expressing some negative feelings, and then I'll see how others in here respond to me. If they are willing to listen to what I don't like, then maybe I can trust them with some deeper feelings." If participants feel they cannot be open about their reactions to the group, including any reservations they may have, then it is highly unlikely that they will feel free enough to reveal personal matters pertaining to out-of-group conflicts. Thus, members are testing the waters at the early sessions to see whether their concerns are taken seriously and whether this group is a safe place for them to express what they think and feel.

Ways of Creating Trust During the Initial Stage

There is not a single technique or even a set of techniques that alone creates trust (Corey, Corey, Callanan, & Russell, 1982). Using techniques without first establishing a good relationship with group members is likely to result in suspicion and holding back on the part of members. If you are interested in eventually leading a group, I hope that you give consideration to thinking about how *you* can be your most important technique in fostering trust. The person that you are and especially the attitudes toward group work and toward people that you demonstrate by the way you behave in the sessions may be the most crucial factors in building a trusting community. You teach most effectively through your example. If you trust in the group process and have a faith in the members' capacity to make significant changes in themselves, they are likely to see value in this group as a pathway toward personal growth. If you listen nondefensively and respectfully and are able to convey that you value members' subjective experience, they are likely to see the power in active listening. If you are genuine and willing to engage in appropriate self-disclosure, you will foster honesty and disclosure among the members. If you are truly able to accept others for who they are and avoid imposing your values on them, your members learn valuable lessons about accepting people's right to differ and to be themselves. In short, what you model through what you do in the group is one of the most potent ways to teach members how to relate to one another constructively.

Whereas trust is the major task to be accomplished at the initial stage of a group's development, it is a mistake to assume that once trust has been established, it is taken care of for the duration of the history of that group. Trust ebbs and flows, and new levels of trust must be established as the group progresses toward a deeper level of intimacy. A basic sense of trust and safety is essential for the movement of a group beyond the initial stage, and yet this trust will be tested time and again and take on new facets in later stages.

One of the best ways of creating a trusting climate is for the leader to encourage members to express openly any feelings of mistrust or absence of trust they might be experiencing. If work is to proceed, mistrust must be first recognized and then dealt with in the group. If it is not, a hidden agenda develops, the lack of trust is expressed in indirect ways, and the group ceases to progress to a more advanced stage of development. If a basic sense of trust is not established at the outset and the group leader tries to push an agenda too soon, serious problems can be predicted: lack of energy, awkward silences, and the development of hidden agendas.

When trust is present in a group, the members express their reactions without fear of censure, they are actively involved in the activities, they are willing to make themselves known to others, they take risks both in the group and in everyday life, they disclose persistent feelings that pertain to the group itself, and they both support and challenge others in the group.

Helping Members Define Goals

As a group leader, one of your tasks at the initial stage is to help members establish their own goals. In most of the groups that I lead, members typically come to the group with unclear and abstract goals. When I ask participants what they most want for themselves from the group or what kinds of behaviors they most want to change, I typically receive vague answers such as "I just want to be able to communicate with others," "I hope I can get in touch with my feelings," "I'd like to become self-actualized." These vague ideas need to be translated into specific and concrete goals with regard to the desired changes and to the efforts the person is actually willing to make to bring about these changes. Since such global goals are hard to work on, leaders can help a member who is vague by encouraging the person to narrow down some statements. For example, if a member says "I would like to learn to express my feelings," the leader might ask: "What are some particular feelings that you have the most difficulty in expressing? To whom do you experience problems in expressing feelings? What are some situations in which you find it most difficult to express a certain feeling? How would you like to be different?"

Developing *contracts*, both orally and in writing, can help members develop concrete goals that will guide their participation in the group. This need not be accomplished in one meeting, and it might well take several sessions to develop realistic contracts for all members. I find that asking members to write down their goals is valuable, for taking an active role in doing something to bring about the changes they say they want to make increases their commitment level.

Major Member Functions and Possible Problems

Early in the course of the group some specific member roles and tasks are critical to the shaping of the group. Some of the member functions are the following:

- Taking active steps to create a trusting climate in the group.
- Learning to express one's feelings and thoughts, especially as they pertain to in-group reactions.
- Being willing to express fears, hopes, expectations, reservations, and personal concerns as they pertain to the group.
- Being willing to make oneself known to others in the group.
- Being a part of the creation of group norms.
- Establishing specific and personal goals that will govern group participation.
- Learning the basics of group process, especially how to involve oneself in the interactions in the group.
- Recognizing and expressing any negative reactions and learning to pay attention to one's own resistances.

These are problems that can arise with members:

- They might wait passively for "something to happen."
- They might keep to themselves feelings of mistrust or fears pertaining to the group and thus entrench their own resistance.
- They might choose to keep themselves hidden and reveal only safe parts of themselves.
- There is the danger of slipping into a problem-solving and advice-giving stance with other members.
- They may be content to put up with superficial interactions.

Major Leader Functions

The major tasks of group leadership during the orientation and exploration stage of a group are these:

- Teaching participants some general guidelines that will increase their chances of having a productive group, and continuing to teach them ways to participate actively.
- Developing ground rules and norms and helping members see how these are related to an effective group.
- Assisting members in expressing their fears and expectations and working toward the development of trust.
- Modeling basic conditions such as genuineness, respect, attentiveness,

concern, acceptance, active listening, support, and caring confrontation (or challenge).
- Being open with members and being psychologically present for them.
- Clarifying the division of responsibility.
- Assisting members to establish concrete and meaningful goals.
- Helping members see how they might practice what they learn in the group in and out of group situations.
- Dealing openly with members' concerns and questions.
- Providing a degree of structuring that will neither increase member dependence nor promote excessive floundering.
- Assisting members to share what they are thinking and feeling as it pertains to what is occurring within the group.
- Helping members learn basic interpersonal skills, such as listening and responding nondefensively.
- Assessing the needs of the group and facilitating in such a way that these needs are met.

Stage 2—The Transition Stage: Learning to Deal with Conflict

Before a group progresses to a working stage, it typically goes through a transition stage, which is characterized by anxiety, defensiveness, resistance, the struggle for control, intermember conflict, conflicts with or challenges to the leader, and a variety of problem behaviors. To move from the initial stage to the working stage, a group must deal successfully with certain critical developmental tasks at the transition stage.

Characteristics of the Transition Stage

Some groups remain stuck at the transition stage because resistance is bypassed or because conflict is ignored or smoothed over. At this point in the evolution of a group, feelings of anxiety and resistance to this anxiety are common, and members often are—

- Experiencing anxiety over what they will think of themselves if they open themselves up, as well as being concerned over others' acceptance or rejection.
- Testing the leader and other members to determine how safe the environment is.
- Struggling with wanting to play it safe versus wanting to risk going beyond safety and getting involved.
- Experiencing some struggle for control and power. Conflict among members and between members and leaders is common.
- Being challenged with learning how to work through conflict and confrontation.
- Being reluctant to get fully involved in working on their personal concerns because they are not sure others will care.

Anxiety. Anxiety grows out of the fear of letting others see us on a level beyond the public image. Anxiety also results from the fear of being judged and misunderstood, from the need for more structure, and from a lack of clarity about goals, norms, and expected behavior in the group situation. As participants come to trust more fully the other members and the leader, they become increasingly able to share of themselves, and this openness lessens their anxiety about letting others see them as they are.

Common Fears Associated with Resistance. If fears are kept inside, then all sorts of avoidances are bound to occur. Although group leaders cannot pry open members and force them to discuss their fears that could inhibit their participation, leaders can sensitively invite members to recognize some of these fears, which often include fear of making a fool of oneself, fear of rejection, fear of discovering that one is empty, fear of being left hanging, fear that one will not like what is discovered, fear of self-disclosure, fear of being attacked and being left without defenses, and fear of getting intimate with others.

It is important that the group leader understand and appreciate the anxiety and resistance of members. Resistance must be respected, for it is to be expected that members will have doubts, reservations, and fears. The central task of the leader at this time is to help the members recognize and deal with their resistances and defenses against anxiety.

Learning to Recognize and Deal with Conflict

The transition stage is characterized by conflict and the expression of negative feelings. The initial business of getting acquainted, establishing trust, and beginning to get a sense of the purpose of the group gives way to testing the water by expressing negative feelings. Members challenge other members and the leader. Some statements that indicate intermember conflicts are "Why do we focus so much on the negative in this group?" "I don't belong here because my problems aren't as great as most of the others' in here." "Some people in here sound like they have it all together." "I feel threatened by Sally."

Conflicts with leaders are not uncommon at the transition stage, for a key task of members is to learn how to challenge the leader in a direct and constructive manner. This can be a sign that the members are moving toward greater independence. The way the leader handles this challenge is crucial to the future of a group. If leaders are excessively defensive and refuse to acknowledge criticism, they inhibit the members from confronting each other in a constructive manner, thus impairing the level of trust within the group.

At this stage of the group's development, the leader's major function is to help members move from conflict to a level of relating openly. Some other tasks are teaching members the value of recognizing and dealing with conflict, teaching them to respect and work with their resistance, providing a model for members by dealing directly with any challenges they receive, and encouraging members to express their reactions to what is happening within the group.

Stage 3—The Working Stage

During the initial stage, the group is characterized by tentativeness, for the members are finding out what a group is about and their place in it. During the transition period, there is an expression of feelings pertaining to interactions within the group, as well as individual personal problems. The working stage is characterized by the commitment of members to explore significant problems they bring to the sessions.

One of the main characteristics of the working stage is that participants have learned how to involve themselves in group interactions, rather than merely waiting to be invited into an interaction. In a sense, there is a sharing of the group leadership functions, for the members are able to assume greater responsibility for the work that occurs in the group.

A central characteristic of the working stage is group cohesion, which results when members are willing to become transparent with one another. Cohesion is necessary for the success of a group. Some indicators of the level of cohesiveness (or "togetherness") in a group are the extent of cooperation among group members, the degree of initiative shown by the participants, attendance rates, punctuality, the level of trust shown, and the degree of support, encouragement, and caring that members demonstrate in their interactions.

How does group cohesion come about? Group cohesion and authentic positive feelings within a group typically occur after negative feelings are recognized and expressed, for expressing such negative feelings is one way of testing the freedom and trustworthiness of the group. Participants soon discover whether this group is a safe place to disagree openly and whether they will still be accepted in spite of having negative feelings. When negative feelings are constructively dealt with, members learn that their relationships are strong enough to withstand an honest level of challenge. My experience continues to teach me that cohesion occurs when participants open up and take risks by making themselves known. It is the honest sharing of significant personal struggles, as well as discussing reactions to one another, that brings a group together. Cohesion, which is a process of bonding, and genuine trust are things that the group *earns* by a commitment to be honest in the sessions. At this stage the members are able to see commonalities, and they are quite struck by the universality of their life issues. For example, in a number of adult groups that I have led, it becomes apparent that there are some common human themes that most of the members can relate to personally, regardless of their age, social/cultural background, and line of work. Although in the earlier stages members are likely to be aware of their differences and at times feel separated, these differences recede into the background as the group achieves increased cohesion. Members comment more on how they are alike than on how they are different. A woman in her early twenties sees that she is very much like a man in his fifties, in that both are still striving for parental approval and measure their worth by standards set by their parents. A man learns that his struggles with masculinity are not much different from a woman's struggles with her femininity. An older person who suffers from guilt because of the experiences he missed with his daughter as she was growing up finds that he is deeply touched by a young woman who expresses her hurt of never really getting to know her father. A woman learns that she is not alone when she discovers that she is not strange for feeling resentment over the many demands her family makes on her. Other common themes evolving in this stage that lead to an increase in the level of cohesion and trust are feelings of loneliness and abandonment, feelings of inferiority and living up to others' expectations, painful memories of childhood and adolescent experiences, guilt and remorse over what members have and have not done, discovering that their worst enemy often lives within them, becoming aware of the need for love and the fear of love, feelings about sexual identity and sexual performance, conflicts with significant others, unfinished business with parents, and searching for a meaning in life. This list is not exhaustive; it is merely a sample of the universal human issues that participants recognize and explore together as the group progresses to a working stage.

In addition to the characteristics mentioned, there are some other ways to determine whether a group has progressed to the working stage. Some factors that indicate that the group has come together for a common purpose and that the members are engaged in productive and meaningful work are as follows:

- Communication within the group is open and involves an accurate expression of what is being experienced.
- Leadership functions do not rest solely with the group leader, for now the members interact freely and directly, and they initiate the direction they want to move toward, rather than relying on the leader for direction.
- There is a willingness to risk dealing with threatening material and to make oneself known in significant ways, and members bring personal topics to the group for discussion.
- When conflict is present, it is recognized and dealt with directly and effectively, and hence hidden agendas and indirect expressions of hostility do not become a pattern.
- Feedback is given freely and is received in a nondefensive manner.
- Confrontation occurs without members' slapping judgmental labels on others.
- Members are willing to work and practice outside the group to achieve behavioral changes.

- Participants are willing to risk new behavior, for they feel supported in their attempts to change.
- Members are willing to offer *both* challenge and support to others, and they engage in self-confrontation.
- Participants continually assess their level of satisfaction with the group, and they take active steps to change matters if they see that the sessions need changing.
- Members feel hopeful that they can change if they are willing to take action, and they do not feel hopeless.

Stage 4—The Final Stage: Consolidation and Termination

During the final stage a number of characteristics can be expected, all of which are associated with successfully accomplishing the difficult processes of consolidation and termination. These include the possibility of sadness and anxiety over the reality of separation, a tendency of members to pull back and participate in less intense ways in anticipation of the ending of the group, a concern over one's ability to be able to implement in daily life what one learned in the group, and decisions about what courses of action to take and the development of action programs. And there may be some talk about follow-up meetings or some plan for accountability, so that members will be encouraged to carry out their plans for change.

The final stages of group evolution are vital, for during this time members have an opportunity to clarify the meaning of their experiences in group, to consolidate the gains they have made, and to revise their decisions about what newly acquired behaviors they want to transfer to their everyday life. As group members sense that their group is approaching termination, there is a danger that they will begin to distance themselves from the group experience and thus fail to closely examine the ways in which their in-group learning might affect their out-of-group behavior. Other possible problems that can occur at this time include the tendency for some members to avoid reviewing their experience and failing to put it into some cognitive framework, thus limiting the generalization of what they have learned to their everyday existence. Further, members might consider the group an end in itself rather than a laboratory for interpersonal learning. For these reasons, group leaders must learn to help the participants put into meaningful perspective what has occurred in the group. If leaders handle the consolidation and termination stage poorly, the chances are greatly reduced that members will be able to use what they have learned. Even worse, participants can be left with unresolved issues and without any direction to bring these issues to closure. Typically, this is the phase in group work that is handled most ineptly by group leaders, partly because of their own resistance to terminating a group and also because of their lack of training for this difficult stage. Some specific functions of group leadership and some tasks that need to be accomplished during the final stage are as follows:

- Members can be encouraged to face the inevitable ending of the group and to discuss fully their feelings of separation.
- Members can complete any unfinished business they have with other members or leaders.
- Members can be taught how to leave the group and how to carry with them what they have learned.
- Members can be assisted in making specific plans for change and for taking concrete steps to put into effect in their daily lives the lessons they have learned.
- Leaders can help members develop specific plans for follow-up work, evaluations can be made, and leaders can help members create their own support systems after they leave a group.

Members need help in facing the reality that their group will soon end. Feelings about separation, which often take the form of denial or avoidance, need to be fully brought out and explored. Members can be helped to face separation by the leader's disclosure of his or her own feelings about terminating the group.

During the initial stage, members are often asked to express their fears of *entering* fully into the group. Now they should be encouraged to share their fears or concerns about *leaving* the group and having to face day-to-day realities without the group's support. Members typically express concerns of not being able to be as trusting and open with people outside the group. The leader's task is to remind the participants that they had to work at developing the trust they valued and that trust did not automatically happen *to* them. Therefore, they can make similar choices and commitments, and be equally successful, in their relationships outside the group.

During the consolidation stage, leaders need to prepare participants to deal with those with whom they live and work. Role playing can be extremely helpful for practicing ways of responding to the significant people in one's life. In role playing, members can practice new behaviors and receive feedback from other members on their impact, as well as suggestions for alternative behaviors they may not have thought about. The feedback from the group can help members concentrate on changing themselves rather than making plans to change others.

Postgroup Issues: Follow-Up and Evaluation Procedures

There are some techniques and strategies that can be used after the termination of a group, mainly for the purpose of a follow-up to assess outcomes. These techniques can introduce a sense of accountability into group work, for the group's having come to an end does not mean that the leader's job is finished or that members' work ceases. In our book *Group Techniques* (Corey, Corey, Callanan, & Russell, 1982) we describe some specific approaches for leaders in helping members evaluate the effectiveness of their group experience.

Conducting Follow-Up Interviews

As a safety check and as a method of assessment, leaders can try to arrange a private interview with each group member a few weeks to a few months after the group terminates. Such an interview can be beneficial to the member as a "booster shot" and to the leaders as a way to evaluate the effectiveness of the group.

The individual screening interview at the pregroup stage is generally partly devoted to ascertaining why people would like to join a group, helping them identify personal goals, and discussing their expectations. The postgroup individual interview can be used to determine the degree to which members have accomplished their stated goals and to which their expectations were met, and participants can discuss what the group meant to them in retrospect. If members are having problems applying what they learned in the group to everyday life, this individual contact is an opportunity to explore ways of dealing with these difficulties. It is also an excellent opportunity for leaders to suggest other groups, individual counseling, marital and family counseling, or some other type of workshop or class—if they seem appropriate. This practice of arranging for a follow-up interview is in keeping with the *Ethical Guidelines for Group Leaders*, as designed by the Association for Specialists in Group Work (1980). One of the guidelines states: "Group leaders shall provide between-session consultation to group members and follow-up after termination of the group, as needed or requested."

Encouraging Contact with Other Members

A technique that can lend support to members as they are practicing new behavior or completing an action program is to contact another member from the group periodically after termination. This contact can be especially important when members find that they are not pushing themselves to do much now that the group is finished. This is a method of accountability, and it is a way for people to learn how to establish a support system.

Arranging a Follow-Up Group Session

A follow-up group meeting can take place a couple of months after the end of the group to assess the impact of the group on each member. Having such a session is one more way of maximizing the chance that members will receive lasting benefit from the group experience. Many people have reported that simply knowing that they would be coming together as a group in the future after the group's termination was the motivation they needed to stick to their commitments to carry out their action programs. Finally, the follow-up session offers leaders another opportunity to remind participants that they are responsible for what they become and that if they hope to change their situation, they must take active steps to do so.

Ways of Carrying One's Learning Further

Assisting members to carry their learning into action programs is one of the most important functions of the group leader. If a group is successful, it may mark the beginning of growth for many members. Even though some members may appear to get little from their first group, it often readies them for future growth experiences. Thus, during the final session, the follow-up interview, or the follow-up group session, leaders might give a number of suggestions to those participants who wish to continue the work they have begun. Because members may be ready to consider another group or individual counseling only after some time has elapsed, the follow-up session is an excellent place to reinforce the value of getting involved in various types of growth projects.

In many ways, the ending stage of a group is really a *commencement,* for members now have some directions that they can begin to take in dealing with problems as they arise. Members should now have additional tools and skills to cope with personal difficulties, and they are likely to be open to using resources for continuing the process of personal growth and change.

A Commentary on the Group Leader's Competence

Having seen the various stages that a group moves through, you might be asking yourself what it takes to be a leader of a group. Unfortunately, during the 1960s and to a lesser extent the 1970s, many groups were quickly put together and were conducted by unqualified people. Some people assume that merely having been a member of a group or attending a few weekend encounter groups or workshops qualifies them to organize and facilitate their own group. The issue of group-leader competency is a broad one that cannot be fully addressed here. However, I can outline the personal and professional skills, attitudes, knowledge, and background of education and training that I deem essential for professional counselors who lead groups.

Determining One's Own Level of Competence

Different groups require different leader qualities. For example, you may be fully competent to lead a group of relatively well-adjusted adults or of adults in crisis situations and yet not be competent to lead a group of seriously disturbed people. You may be well trained for, and work well with, groups for the elderly and yet not have the training or skills to work with children or adolescents. You may be successful in leading groups of substance abusers and yet find yourself ill prepared to work successfully with family groups. In short, you need specific training and supervised experience for each type of group you intend to lead; competence in *some* areas of group work does not imply competence in *all* areas.

Some Paths toward Becoming a Qualified Group Leader

As I have mentioned elsewhere (Corey, 1981), there are numerous paths that can lead one to become qualified as a group leader. Most practitioners have had their formal training in some branch of the mental-health field, such as psychiatric social work, clinical or counseling psychology, psychiatry, psychiatric nursing, marriage and family counseling, or educational psychology. Generally, however, those who seek to become group practitioners find that formal education, even at the graduate level, does not give them the practical grounding they require to lead groups effectively. Consequently, they find it necessary to take a variety of specialized group-therapy training workshops and in-service programs dealing with the theory and practice of group work.

In addition to formal academic study, workshops, and supervised experience, I think it is essential that practitioners participate as *members* in a variety of groups and that, if possible, they also experience individual counseling as a *client*. Being a member in various groups can be an indispensable part of training for group leaders, for it allows them to experience what it is like to be a working member of a group. All the stages described in the previous section can be actually experienced. Being in a group *as a member* will allow you to experience your own resistances, fears, and uncomfortable moments in a group; by being confronted and by struggling with your own problems in a group, you can receive practical experience concerning what is needed to build a trusting and cohesive group.

Some Dimensions of the Education and Training of Group Counselors

Speaking in broad terms, I see the following as important components of the training and education of counselors who want to lead various types of counseling groups: foundations and course-work background, observation of professional group leaders, didactic course work, supervised practice, and individual and group counseling experience as a client.

1. *Foundations and course-work background.* Course work that most writers in the group field describe as a basic requirement for an effective

group-leader training program includes group dynamics, family dynamics, human growth and development, personality theory and psychodynamics, psychopathology, theories of counseling, principles of individual counseling and therapy, human socialization, cultural and social factors of human behavior, and practicum and internship in counseling. I think that experience in and knowledge of individual-counseling approaches are essential parts of the didactic and experiential training of group counselors. However, I also think that specific course work in *group* counseling is essential, for the fact that a person is competent to do individual counseling does not mean that this person will necessarily be able to lead a group effectively.
2. *Observation of professional group leaders.* Highly competent leaders can serve as excellent models to imitate. Observing and experiencing a skilled group leader in action is one way to learn how to facilitate a group.
3. *Didactic course work.* Gazda (1978) has found that students receive the most from a course in group-counseling theory when they have an opportunity to try out the theory and some of the techniques suggested by the model. Gazda believes, as I do, that the best preparation for group leadership requires the student leader to master a number of group models rather than buying one single approach. I think that a comprehensive course in the theories of *group* counseling, with an emphasis on application of techniques based on the various theoretical approaches, is a must in the background of those who want to lead groups. Readers who wish to study the practical applications of various theoretical models relating to group work might consult Corey (1981).
4. *Supervised practice.* In my view, the heart of a training program for group leaders is practice in leading groups under adequate supervision with a coleader. Feedback from the supervisor and from the coleader can help trainees recognize mistakes and detect areas they are overlooking. Feedback can also call attention to the trainees' strengths so that the student leaders can build on them. The Association for Specialists in Group Work is presently working on guidelines for the preparation of group counselors. In tentative form, these guidelines suggest that supervised experience should include critiquing group tapes, observing group-counseling sessions, participating as a client in a group, coleading a group with a supervisor, coleading a group with a partner, and receiving critical feedback from the supervisor.
5. *Individual counseling and personal group experience.* As mentioned earlier, some form of personal therapy—be it individual, in a group, or a combination—is, to me, an essential part of the group counselor's training program. I believe that undergoing therapeutic experiences as a client increases the chances that trainees will become aware of their motivations for becoming group counselors, as well as helping them see how their needs and values might either facilitate or inhibit them in their

role as a leader of a group. One guideline in the ASGW's *Ethical Guidelines for Group Leaders* (1980) is "Group leaders shall refrain from imposing their own agendas, needs, and values on group members." Experience in personal or group counseling, as a client, can be instrumental in helping the trainee to become aware of the tendency to use the group leader's role as a way of meeting personal needs at the expense of the members.

The training program for group therapists designed by the American Group Psychotherapy Association (1978) requires a minimum of 120 hours' participation as a member in a therapy group. Although some limited substitution in group process is allowed, the association's guideline is based on the conviction that a therapist should have an experience comparable to that of a client in an ongoing group.

6. *The person of the group leader.* I think that the personal characteristics of a counselor who wants to lead groups are crucial. A few such characteristics are self-awareness, ability to relate effectively with people in groups, willingness to take risks, ability to look at one's life and be willing to do for oneself what one would expect of one's clients, and belief in the value of group process as an agent of change.

Perspectives for the '80s

From the workshops I have done, I have become aware of the great interest in group counseling. I have also learned that many counselor education programs in this country are weak in formal course work in group counseling and in providing quality supervised experience in group work. Although the interest in groups seems evident, a major challenge facing the group field is to develop good theory courses and supervised internships in group work. This increased and renewed interest in group counseling and group psychotherapy is reflected in an increasing number of books published that deal with group therapy (Silver, Lubin, Miller, and Dobson, 1981).

What are some of the challenges for those interested in group work? Although I cannot accurately predict trends in the 1980s in the field of group work, let me mention a challenge facing those of you who want to become group counselors. This challenge is to become sensitive to the ethical aspects of group practice. In 1980 the Association for Specialists in Group Work published *Ethical Guidelines for Group Leaders*. Ideally, this event signaled an increasing interest in organizing and conducting groups ethically. Much of the poor reputation of groups is due to sloppy and unethical practice that characterized some groups during the group movement in the 1960s and 1970s. In my view, the negative reputation of groups is partly due to inept practitioners and has thus been earned. My hope would be that group practitioners will pay increasing attention to sound practices in organizing, conducting, and evaluating groups.

Summary

What is group counseling about? Surely it is more than can be presented in a single chapter. My attempt has been to discuss some of the values and advantages of group counseling in working with various age populations. The bulk of the chapter has focused on the stages in the life history of a group, with special attention given to characteristics of each stage, member functions and roles, tasks and functions of the group leader at each stage, and group-process concepts associated with each phase in the evolution of a group. The stages in the life of a group do not generally flow neatly and predictably in the order described in this chapter. In actuality there is considerable overlap between stages, and once a group moves to an advanced stage of development, there may be temporary regressions to earlier developmental stages.

Certainly you will not be ready to lead a group by reading this chapter alone (or even by reading many of the books I suggest at the end of this chapter). My intent has been to give you a general picture of the course of a group in action—from its beginning to its end—and to stimulate you to think about how groups can be a valuable tool and approach in professional counseling.

Now It's Your Turn

For the following exercises, I suggest that you form small groups in class and discuss the issues involved in each of the questions or situations. The purpose of these exercises is to stimulate your thinking about groups as well as spark your interest in learning more about them. Another purpose is to encourage you to share your ideas, reactions, and experiences as they pertain to some of the ideas in this chapter. In your small groups, select a few of the following exercises that have the greatest degree of interest. If you are unable to discuss some of these exercises in class, you might think about them and talk with another student.

1. What were your reactions to this chapter? What stood out as being most significant to you, and why? Discuss the ideas that you found most useful and interesting. What are some other things you would like to know about groups?
2. Assume that you were going to join a group *as a member*. What are some questions you would like to ask of the leader before you joined the group? How would you determine whether this group was right for you? What would you most be looking for in a group leader?
3. When you think of group counseling or group therapy, what comes to mind? Discuss with others in your small group things you've heard about groups, possible misconceptions, and any experience you've had with groups.

4. What are some values that you can think of pertaining to the use of counseling groups with children? Adolescents? College students? Middle-aged adults? The elderly? What are some advantages, if any, in using group approaches over individual-counseling approaches?
5. Assume that you are asked by the director of the agency that employs you to organize and lead a group. Your boss tells you that because of the large number of people seeking psychological counseling, a group approach will be a good way to reach increasing numbers. What will you say to your boss?
6. Assume that you want to organize a group with some population that you are working with, and assume that you begin by developing a proposal for such a group. Discuss some of the things you will consider in setting up such a group, including how you might structure the group, topics to be covered, methods of screening and selecting members, and how you might begin the group.
7. What are some of the challenges that you see for the 1980s pertaining to the future of group work?
8. Discuss your own views on requiring personal group-counseling experience for any counselor who expects to lead groups. Do you think that group leaders should have first been members of a group? Why or why not?

References and Suggested Readings

American Group Psychotherapy Association. *Guidelines for the training of group psychotherapists*. New York: American Group Psychotherapy Association, 1978.

Association for Specialists in Group Work. *Ethical guidelines for group leaders*. Falls Church, Va.: Association for Specialists in Group Work, 1980.

Burnside, I. M. (Ed.). *Working with the elderly: Group processes and techniques*. North Scituate, Mass.: Duxbury Press, 1978.

Corey, G. *Theory and practice of group counseling*. Monterey, Calif.: Brooks/Cole, 1981.

Corey, G. *I never knew I had a choice* (2nd ed.). Monterey, Calif.: Brooks/Cole, 1983.

Corey, G., & Corey, M. *Groups: Process and practice* (2nd ed.). Monterey, Calif.: Brooks/Cole, 1983.

Corey, G., Corey, M., & Callanan, P. *Professional and ethical issues in counseling and psychotherapy*. Monterey, Calif.: Brooks/Cole, 1979.

Corey, G., Corey, M., Callanan, P., & Russell, J. M. *Group techniques*. Monterey, Calif.: Brooks/Cole, 1982.

Duncan, J. A., & Gumaer, J. (Eds.). *Developmental groups for children*. Springfield, Ill.: Charles C Thomas. 1980.

Gazda, G. M. *Group counseling: A developmental approach* (2nd ed.). Boston: Allyn & Bacon, 1978.

Gazda, G. M. (Ed.). *Innovations to group psychotherapy* (2nd ed.). Springfield, Ill.: Charles C Thomas, 1981.

Oaklander, V. *Windows to our children.* Moab, Utah: Real People Press, 1978.

Shapiro, J. L. *Methods of group psychotherapy and encounter: A tradition of innovation.* Itasca, Ill.: Peacock, 1978.

Silver, R. J., Lubin, B., Miller, D. R., & Dobson, N. H. The group psychotherapy literature: 1980. *International Journal of Group Psychotherapy,* 1981, *31*(4), 469–526.

Yalom, I. D. *The theory and practice of group psychotherapy* (2nd ed.). New York: Basic Books, 1975.

CHAPTER **6**

Consulting

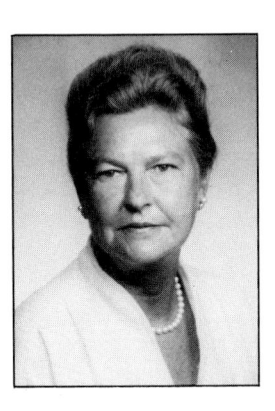

Jeannette A. Brown

Jeannette A. Brown is a professor of counselor education at the University of Virginia. She designed a nationally validated Title III ESEA elementary school guidance project based on a consultation model. Dr. Brown is the author of a text on elementary school guidance services and teaches courses on the use of counseling skills in the varied settings in which counselors work.

The consulting sessions were progressing reasonably well. The day included its usual quota of unexpected difficulties and required a high degree of flexibility. Also demanded were extreme perception and sensitivity, as well as creativity and a high tolerance for ambiguity. Helping people learn how to learn is discouraging and often ego-deflating, particularly in the early stages of consulting. But dealing with conflict, confrontation, and the unexpected is, after all, the life of a consultant.

Nevertheless, she was totally unprepared for the administrator's question. As he held the door for her, he asked whether she knew the definition of a consultant. "A consultant," he announced, "is someone who blows in, blows off, and blows out!"

It is not known when people decided they needed someone outside themselves to change the circumstances of their lives. The Greeks had an oracle, Native American tribes had a shaman, and in modern society business, industry, educational institutions, and community agencies have a consultant. Oracle, shaman, consultant, palmist, guru, or seer—each of these titles has been reserved for someone uniquely qualified to intercede against all the troublesome affairs of life.

By virtue of the power attributed to them, consultants have created solutions for improved organizational behavior, interpersonal relations, program content, worker efficiency, and financial management. They are all-knowing and all-powerful. Or are they? Are they all-powerful because they are all-knowing, or are they presumed to be all-knowing because others have given them all power over their lives?

Generally, the perfectly normal abnormalities of human beings do not include relinquishing power over their own lives. Most healthy people reserve the right to solve their own problems. They may discuss their problems with others, but they almost never accept someone else's solution to their problems. Over time they may arrive at a similar solution, but unless they do, they rarely follow a course of action prescribed by someone else. How, then, has the consultant continued to prosper? There are many reasons, and the consulting process, as we define it for professional counselors, has tried to capitalize on the most prominent among them.

Why Counselors Consult

As you know, your professional organization endorsed a statement of standards for professional counselors (American Personnel and Guidance Association, 1979). The standards stipulated *counseling* as the counselor's primary function and consulting as a necessary correlate of the counseling process. Despite the professional counselor's depth of knowledge in the dynamics of human behavior and personality, or perhaps because of it, counselors have a deep appreciation for human fallibility. The critical nature of the counseling process makes it mandatory for counselors to exhaust all known sources of information and to solicit the assistance and support of a variety of persons who may be able to help counselees help themselves.

Because the counseling process includes a continuing effort toward more satisfying interactions of counselees with their environments, the effectiveness of counseling is directly proportional to the amount of information brought to, and shared in, the relationship. This is why effective counselors do not work in isolation from all those others who live and work with the counselee. This is why effective counselors consult. Counseling effectiveness requires consulting effectiveness. As professional counselors, you can't have one without the other.

Definitions and Approaches

How can we define *consulting*, and how can we arrive at an appropriate approach to the consulting function? As implied, there are a variety of answers to both questions, but our quest is made easier because the answer to either question is intimately related to the answer to the other. Definitions create approaches and approaches create definitions. As with the counseling process, how you define your own and your counselees' needs, capabilities, and attributes will necessarily define your approach to them.

This interrelated and interdependent nature of definitions and approaches might be demonstrated by an examination of four definitions offered below. A consultant is someone—

1. to whom problems are given
2. who defines problems and creates solutions
3. who designs and manages a system for the problem-solving efforts of others
4. who helps others "learn how to learn" what their problems are and how to solve them.

Inherent in each of these definitions are certain consequences for you and those for whom you will provide consulting services.

If it is true that our attitudes, values, and beliefs direct our behavior, then the search for a definition of *consulting* requires self-searching. What do you believe about yourself—your talents, your power, and your competencies? What do you believe about your working associates—their talents, their influence, and their competencies? More to the point, what do you believe about your responsibility to people with whom you are interacting? Are you and your skills sufficient resources for people in need of help? More bluntly put, are *you* all they need? Perhaps, but keep these questions in mind as we examine four proposed modes of consulting, which seem related to the four definitions offered above.

The consulting process is represented as a three-party system including (1) a consultant, or person providing the consultation, (2) a consultee, or person(s) requesting the consultation, and (3) a target, or person(s) or circumstance(s) precipitating the consultation (Kurpius & Brubaker, 1976). For example, you are a professional counselor (consultant). A residence-hall counselor (consultee) can no longer cope with the disruptive behavior of students in the dorm (target) and comes to you because he wants to solve the problem. Depending on your definition of a consultant, you would respond to this plea for help by implementing one of the four consulting modes identified by Kurpius and Brubaker (1976): (1) provision, (2) prescription, (3) mediation, and (4) collaboration. As we discuss them, you might try matching each of them to one of the four definitions offered above.

Provision

The provision mode suggests that a consultant provides a service to consultees who have neither the time, inclination, nor perceived skill to deal with the target, or problem. The consultee simply refers the problem to the consultant. The consultant's responsibility in this approach is to bring about changes in the target that will satisfy the consultee.

For example, you are a drug-abuse counselor (the consultant), and you are sought out by parents (the consultees) of an adolescent who want you to cure their daughter's drug habit (the target). As the consultant, you are responsible to the counselees, and you are expected to bring about the desired change in the target without the participation of the consultees. Their responsibility ended when they identified the problem to you.

Prescription

The prescription mode doesn't require the consultant to bring about the cure. As a prescription consultant, you would be expected to advise your consultee what is wrong with the target and what should be done about it. As its label implies, the prescription mode consists in diagnosing a problem and prescribing a cure.

An example might be found in a community agency. You are a professional counselor in a mental-health clinic. The juvenile court has suspended sentence on a 16-year-old involved in an attempted-rape incident and has consulted you regarding the disposition of the juvenile's case. When you meet with the young man, you make various observations of his behavior; gather other information relative to his home life, friends, school life, previous encounters with the law, and so on; diagnose his problem; and advise the court how his problem should be solved. As a prescription consultant, your responsibility to your consultee, the court, is to let the court know what is wrong with the young man and what to do about it. Generally, your responsibility ends when you have diagnosed the problem and prescribed its cure.

Mediation

The mediation mode requires a consultant to coordinate the services of a variety of persons who are trying to solve a problem. By virtue of their differing perceptions of "the problem," they each may have created differing "solutions" that are being independently implemented. The work of a mediation consultant would include either an effort to coordinate the various services being provided or the creation of an alternative plan of services that represents a mutually acceptable synthesis of the several "solutions." Finally, the plan of action must be adopted by everyone.

An example of this approach might be found in a school setting wherein a school psychologist, speech therapist, curriculum specialist, probation officer, special educator, and school counselor are all providing services for a student either without concern for, or perhaps without knowledge of, one another's effort. If you were a professional counselor in such a setting, then you might have been appealed to by a distressed parent who felt that her child was being pulled in too many directions. The parent (consultee) asks you (consultant) to get all the specialists (mediators) to stop working independently and start working together to solve the child's (target's) problem. As a mediation consultant, you would be responsible for coordinating the multiple efforts of the mediators into a comprehensive, cooperative, single thrust. Sometimes this would require you to create, and persuade the mediators to adopt, an alternative plan for their intervention efforts.

Collaboration

The collaboration mode requires the consultant to facilitate the consultees' active involvement in the problem-solving process. The consultees must analyze their own problem, design their own solution, and implement and evaluate their self-determined plan of action. Consultants facilitate this level of consultee involvement by utilizing all their counseling skills and intellectual abilities. They must have the insight and perception to understand the vested interests separating the problem solvers. But they must also have the interpersonal skill and conceptual sophistication to emphasize to the consultees only those vested interests they share. Obviously, consultants using this mode must understand how people learn and under what conditions they are willing to change. It is vital that consultants be optimistic and able to generate optimism and self-confidence in others. Incidentally, a bit of charisma wouldn't hurt, either.

For example, you are an organization development counselor for an industrial company. Profits are down, and an ultimatum has come down from the board of directors: the profit margin must be increased. The president of the corporation has called a meeting of the comptroller, sales manager, union representative, production-line foreman, a sales representative, and you. Each of these participants in the meeting defines the problem differently, and the solutions they propose also differ, as shown in Table 6-1.

TABLE 6-1. Problems and solutions as perceived by different participants

Participant	Problem	Solution
President	Profits are down	Find out why
Comptroller	Payroll is too large	Lay off employees
Union representative	Morale is down	Increase wages
Sales manager	Territories are too large	Hire more sales reps
Foreman	Work environment is bad	Install new lighting
Sales representative	Travel expenses are too high	Increase commissions

The consulting service you would provide this group would include (1) creating an environment within which each participant could begin to understand the vested interests of the others; (2) providing opportunities for each to understand their shared vested interest, namely, increased profit margins; (3) helping all the participants pool their differing talents and resources in a redefinition of the problem; (4) assisting the group as they formulate a plan of action; (5) coordinating the efforts of the differing participants during the implementation of the plan; and (6) assisting them in their evaluation processes. As a collaboration consultant your responsibility is not only to help the participants learn about the differences that separate them but to help them discover those areas of common agreement that unite them. Having accomplished this they will be able to create a solution to the problem that will be a comprehensive, coordinated plan of action that can be cooperatively implemented and evaluated.

Before we began this discussion of Kurpius & Brubaker's (1976) four consulting modes I suggested you try to match each with one or another of the four *definitions* proposed. I have no illusions that the exercise was either difficult or taxing. But I beg your indulgence. Perhaps your next task will be a bit more challenging.

A Critical Analysis

Implicit in the APGA Standards (1979) is the conviction that consulting is not only an appropriate, but an expected function for professional counselors. Nevertheless, this vital component of the counselor's professional role description has been generally neglected. Only recently have professional counselors begun to give more than lip-service to the function. Many reasons could be postulated for this state of affairs but none are currently viable.

Societal Considerations

During recent years various societal concerns combined to force serious attention on the consulting function. One of the more powerful influences was the accountability movement. Counseling centers, human service agencies, and educational institutions all felt the impact of the taxpayers' rebellion. Counselors' budgets were difficult to justify, not only because of our limited and/or less than definitive research, but also because of the small number of people for whom counselors provided services. The number of counseling sessions, individual and group, held in a given day necessarily limited the numbers of people receiving help in a given day, week, or month. The year's total, as a consequence, was small. The total budget, though not excessive from the perspective of some counselors, was considered so by the taxpayer when averaged out for a per counselee/counselor cost.

Professional Considerations

Counselors in all settings from coast to coast were subject to the taxpayers' revolt. Because counseling was perceived as a frill to be added only after basic needs were supplied, radical reductions in counselor staffing occurred. These were anxious times for professional counselors. No one likes ultimatums, nor are they accepted gracefully. At such times at least three options are available responses: (1) attack, (2) retreat, or (3) reconnoiter. Professional counselors exercised all three.

Some professional counselors formulated rebuttals that attacked the legitimacy of the taxpayers' accusations with arguments that had more sound and fury than substance. Their attack failed because they had failed to address the issue. A period of retrenchment followed during which the crisis was examined more rationally and counselors saw that among the many available options was the implementation of the professional counselor's consulting function. But how was it to be performed?

Among the variety of recommendations made by various writers were one or another of the four modes just described. But at this point in our discussion we know only *what* each task is, not what the *implications* of each include. Your task during our reexamination of the four modes is to make a decision. You must choose, not expediently but with reasoned judgment, which mode you would be committed to as a professional counselor. Remember, commitments, personal or professional, are accompanied by a host of considerations not always originally perceived and a set of consequences often more critical than initially predicted. So, choose carefully and withhold final judgment until the reexamination has been completed.

Reconsiderations

It might be useful to examine the four modes for their viability as consulting approaches for professional counselors. Viability, in this instance, would be measured by the mode's legitimacy and its predicted effectiveness. For example, does the process described for the mode conform to accepted consulting definitions? And what is the probability that the desired changes would occur when using that mode? Keep these considerations in mind as we reconsider the four modes.

Provisional consulting might be assessed as an illegitimate as well as an ineffective approach on several counts. First, we could agree with Kurpius and Brubaker (1976) that it may not qualify as consulting, since it could be more accurately described as counseling. Remember those parents who were having a problem with their drug-taking daughter? They sent her to you, and you were expected to solve the problem by providing a direct service to the daughter. Is this *consulting*? Perhaps, but to us it certainly does not seem to be an effective definition of the process. Consulting is defined as a triadic relationship, and so we might question the limited participation of the parents in the process. Whose problem is it—the parents', the daughter's, or both? If both, then can we expect a more harmonious interaction of the daughter with her parents in the absence of mutual understandings and shared concerns? Perhaps we cannot.

Consulting is often differentiated from counseling as an *indirect* versus a *direct* process (Dinkmeyer & Carlson, 1973; Faust, 1967; Nelson, 1972). The desired behavior changes are facilitated in counseling by providing help directly for the person in need of it. In the consulting process, the needed help is provided indirectly. Applied to the case at hand, this criterion means that our drug-abuse counselor would be expected to consult with the parents about their daughter's problem to discover how they, the parents, could help their daughter change her drug-taking behavior. The counselor-as-a-consultant would solicit information from and share information with the parents. Collaborating as equals, the parents and the consultant would examine a variety of alternative responses to the problem and select one, and the parents would test it out by implementing it. Considering this dimension of the consulting process, does the provision mode qualify as consulting?

But what about the prescriptive mode? Was the mental-health-clinic counselor behaving as a consultant? Recall that the juvenile court had asked you to assist it in the disposition of an attempted-rape case. The court had not asked you to solve its problem; it had asked you to help it solve its problem. *On this level* we might decide that the prescription mode is a legitimate and effective consulting approach. However, we might not. Do consultants help others solve their problems, or do they help others *learn how* to solve their problems (Lippitt & Lippitt, 1978)? There is a difference. The latter option requires the consultees' active participation in the decision making. Was the problem solving shared by the juvenile court? Not if *you* made the diagnosis and prescribed the cure. Viewing the example in this manner, we might conclude that the prescription mode is neither a legitimate nor an effective consulting approach for professional counselors.

The mediation mode is rich with excellent opportunities for professional counselors to apply their human relations skills, interpersonal competencies, and organizational and management talents and to provide a much-needed service. In this era of specialization someone must assume the responsibility for integrating the independent pursuits of the various experts and for organizing their efforts into a comprehensive, coordinated thrust. Professional counselors have the skills and the opportunity to respond to this need and perform this function. But what function? Is mediating consulting? Perhaps not.

Many of the same problems that exist for the provision and prescription modes are present in the mediation mode. As in the provision mode, the consultant provides a service for someone who does not participate in the consultation process. Remember, it was a distraught parent who came to the school counselor for help, but you met and worked with all those others who were the object of her concern. You provided a direct service to the various school specialists for your consultee, the parent.

Of course, the service you provided in this instance was not *counseling*. At one *level* it might even qualify as consulting, because your service to this group did permit an exchange of information among equals who shared a common problem, explored its dimensions, agreed on a solution, and implemented it. But examine this analysis a little more closely. They did, in fact, share a common problem, but it seems obvious that they did not perceive it as a problem. Otherwise, one or all of them, rather than the parent, would have come to you for help.

Perhaps you noticed another omission in the analysis. It was not stipulated that the participants designed their own solution. You will recall that the mediation mode leaves this option open—that often it is necessary for the consultant to present a plan that takes into consideration all the vested interests of the various participants. Often the mediation consultant must coordinate the various interests and activities, goals and objectives of the different specialists and, having organized them, manage the implementation process. For these reasons, we might conclude that professional counselors using the mediation mode are not consultants. They are coordinators.

Finally, what kinds of conclusions can be drawn for the collaboration mode as a consulting approach for professional counselors? In this mode consulting services are provided indirectly. The consultant does not do something *to* someone; rather, the consultant does something *with* someone. Moreover, this mode requires active involvement of all the participants in planning, implementing, and evaluating their solution to their problem (Arensberg & Niehoff, 1964; Goodenough, 1963; Miles & Schmuck, 1971).

In addition, equal status is attributed to all the participants during the information-sharing and problem-solving process. The consultant does not judge the worth of one point of view versus another; the participants do. But the consultant does facilitate the sharing of ideas and information. And the consultant facilitates the vital process of combining knowledge into new patterns so that mutually agreed upon decisions can be made (ACES-ASCA, 1966). The consultant in this mode is not counseling, dictating, or coordinating. In this mode the consultant is consulting.

One last comment should be made about the four modes—namely, that these categories or labels are not etched in stone. They are one classification system for creating order out of a diffuse and currently unsystematic body of knowledge. You should be aware that differing consulting approaches will be variously referred to by different writers. You will also discover that different terms will be used to describe the triadic relationship. The labels are unimportant. It is the *process* that is consequential for your effectiveness as a consultant. And this returns us to the task set for you at the beginning of this section. Which consulting approach would you adopt as a professional counselor? And why?

Practical Considerations

Certainly, at this point you have discovered which consulting mode I believe could be an appropriate consulting approach for professional counselors. I am, personally and professionally, committed to the notion that individuals are capable of solving their own problems but that occasionally they need a little help. I am also committed to the notion that the kind of help they need is an opportunity to "learn how to learn." Finally, I am committed to the notion that people learn by doing. Because I am committed to this belief system, I am committed to a consulting approach that permits the active involvement of consultees in the resolution of their problems. I am committed to a collaboration consultation approach.

The approach is not haphazard. Its system is based in principles generated by innovation and change theory (Arensberg & Niehoff, 1964; Goodenough, 1963; Miles & Schmuck, 1971). Primary among these principles is the proposition that successful change requires active involvement of the consultees during all stages of the change process: (1) problem identification, (2) planning, (3) implementing, and (4) evaluating. This means that all the persons who will be affected by the change must be involved in effecting it. It also means that a willingness to become involved requires awareness of the problem and a conscious need to solve it cooperatively.

Successful change cannot occur if people either do not know they have a problem, do not feel the need to solve it, or are unwilling to work together in discovering its solution. If any one of these conditions exists, then the change effort will fail. But the consultant can facilitate the necessary and critical involvement and the consultees in their own change process.

People resist change for a variety of vested interests, including workload, power and prestige, and income or job security. They *accept* change for the same reasons. If individuals or groups can be shown that any one of their vested interests is being jeopardized by an existing state of affairs, then their awareness of the problem and need to solve it cooperatively will be increased. They will become involved. So, the first and most vital step to be taken by a consultant is to *involve* the consultees by helping them identify *with* the problem, not by describing the problem to them but by describing to them how their vested interests are not currently being served.

The second step is to provide an opportunity for everyone to express individual views of the problem and its solution. Having provided this opportunity, the consultant must discover and identify to everyone all the *areas of common agreement.* But more important, the consultant must discover and identify to everyone a superordinate goal that would serve all the individual goals that surfaced during the problem-analysis and problem-solving sessions.

Admittedly, this is not an easy task, but once it is accomplished, the tasks remaining are relatively simple. After the unique needs that divide the participants are organized into a single-focused view of the problem, the consultant assists the group in the formulation of a plan of action and in the design of its evaluation, and supports the group through both the implementation and evaluation stages. If the evaluation indicates the planned change was effective, then the consultant is phased out. This means that the consultant does not withdraw immediately. The consultant continues to provide support until the planned change is a fully functioning, integrated part of the on-going system. If the evaluation failed to confirm the effectiveness of the planned change, then it's back to the drawing board for a new plan of action.

How often do you suppose such plans are found not to be effective? Not very often. Whenever people create something, it becomes theirs. They own it, nurture it, and protect it. They will go to great extremes for its survival and welfare. If it is theirs, then they will make sure it works by defending it against all obstacles. People are very resourceful and creative in dealing with emergencies that threaten something that belongs to them.

So, we are back to where we started. Successful change efforts require the active involvement of the consultees in identifying the problem, planning the intervention, implementing the plan of action, and evaluating it (Arensberg & Niehoff, 1964; Goodenough, 1963; Miles & Schmuck, 1971). In short, change requires that the consultees be allowed to create something that is *theirs*. More to the point, it requires consultants to facilitate, support, assist, and let go and let their consultees "learn by doing." The ultimate measure of the consultant's success comes when the accolades are handed out. If the consultees are praising themselves and no one asks the consultant to take any bows, then the consultant did an excellent job.

We can examine this process in action by using the example cited earlier for the organization development counselor. You were advised that profits are down. The president of the corporation consults with you because there is an urgent need to know why the profit margin has been reduced, and you are told to take care of it.

You express your appreciation for the faith placed in you, but you also suggest that problems rarely have a single cause. Multiple influences usually combine to create any given set of circumstances, functional or dysfunctional. Then you recommend that representatives from each of the divisions be invited to meet together and explore the problem. The president thinks this is a waste of time but tells you to go ahead and meet with them. At this point you remind the president of her power, and your lack of it, and the consequences of her absence for the productivity of the meeting. She protests because she can't spare the time and also because she doesn't believe the meeting will be productive anyway. But eventually the president's pride in the power of her office persuades her to acquiesce to your request.

Now, there are many other of the president's vested interests that could be used to provoke participation and involvement. Power and prestige were selected merely to demonstrate the *utility* of vested interests for precipitating involvement. Effective consultants must never neglect this vital dimension of their work. Attention to vested interests is critical to consulting success. The problem of active involvement is solved not by asking "*Which* vested interest do I use?" but by asking "*How can I use* the vested interests?" The way you answer the former is consequential only as it directs your attention to the latter.

Now, do you, as the OD counselor, call the meeting? You do not. You are a congruent professional counselor. You have told the president that it is presidential power that spells success for the effort, and so you ask the president to summon the comptroller, the union representative, the sales manager, the production-line foreman, and the sales representative. And it is the president who must chair the meeting.

There are several reasons for persuading the president to assume this role. The one you tell her about is the power reason. Another, which you do not tell her about, is the need for the president's active involvement and participation throughout the entire proceedings. Things don't run, at least not very far, in the absence of the chair. And chairpersons don't, generally speaking, jump up and run out of meetings they are chairing. Moreover, in assuming the chairperson role, the president also assumes responsibility for the productivity of the meeting. The probability of success for the meeting is greatly increased when the power and prestige of the president's office are at stake.

One last reason is offered for why the consultant must not chair meetings. Generally, the effectiveness and success of the change effort are directly related to how dominant the consultant is perceived to be in the process. If the consultant is perceived to be running the show, then your consultees will *let* you run the show. They will become uninvolved. The change effort will become yours, not theirs, and the changes you implement will last only so long as you are there to monitor them. Once you are out of their way, your consultees will return to their old ways of doing things.

In addition, the consultant who takes charge has lost the opportunity to help people learn how to solve their own problems. By becoming actively involved in the problem-solving process, we learn that we do *know how*. It is our thesis that the ultimate goal of consulting is to provide these learning opportunities. It is also our thesis that the teacher/learner relationship is a cooperative relationship. Ideally, the teacher is something of an authority on the problem being explored, but we are dedicated to the proposition that the learning climate is enhanced when teachers do not behave as authorities.

This means that the president chairs the meeting and that you create opportunities for *all* the participants to learn how competent and resourceful *they* are. It means that while the president is running the show, on a perceptible level, you are orchestrating it on an imperceptible level. It means that you are using all your knowledge of human behavior and all your professional-counselor interpersonal skills to facilitate a harmonious interaction of everyone in the meeting. It means that your "leadership" must be insidious.

Incidently, do you think *insidious* is a dirty word? Its earlier definitions did include ugly connotations that ranged from "deceitful" and "treacherous" to "sly" and "wily." But the plotting and scheming quality of the word belongs to its archaic definition. Today, *insidious* means only "below the level of perception." It is a quality of teaching behavior we endorse, because we believe learning climates are enriched when the teacher's influence does not dominate the learning process. Similarly, it is our thesis that a consultant's "leadership" should be insidious, not obvious. But back to your meeting.

The comptroller is arguing that costs can be cut by payroll reductions and cutbacks in employee fringe benefits, while the union representative is demanding wage increases and the production-line foreman is insisting that the lighting fixtures are museum pieces and need replacing. Although the sales manager is pushing for territorial splits, the sales representative is adamant for increased commissions. All the president wants is to know why the profit margin has narrowed.

What do you do? Nothing. You let them express their individual vested interests. Well, not quite *nothing,* because as they express their interests, you acknowledge them—nonverbally. Your concern is to support *everyone* and understand everyone's concern—that is, vested interest. Why? Because you are an indecisive, mealymouthed coward? Nope, because you are a consultant with professional-counselor skills. You know that people must have a chance to "ventilate" and that once the complaining is over—and it will terminate if it is allowed to proceed unchallenged—everyone will settle down and attack the problem more rationally.

During the heated exchange you indicate your acceptance of each argument *nonverbally* because you are a consultant who knows the importance of interacting on an imperceptible level. Your eyes are unequaled in eloquence, and so are your smile and gentle nod. A word of caution: do not develop the habit of letting your head bob up and down like that foolish bird on the edge of a water glass. Professional counselors behave less perceptibly.

If you have listened carefully, you will have indentified the vested interests expressed, and you will be able to organize them into a comprehensive statement of the problem that respects all the expressed concerns. But your statement is offered as a *question.* You acknowledge the high cost of travel, the soaring cost-of-living index, and the consequences for production costs. You agree that worker effectiveness is related to effective working environments, and you admit that presidents of corporations who must maintain a profit line do not have an easy task.

You conclude this *very brief* statement by "wondering whether" it would help if (1) the sales manager, rather than reducing the sales territories, offered a bonus commission for sales in excess of the current volume written by each sales representative, (2) the production-line foreman explored the feasibility and cost of new lighting, (3) the union representative could meet with the workers and explain the need for increased daily production, and (4) the comptroller would delay the proposed layoffs until the effect of these efforts was observed.

Then you casually observe that "it might" be wise to test these efforts before instituting mass layoffs and territorial splits. In doing so, you have identified to your consultees a superordinate goal around which all their individual vested interests can be rallied. You have subtly, but conclusively, pointed out that the consequence of not giving a little is the loss of everything. Since the company's financial well-being is intimately tied to employee well-being, all of them must unite their resources and influence in a genuine cooperative effort to solve the "big" problem.

Now, don't be misled. The proposals you suggested will *not* be the ones ultimately tested. Each of your consultees will want to alter them in some way. And *you* will want them altered because you want the plan of action to be theirs, not yours. Your proposals were offered only as a stimulant to their problem analysis. Moreover, your suggestions were aired not only to help them discover an area of common agreement but to provide them with a model for their subsequent interactions. Your proposal had taken into consideration the unique needs of the differing consultees, hopeful that their future discussions would be characterized by an exchange of information between persons attributed equal status.

Rarely is your initial equal-status effort sufficient. Yours must be a constant and continuing concern to help your consultees learn how to consider the ideas and suggestions of everyone before drawing conclusions about a plan of action, the way it will be implemented, and the criteria by which it will be evaluated. But your most critical concern is to discover how to do all this *imperceptibly*—how to ask questions rather than provide answers, how to facilitate rather than dictate, and how to be unobtrusive so that they will know that they, not you, solved the problem.

Perspectives for the '80s

The '60s were a "heyday," the '70s were a "transition," and the '80s are a "challenging opportunity." In contrast to the '60s, when society was willing to support any professional group that might help the "Sputnik catch-up" effort, taxpayers of the '70s were disillusioned with, and critical of, our tentative strivings to discover what we were supposed to do and how we were supposed to do it. But those days are done. In the '80s we will have the professional maturity to understand that our most effective way of responding to the needs of individuals is by responding to the needs of society.

In the '80s counselors will realize that their client is the entire social environment (Wrenn, 1979). In the '80s counselors cannot be confined by a limited view of their goals and objectives. Since the Carnegie Council on Policy Studies in Higher Education examined its policies within the entire social milieu, then it might be wise for counselors to do the same. Perhaps what is being called for now is an admission by all professional groups that an insulated, narrow view of themselves and their own vested interests is no longer sufficient—that self-serving goals and objectives are self-destructive.

In the '80s we will describe goals and objectives for ourselves that are in concert with the superordinate goals and objectives of society, a citizenry that is literate, orderly, and productive. As servants of society, we have a responsibility to respond to the needs of society. Better still, we have the opportunity to join forces with others and provide a comprehensive, rather than a piecemeal, response to society's needs. This opportunity has been realized through our *consulting* activities.

Educational Goals and Objectives

If illiteracy and reduced academic performance pose a threat to society and the individual, then in the '80s we will become more directly involved in the business of education. As Jim MacKay wrote after 60 years as a counselor, "I do not apologize for being a teacher." The counseling process includes a teaching function (MacKay, 1979, p. 8). And through our consulting activities we will find even more effective ways of not only teaching but "giving away" our interpersonal skills.

What counselors of the '60s and '70s failed to learn was that the school was not the only institution responsible for, or in the business of, education. Just when counselors were so anxious to disavow affiliation with this low-status occupation, every other dimension of society was becoming increasingly involved with educational efforts. Education now is the province of the communications media, business and industry, the armed forces, libraries, museums, health and welfare agencies, community agencies. In the '80s counselors, through their consulting activities, will join forces with all of these to discover new, exciting, and creatively inventive opportunities for the academically unachieving to become contributing adult members of society by—

1. collaborating with school specialists, community and federal agents, and others, by serving as resource persons, referral agents, and consultants to special learning projects for individuals with special needs.
2. creating, implementing, and serving as a consultant to remedial and preventive intervention programs that can be led by parents, teachers, senior citizens, and other members of the community.
3. organizing and consulting with parent study groups, dealing with such

topics as how they can help their young people cope with homework, improve their study skills, and discover the relevance of what they are learning now to what they will need to know later.
4. organizing and serving as a consultant to teacher-training projects on (a) the identification of learning problems, (b) differing learning styles, and (c) available help and how to avail themselves of it.
5. enlisting the help of business and industry representatives, implementing study programs for neighborhood youth who are potential dropouts.
6. consulting with anyone and everyone in all aspects of society for the purpose of creating innovative educational experiences for individuals who have failed to learn in traditional educational environments.

Implied here is that counselors, regardless of their work settings, will not fight against the "back to basics" movement because rational, civic-minded members of society *cannot* argue against a literate society. We will not, as in the past, provide succorance to individuals who place the blame for their failure outside themselves. Nor will we provide them a safe haven in which they can absolve themselves of all blame. Instead, we will provide them with systematic opportunities to learn what they failed to learn.

Social Goals and Objectives

Also implied here is a weightier question unresolved by counselors of the '60s and '70s. Can we expect to respond to the needs of *the individual* in isolation from all those others with whom the individual interacts daily? Counselors of the '80s will resolve the question by involving all those others, as equal partners, in the solution of the problem, which accrues not merely to the individual but to society at large. And counselors of the '80s will be able to resolve the question because they will have the *consulting skills* necessary to resolve it.

If the quality of life is being threatened by the disorderly behavior of a particular segment of society, then counselors of the '80s will discover and provide systematic opportunities for individuals to learn one of the most necessary attributes of living—self-discipline.

Counselors of the '60s and '70s wasted a lot of time and psychic energy protesting responsibility for discipline. They were not disciplinarians, they were advocates. Some would also say that these counselors were foolish. *Discipline* isn't a dirty word. It means training that corrects, molds, strengthens, and perfects. *Advocate*, however, is a dirty word, for all except those in the legal profession. It means one who defends, vindicates, or espouses any cause—right or wrong. Counselors of the '80s will have the professional maturity to admit that "advocate" counselors don't help people. They rob them of the chance to learn how to defend themselves. They rob them of the chance to learn how to win when they are right and to

THE WILDEST RIDE OF YOUR LIFE

They're no longer children, and yet they are only in the process of becoming adults. They are inconsistent, curious, insecure, impatient, sensitive, and misunderstood. Some are sexually active; others still believe the stork brings the babies. Some have trouble passing state competency exams for graduation, while others get SAT scores that would make college students envious. The preteen teen is the biggest challenge I've ever faced in my life.

But so is the school and how it's run. Dealing with the middle years of a kid's growing up time means middle schools have to middle-of-the-road it, too. It's half elementary—the kids don't change teachers for their different subjects. And half high school—they do have more than one teacher for their different class periods. They have extracurricular activities, but not as many as a high school has. And they don't have competitive athletic programs.

If you think diversity is the name of the middle-school game, then you are right. The kids are diverse, and the counselor has to be. You've got to be able to counsel individually with kids who bring you their "growing up" problems. You've got to be able to work with them in groups, and you've got to try to become an expert on educational programs so that you don't add to their "growing up" concerns. You've got to work with teachers and be willing and able to let them deliver some of your services. And you've got to provide services for parents. Don't make the mistake of thinking parents aren't interested. They are, and they want in on your act.

Middle schools are the most exciting places in the world because they are full of middle-school kids. Someone said it's like being on a roller coaster, but the emotional ups and downs don't belong just to the kids. As a counselor, you'll have plenty of them. But the "downs" won't get you down, because after each one there's another "up" coming up fast.

—A Middle-School Counselor

---

suffer the consequences when they are wrong. People in trouble aren't always right, and even they know it and secretly resent anyone who does not.

In the '80s counselors will, through their consulting activities, help all of society and each of their counselees acquire the three most important skills of life: self-discipline, self-respect, and a sense of responsibility. The consulting services they will provide will increase not only a sense of orderliness in the life of each individual but the quality of life for all members of society. Counselors will be—

- serving as consultants to parole and probation agents in small- and large-group training sessions on (1) social skills, (2) tolerance for ambiguity,

(3) the assumption of responsibility, and (4) respect for the rights and property of others.
- organizing and conducting parent and teacher group consultation sessions on (1) disruptive behavior, its multiple influences, and available interventions, (2) developmental tasks and child-rearing practices, and (3) risk taking, autonomy seeking, conformity and deviance, behavior modeling, monitoring, and supervision.
- organizing group consultation sessions with children and young adults on (1) social norms and behavior norms, (2) law and order and a social consciousness, (3) cooperation and conflict and their differing outcomes, and (4) the acceptance of responsibility.

Implied here are some notions near and dear to the hearts of all counselors in all decades—namely, that people do not mean to be mean; that no one deliberately chooses to disrupt society and that persons demonstrating antisocial behavior do so because they have not had opportunities to learn any other way of behaving. And our response, in the '60s and '70s, was remedial. We provided counseling services that yielded few, if any, positive results. In the '80s we will provide consulting services that are both preventive and remedial.

We will provide individuals opportunities to learn socially approved behavior and examine the differential consequences of alternative responses to their environment. And when they have mastered the new behaviors, we will let go and let them decide whether or not they want to use them. The choice will be theirs, and so will the consequences.

Economic Goals and Objectives

Finally, if society is suffering from a loss of productivity because many of its young people are ill prepared for the job market, then we will collaborate with business and industry, schools, federal and state institutions, and all others who can help our young people help themselves contribute to the world of work. Counselors of the '80s will be actively involved in consulting activities as resource persons, referral agents, and coordinators of the transition between education and work by—

- providing consulting sessions on career development, job-market opportunities, job-seeking and job-finding skills, and so on.
- organizing, helping to implement, and coordinating work-study programs with business and industry representatives.
- coordinating vocational training and alternative education programs envisioned and proposed by the Carnegie Council on Policy Studies in Higher Education (1980).

Implied here is that counselors of the '80s will accept their professional responsibilities to help people *learn how* to help themselves—not just some people with certain problems but all people, regardless of the difficulties they are experiencing or will run the risk of experiencing. Counselors of the '80s will provide consulting services that will meet individual needs not only when the needs arise but, more important, *before.*

Committing ourselves to new behaviors is always difficult and frustrating. That is why the "transition" period of the '70s was so difficult for so many counselors. Our tentative strivings to adopt the unfamiliar were accompanied by our reluctance to give up the familiar. This usually resulted in our doing both—badly. But in the '80s we will have moved out of our transitional period and into a period of challenging opportunities to join forces with other agents of society and provide consulting services that will improve the quality of life for everyone.

Summary

During our relatively short professional evolution the consulting function of professional counselors has been generally neglected. Perhaps we were so busy learning about our counseling function that we failed to provide training for consulting. Or we may have neglected this vital aspect of a professional counselor's training because we did not know *how* to provide it. But recent societal and professional concerns have made the consulting function a professional imperative.

Consulting is not a systematic body of knowledge. It is a process guided by principles and concepts generated by other disciplines, including theories of learning, human behavior, and innovation and change. We examined four possible modes in our search for an appropriate and effective consulting approach. Only one of these was judged to be viable for professional counselors. Finally, an example of how this approach could be implemented was offered.

Now It's Your Turn

1. What do you believe about human behavior? Are people, generally speaking, self-directed and autonomous, or are they indecisive and dependent? Do they want to be told how to behave, or do they want to make their own mistakes?

    The world has some of both kinds, of course, but professional counselors work with perfectly normal people who occasionally need help with "perfectly normal abnormalities." So, what are your beliefs about human nature? Remember, the onus of demonstrating the effectiveness and contributions of counseling is not merely on you but on us, your professional colleagues.

2. What do you know about human beings? Do people tend to perform those behaviors that are satisfying and productive? Do they tend to repeat past failures if they are not given opportunities to learn new coping skills? Do people learn by doing, or does sufficient learning result from talking about problems?

   Not all the answers about human behavior are available to us yet, but there is some reason to suspect a discrepancy between a person's skill in talking about something and his or her ability to perform that thing. So, what learning opportunities should professional counselors provide? Remember, the changes we are expected to facilitate are ultimately a measure of our professional stature. It is by our works, not our words, that society will judge us.

3. What do you know about yourself and your motives for becoming a professional counselor? Do you have a need for power and public acclaim, or do you have a high regard for humility and its influence on your interactions with others? Do you need to learn how to help others insidiously so that they can finally say they did it themselves? Or have you already experienced that special joy that comes from *not* being acknowledged?

   Motives matter because they provide a sense of direction and also because they are reliable predictors of success. Self-serving motives will not attract either the interest or the support of others, whereas a desire to help others learn how to help themselves has always enlisted the cooperative involvement of others. Just remember, successful consulting not only requires your most effective counseling skills; it also requires that you give these skills away. Consulting isn't merely helping others "learn how to learn." And it isn't easy—without right motives. So, what are yours? And why?

4. You are a human services counselor. You have a warm, accepting, unconditional positive regard for the young man who sits in front of you and tells you that his mother and father threw him out of the house because he had been accused of stealing by his employer. It wasn't his fault. He didn't want anything to do with the gas-station robbery. A street gang made him do it. He was outnumbered and he had to go along. What do *you* have to do? And *how* do you do it?

5. You are a counselor in a child-abuse center who is visited by a social worker who tells you of a child who has been severely burned. The parents' explanation is that the child was ill and suffering from extreme chills. To warm the child, they had placed a heating pad in the child's bed. The heating pad was many years old, and the wiring must have been defective, because the bed caught on fire. They were unaware of

the accident until they heard the child's screams. By the time they were able to reach the child, third-degree burns had been inflicted.

The social worker also explains that this is the third in a series of terrible accidents sustained by the child within two months. So you—

a. call the police and have the parents locked up.
b. tell the social worker to stop being so suspicious—accidents are not unusual in the lives of children.
c. tell the social worker the parents need intensive counseling.
d. thank the social worker and "wonder whether" it would help to meet with the parents and the social worker and discuss the child's accident-prone problem.

Did you choose "d"? Of course you did. That problem was easy to solve, but this one requires more resourcefulness. Assume that the meeting was arranged and the parents and the social worker arrive. What do you do then? And how?

6. Your high school has been vandalized. Your principal assigns the problem to you. So you—

a. remind the principal that counselors are not disciplinarians.
b. collaborate with the police in apprehending the culprits.
c. address the student body and ask the miscreants to identify themselves because you are a "student advocate" and will protect them.
d. take up a collection to pay for the damages.
e. or—
   1. involve the principal (how?).
   2. suggest a meeting that includes one representative from each of the relevant and influential groups (parents, taxpayers, students, teachers, community agents, school administrators—all groups that have a vested interest in the school and its maintenance).

Right again! "e" is your answer. But what do you do then? And how?

7. The "hotlines" at your mental-health clinic are always busy. Your callers, when they reach you, are distressed by their unsuccessful attempts to reach you. So you—

a. increase your annual budget request to accommodate additional trunk lines.

But you discover you do not have enough counselors to answer the phones. So you—

b. increase your budget request to accommodate additional staffing.

But your budget request is denied because evidence of the influence of your clinic on the welfare of the community is inconclusive. So you—

c. realize that as a lone voice crying in the wilderness your hope for success is slim.

But your motives are right. Yours is a sincere desire to help others—not merely the troubled members of the community but the entire community by virtue of having helped the troubled members. So you—

d. remember that two heads are better than one and that many heads are even better. Also, you know that when people decide to solve everyone else's problem, everyone else will let them. You are annoyed with all those others who are not interested in solving a community problem.

But you realize that they have had no opportunity to learn that they have a problem. Therefore they have no concern to solve it or to cooperatively design a plan of action that might intervene against it. So you—

e. ? It's up to you. What do you do now? And how?

References and Suggested Readings

ACES-ASCA Joint Committee on the Elementary School Counselor. Report of the ACES-ASCA Joint Committee on the Elementary School Counselor, April 2, 1966 (Working Paper). Washington, D.C.: American Personnel and Guidance Association, 1966.

American Personnel and Guidance Association. *Standards for preparation in counselor education.* Falls Church, Va.: American Personnel and Guidance Association, 1979.

Arensberg, C. N., & Niehoff, A. H. *Introducing social change: A manual for Americans overseas.* Chicago: Aldine, 1964.

Caplan, G. *The theory and practice of mental health consultation.* New York: Basic Books, 1970.

Carlson, J., Splete, H., & Kern, R. *The consulting process.* Washington, D.C.: APGA Reprint Series/Seven, 1975.

Carnegie Council on Policy Studies in Higher Education. *Giving youth a better chance: Options for education, work, and service.* San Francisco: Jossey-Bass, 1980.

Cowley, W. H. A tentative holistic taxonomy applied to education. In E. L. Jones & E. Westervelt (Eds.), *Behavioral science and guidance: Proposals and perspectives.* New York: Bureau of Publications, Teachers College, Columbia University, 1963.

Dinkmeyer, D., & Carlson, J. *Consulting: Facilitating human potential and change processes.* Columbus, Ohio: Charles E. Merrill, 1973.

Dinkmeyer, D., & Carlson, J. *Consultation: A book of readings.* New York: Wiley, 1975.

Faust, V. The counselor as consultant to teachers. *Elementary School Guidance and Counseling,* 1967, *1* (2), 112–117.

Goodenough, W. G. *Cooperation in change.* New York: Russell Sage Foundation, 1963.

Hausser, D. L., Pecorella, P. A., & Wessler, A. L. *A manual for consultants.* La Jolla, Calif.: University Associates, 1977.

Kleiman, D. "Keeping discipline in the schools is the no. 1 educational headache." *New York Times,* October 28, 1979, p. 6E.

Kurpius, D. J. (Guest Ed.). Consultation I ... definition-models-programs. *Personnel and Guidance Journal,* 1978, 56(6), 320–373.

Kurpius, D. J. (Guest Ed.). Consultation II ... dimensions-training-bibliography. *Personnel and Guidance Journal,* 1978, 56(7), 394–448.

Kurpius, D. J., & Brubaker, J. D. *Psychoeducational consultation: Definition-functions-preparation.* Bloomington: Indiana University Press, 1976.

Lawrence, R. S. "Teacher biz needs a little show biz." *New York Times,* January 6, 1980, p. Educ 23.

Lippitt, G., & Lippitt, R. *The consulting process in action.* La Jolla, Calif.: University Associates, 1978.

MacKay, J. L. "MacKay assays field: Excerpts from 60 years on the counseling scene ..." *Guidepost,* November 15, 1979, p. 8.

Meyers, J., Martin, R., & Hyman, I. (Eds.). *School consultation.* Springfield, Ill.: Charles C Thomas, 1977.

Miles, M., & Schmuck, R. (Eds.). *Organization development in schools.* Palo Alto, Calif.: National Press Books, 1971.

Nelson, R. C. *Guidance and counseling in the elementary school.* New York: Holt, Rinehart & Winston, 1972.

Parker, C. A. *Psychological consultation: Helping teachers meet special needs.* Minneapolis: Leadership Training, 1975.

Wiggins, J. D. "Know how to help: To the editor." *Guidepost,* November 15, 1979, p. 2.

Wrenn, C. G. "Proposed changes in counselor attitudes: Toward your job." *School Counselor,* 1979, 27(2), 81–90.

Yemma, J. "Are U.S. schools good enough?" *Christian Science Monitor,* October 18, 1979, p. 2.

CHAPTER 7

Assessment and Information Giving

Robert H. Pate, Jr.

The focus of this chapter is counselee assessment. The term *assessment,* rather than *testing,* was deliberately selected because I believe counselee assessment to be a more appropriate and vital dimension of the work of the counselor. Moreover, I believe assessment and information giving to be a more accurate definition of the counselor function discussed in this chapter. To me, assessment and information giving are interrelated and interdependent because the purpose of tests and the issues surrounding the use of their scores are remarkably similar to issues surrounding the use of other types of information by counselors. In fact, it might be concluded that what we are actually considering in this chapter is the role of information in the counselor's work.

This view of the counselor's *testing* function may require some readers to turn themselves upside down in order to critically examine and understand the propositions offered, because they depart from the traditional view. Historically, counselors have embraced notions more closely identified with psychometrists than with the goals of developmental counselors. But this is a new era and a time for counselors to rethink some of their old thoughts.

If open-mindedness is a necessary prerequisite for reexamining the counselor's use of tests, then open-mindedness is even more consequential to your understanding of my propositions about the counselor's *use of the information yielded* by the tests. The heart and soul of the professional counselor's identity is the counseling function, and there are those whose definition of how it should be performed excludes all other counseling definitions and approaches. It is my view that the counseling process cannot be narrowly defined, that it can be variously performed, and that it includes all the counseling approaches currently available and those yet to be successfully implemented. It is hoped that you will give my thesis an open-minded and critical analysis.

Accordingly, you will be given an opportunity to examine in more detail my reasons for combining the assessment and information-giving functions of counselors. After this, we will examine the information-giving and assessment processes. Then we will examine the importance of assessment and information giving in the work of the counselor. A separate section will include a presentation of the social issues related to information giving and assessment.

Assessment, Information Giving, and Counseling

As suggested earlier, I contend that what we are really considering in this section is how information sharing contributes to counseling. For that reason, it seems necessary for me to detail my reasons for proposing that assessment and information giving are intimately related—that you can't *take* one without *providing* the other.

In Chapter 1 you learned that many of your professional roots are in the vocational guidance movement and Frank Parsons's (1909) classic model, which combines information about the counselee and information about the world of work. You will recall that I described the Parsonian counselor as someone who tried to learn the attributes and characteristics of the potential worker, to gain information about the counselee, and, through the counseling process, assist the counselee in making decisions and acting on them. The data base used in the decision-making and action-taking processes was directed by the degree of agreement between the information gained about self and the information gained about the world of work. Put more simply, in the Parsonian model, the counselor helped career counselees to gain and *combine* information about self and external realities. This approach to the counseling process is typically labeled *trait and factor*.

The trait/factor counseling approach is most prominently associated with the work of E. G. Williamson and his *How to Counsel Students* (1939). Those of you who are interested in learning more about the many persons in the counseling profession who have contributed to the variety of approaches to counseling may find the review by Burks and Stefflre (1979) useful. You are also urged to familiarize yourself with the summaries and critical analyses of the major counseling approaches presented by Corey (1982). These supplemental readings may help you to appreciate that a major element in Williamson's trait-and-factor approach is differential diagnosis.

Differential diagnosis includes 3 processes: (1) gathering information about the counselee, or forming a diagnosis of the counselee; (2) gathering information about the counselee's problem, or forming a diagnosis of the problem presented by the counselee; and (3) determining the congruence between the counselee's decision making and external realities. External realities were defined to include the requirements and demands of occupations.

Numerous other theorists whose formulations are related to trait and factor could be cited to demonstrate the close relation between information about the counselee and information about the world, as well as the need for this information to be used in the counseling process. For example, many currently popular counseling approaches, sometimes grouped under the *cognitive* label, place great emphasis on the role of the counselor as a dispenser of accurate information so that the errors in counselee thinking can be corrected (Keller, Biggs, & Gysbers, 1982).

This view, however, is by no means generally accepted. For example, some counselors are dedicated to the proposition that the counseling *relationship* is the essential element in the helping relationship and that client growth can actually be impeded if other elements are injected into the counselor/counselee relationship. Generally, this is the position taken by *client-centered* or *relationship* counselors. This approach to the counseling process was initiated and developed by Carl Rogers (1957), who argued that facilitative conditions—namely, genuineness, acceptance, and accurate empathy—are the necessary and sufficient conditions for counselee change. If you, as a counselor, adhere completely to the notion that the necessary and sufficient conditions for counselee growth and change are limited to the classic Rogerian triad, or even to later extensions of his client-centered thesis, then you will find little substance in my notions concerning the utility of information of any kind in your counseling sessions.

The Rogerian position was endorsed by Arbuckle (1975), who argued that the counselor should not be an information giver. Rather, it was Arbuckle's view that the related processes of testing and information giving are intrusions into the counseling process. By contrast, Patterson (1974), another relationship counselor, argued that counselors should engage in many types of psychological relationships. Patterson included skill training, instruction, reeducation, and behavior modification in his definition of the helping process. But he also argued that the important and necessary condition was the relationship between counselee and counselor: " 'Testing and telling' is not in itself counseling, but where the essential process is the relationship, it is counseling" (Patterson, 1974, p. 12).

In a review of the current status of client-centered theory, Grummon identified the function of information giving as a specific example of a signficant omission in client-centered theory. He stated that it is appropriate and that information giving is a time-honored tool of the counselor (1979, p. 80).

The material presented seems to endorse my notion that information is not only a legitimate inclusion in counseling but an important one.

MONEY, ANYONE?

I really didn't plan to be a financial aid officer; it just happened. I didn't know what to do with my B.A. (English) and decided to go to graduate school. This sounds dumb, but I knew I wanted to work with people, and counselor education was a program I could get in, and I thought I would like it. I knew that jobs would be hard to find and decided to be really flexible. When I went on a field practicum, I found that a financial aid counselor job might be opening up, and I went after it and got it.

OK, what's it like? Financial aid in a community college is handled by a counselor, but the students and faculty identify me as the financial aid officer. Counseling is a part of the job because I have to be able to listen and explain things to students. The whole idea of financial aid is so complicated now with various state and federal programs that most people don't have any idea except that they need money or have heard that maybe I can help them get money.

It sounds funny for a job I just fell into, but I love it. I always needed a lot of structure and like to organize, so all the forms and rules don't bother me. Maybe this is sick, but I really feel good when people see me as an expert; I like it. I remember how I felt at times when I didn't know what was going on, and I try to be really patient, but I have to work on it. Some students come in to talk about other things, so I feel like a real counselor. What don't I like? The odd hours we work for registration. The location of this school. Trying to keep an "open door" and having people drop by when I have reports to file. The upheavals caused by recent administrative changes here make everybody uneasy. Overall it has all worked out well; I wish I had my job somewhere else. I might like to be in a larger, four-year school, but I don't know; I'm in charge here, and I don't know if I would like being one of many.

—*A Financial Aid Counselor*

Counselees will often seek our assistance because they have not accurately assessed their situation. They look to the counselor as a fair and objective source of information about themselves and the world. I believe that such a view of information in counseling is compatible with the counseling process. If, however, you want to define information about clients and their world as separate from counseling, you are free to make your own decisions. Nevertheless, I must be concerned about my own information-giving skill if I have failed to enlarge your view of assessment and information giving in counseling. There are, it is true, only certain uses of assessment and information giving that can be classified as a legitimate part of the counseling process, but we must also recognize that the individual and small-group relationships that we label "counseling" are only one of the functions that define the role of the counselor. In fact, as you review the "Perspectives for the '80s" section in each chapter, you will discover that the expectation for counselors to perform more than their counseling function is increasing.

Counselors use a variety of information when working with their clients. A counselor in a public employment office might supply a counselee with information that a certain business was accepting applications for jobs. A counselor in a family clinic might provide a client information about the effectiveness of various methods of birth control. The list could go on—a school counselor giving information to a group of students about the early decision process for college applicants, a counselor in a substance-abuse clinic leading a group-counseling session for substance abusers. Counselors in virtually all settings are called on to provide accurate and timely information to their counselees, and most counselors probably find dispensing information a legitimate and natural part of their role.

In the examples just cited, questions could be raised about whether these counselors were conducting group counseling or group guidance. Although the distinction I propose is far from perfect, I believe it may be sufficient to facilitate our consideration of information in the work of the counselor.

The basis of the distinction that I suggest is control. Teachers dispense information that is controlled by a curriculum. Although most students recognize the legitimacy of the prescribed curriculum, they have little short-term influence over the material presented to them. The information that counselors dispense is typically controlled by the needs and interests of their counselees. Even most school guidance groups, which in reality may resemble seminar or lecture/discussion classes, are optional and provide no credit for their participants. There are exceptions, such as court-mandated participation in Alcohol Safety Action Programs by persons convicted of drunk driving, in which the curriculum and participation are mandatory. In general, however, counseling information is under the control of the counselee. Supporting evidence is derived from the reports of counselors that counselee resentment and resistance are significant barriers to their helping relationship. It seems quite clear that, regardless of how you define the counseling process, the control of the information introduced is reserved to the counselee. Counselees need it, look to the counselor for it, and reserve to themselves the right to use or refuse it. I am personally secure in believing that information giving is *not* an intrusion on the counseling relationship and that its exclusion from the counseling process does a disservice to our counselees (Senour, 1982).

Gathering and using information about clients is a legitimate part of the counseling process when the information is gathered to address a client need or concern. It is for this reason that the helper and helpee should work together to determine what information, if any, would be useful and at what point in the counseling process the information is needed. The counselor can then assist the counselee in designing a counseling plan in which information that is seen as useful will be seen as only one component.

For example, a client of a vocational counselor in private practice and the counselor both agree that an interest inventory might provide the client with useful information. However, the client should be cautioned against viewing the inventory as the essence of what will result from the counseling relationship. Information of any type should be seen as only one component of a process in which counselees work to achieve some goal which they themselves define as desirable and for which they are responsible.

Nevertheless, the professional counselor is the professional expert who legitimately must provide direction about the best ways to gather the information the client wants. The competent counselor in a family planning clinic would not let misconceptions about the reliability of birth-control methods go unchallenged and would, in fact, supply counselees who wanted such information with the most accurate information currently available. Many counselors who work with adult students find that they have negative perceptions of their potential as students, formed on the basis of tests administered years earlier. The counselor would certainly assist those students in finding more accurate means for assessing their current academic ability.

Counselors also have a responsibility to help their counselees use the best sources of information. Counselees often misinterpret the meaning of their life experiences and are willing to define themselves on the basis of single events. Many high school students believe that the record they have achieved in a ten- or eleven-year school career can be wiped out by a single academic-ability test. Adults who have had numerous paid and unpaid work experiences are willing to "take an interest inventory to discover what I am interested in." The counselor has a responsibility to help clients discover the best source for the information they seek, and the best source is not always a standardized test or a commercially published career, educational, or personal information series. The counselee who is seeking a job in a particular geographic area can get the best data about opportunities in that area from local sources and should not rely on publications that provide only national trends.

Once the needed, relevant, and valid information is acquired, the counselor's role is no less important. The counselor must assist counselees in developing a plan for using the information. If, as I have suggested, both client and counselor have been involved in determining what information is needed, the use of the information is only a logical extension. When the counselor and client have planned the assessment together, the results of a series of roleplays that have shown that the client is not assertive will not be seen as a confirmation that the client is doomed to be a doormat. Rather, the assessment can serve to provide direction for the client's learning to be more assertive.

Finally, the counselor must ensure that the counselee understands the information that has been gathered. Because counselors are trained in the notions of test error and the meaning of percentile ranks, they can easily forget that such ideas are alien to counselees. We must use our best counseling skills to ensure that any information we present is accurately perceived by counselees. Misconceptions about information are not limited to counselees' test results. For example, if we tell counselees that the average combined SAT score of students admitted to a given college is 1100, how many hear us say that you need a score of 1100 to get in and completely miss the fact that half the students admitted actually scored less than 1100?

Environmental Information

Information provided by counselors to their clients is typically categorized as career, educational, or personal/social. The categories are difficult to separate in many instances, but they do provide a useful basis for the organization of information.

Career Information

Career information typically includes all the information about the variety of occupations that exist, statistical data about working and occupations, and information about the process of career choice and obtaining a position after the choice is made. Career information also includes information about the educational and training requirements for various careers, whereas educational information is typically that associated with particular schools and training programs.

Educational Information

Educational information is information about educational and training opportunities. We typically think of information about colleges and universities as synonymous with educational information, but there is also information about private elementary and secondary schools, trade and technical schools, and apprenticeship programs. In addition, information about financial assistance, sources of funds to attend school, is of great interest to some students and their parents.

Personal/Social Information

Personal/social information includes a variety of topics that range from assertive skills to weight control. In many situations the information provides resource material for group activities conducted by counselors. For example, a pastoral counselor might conduct a group for parents in the congregation and use information from one of the numerous parent-training programs as a basis for the group. Some personal/social information and the counseling programs built around these topics create discussion, if not controversy, in communities. Not only have school programs that were labeled "sex education" been questioned, but so have such seemingly noncontroversial topics as "learning to share feelings."

Informational Materials

As you have doubtless noted from the examples, some categories of information are difficult to distinguish from other categories. For example, military materials often stress the training opportunities available in the armed forces, but most would consider military service an occupation, not a training program. The materials that are labeled "personal/social" are often the basis for group programs and become useful as a consequence of the counselor's method of presentation. I am not concerned that you be able to separate material into the three groups, but I do hope you have some idea of the variety of material available to counselors who want to provide information to their counselees.

Published materials provide the greatest variety and depth of topics for counseling information. These include printed material, audio- and videotape presentations, films, slides, filmstrips, microfiche, and data-processing systems. The *Occupational Outlook Handbook* and *Dictionary of Occupational Titles*, discussed in the introductory chapter, are examples of career materials published by the federal government. Various agencies of the federal government and the public employment offices of the states are the best current sources of data about occupations. In fact, many commercial publishers of career material make use of the publicly available data in government publications as a source for their materials.

If information is available from government sources, why then the commercial sources? First, commercial publishers make material available for counselees with varied reading skills. In addition, the commercial materials are packaged in a form easier to store and retrieve. For example, career information on a microprocessor program or a complete career library including a filing system may save more than enough counselor time to justify the cost of the items. Finally, government materials are concentrated in the career area. Very few educational or personal/social materials are published by the government.

One of your degree experiences will be an "Information" course. In it you will study the variety of materials I have mentioned, and you will probably have opportunities to use them in role-playing activities. You will also learn how to evaluate these informational materials, and as you examine the theories of career development usually included in that course experience, you will gain an even greater understanding of the rationale for the use of information in the counseling process.

Assessment Information

The term *assessment* was deliberately selected because I am concerned about counselee assessment as the vital function to be performed by counselors rather than a narrowly defined standardized testing function. Perhaps, in a more specific sense, tests are assessment instruments that have right or wrong answers. They are used to determine the taker's ability, aptitude, and/or achievement on the basis of the number of correct responses. The *Standards for Educational and Psychological Tests* published by the American Psychological Association (1974) states: "Tests include standardized aptitude and achievement instruments, diagnostic and evaluative devices, interest inventories, personality inventories, projective instruments and related clinical techniques, and many kinds of personal history forms" (p. 2). The intent of the standards is clearly stated to apply to a broad range of devices and techniques for gathering information and providing the basis for judgments about people. My discussion of the role of assessment in the work of the counselor examines the broad range of devices and techniques defined by the standards.

There are significant questions about whether ability, aptitude, and achievement tests measure different attributes of the person assessed. Although the recent and widely publicized errors discovered in the Scholastic Aptitude Test (SAT), published by the Educational Testing Service for the College Entrance Examination Board (CEEB), suggest caution, tests are assumed to provide an index of how many correct answers a particular test taker had. More important is how that number of correct answers compares with the number of correct answers achieved by members of some specifically defined group, the norm group. Far less clear is the meaning of the standing of the test taker relative to the norm group.

Counselors also use other standardized instruments that do *not* have right or wrong answers. (To say that an instrument has been standardized means that uniform procedures have been used for the development, administration, and scoring of the instrument.) For example, an interest inventory that requires the taker to indicate "like or dislike" for certain activities can only provide information about the degree of similarity of the taker's responses to the responses of certain groups. Whether scoring high on those items the test maker had defined as determining musical interest, compared with a norm group of high school students, was desirable would depend on the test taker. Likewise, being told that, on those items to which women Air Force officers made different responses than a sample of women in general, "Your responses were very similar to those of satisfied and successful female Air Force officers" may or may not be desired by the person who took the test.

In addition to tests, which have some desirable answer and preferred score, and *inventories*, which only provide information about the relative standing of the taker compared with members of some defined group, counselors use other formal and informal methods to gain information about their counselees. Some counselors use biographical data questionnaires as a routine part of their intake procedures. Others have established through experience a pattern for initial interviews that provide information they believe will be useful in their attempts to serve the client. Elementary school counselors might use a variety of sociometric techniques to determine the patterns of student attraction in a classroom, and a counselor in a business might use a card-sort activity to help employees assess those activities which are vital components of their lives and which must be maintained in a happy and productive retirement.

Just as there is a range of devices and techniques available for assessment, there is also a variety of reasons for making assessments. Cronbach (1970) has cited four purposes of testing: prediction, selection, classification, and evaluation. Counselors might use tests to help a counselee *predict* potential success in some course of study under consideration. A college admissions counselor might use test data to determine whether an applicant should be *selected* for admission to the institution, and an academic counselor might use test data to determine classification as honors students. Another counselor might use a self-concept inventory to evaluate the influence of a special program for physically disabled persons on the participants' view of self. Another often-suggested use of tests is for *placement*. Placement is the assignment of persons to levels within a category of group—for example, the placement of students in levels of sections of a class. It differs from *classification*, which Cronbach defines as arrangement into groups.

There are many who believe that, despite our best efforts, tests can add little to the desired outcomes of counseling. Those who acknowledge the role of tests in the counseling process are exponents of various counseling philosophies. For example, Grummon (1979), as previously cited, argued that information contributes to the client-centered counseling process, and other relationship counselors have also suggested a role for tests. Patterson (1974) specifically proposed that tests are a legitimate part of relationship counseling, and Maples (1977) has even described the compatibility of testing and humanism.

Some of the most telling criticisms of testing have been made not by those who know little of testing and its potential but by people with long-standing reputations in the field of testing. Leo Goldman, author of a widely used text, *Using Tests in Counseling* (1969b), has questioned whether tests contribute anything to counseling. In other writings, Goldman (1969a, 1972a, 1972b) concluded that the potential gain from testing is not worth the possible harm and cautions that counselors may not know enough about tests to make them useful for their clients. Despite the years that have passed since Goldman's articles, his challenge to those who use tests is still valid. Tests certainly should make a difference, and demonstrating that positive difference is still a challenge to those who use tests.

I believe the attitude toward the use of tests that I have suggested provides the greatest opportunity for a positive effect on the counseling process. Those who read Goldman's (1969a) "Tests Should Make a Difference" will recognize the influence it has had on my thinking. I believe entry-level counselors can learn enough about standardized testing to allow them to use tests effectively with their counselees.

What Counselors Must Know about Assessment

The entry-level counselor cannot be expected to become completely proficient in the area of testing, but there are certain critical concepts and ideas each counselor should know and understand. These learnings can be acquired in a graduate course on tests and measurements. The order of presentation will vary, as will the emphasis, but students preparing to be counselors should develop an understanding of at least the following concepts related to assessment.

Counselors must know and understand the range of assessment devices available for their use. A single course in tests and measurements, or even two courses, cannot give counselors the necessary understanding of the variety of assessment devices available for their use. The prospective counselor can learn how to learn about those instruments. The focus of tests-and-measurements courses will not be on specific instruments except as those instruments serve to exemplify essential concepts and principles.

Standardized Tests and Inventories

Counselors should know about representative ability, achievement, and aptitude tests. Knowing how these instruments are constructed and standardized is the key to understanding tests not covered in courses or those tests that will be published in the future. The same is true of standardized interest and personality inventories. Although the specific titles vary, I am using the category "personality inventory" to cover instruments ranging from attitudes to values. One leader in the field of interest assessment, John Holland (1966), has even suggested that interest inventories are actually personality inventories.

For our purposes, perhaps a simple classification is best. There are assessment instruments that have right or wrong responses. Some of these are designed to determine the taker's mental acuity and learning potential and are called "general-ability tests." The formerly widely used term *intelligence test* is now being questioned because its use and the meaning attributed to it contribute to much of the controversy

THE VARIETY PRESERVES YOUR SANITY

Career counselors do much more than counsel. You must be salespersons and public-relations managers because you must continually reach out to others and convince them that your product, career planning, is worth their involvement. You must be a coordinator because you are the liaison between your counselees and the company recruiters. You must be an educator because you are your counselees' source of information. At least you are the resource person who guides them to the information they need by conducting workshops or programs for special groups at a variety of locations. You must have well-developed public-speaking skills. You have to be able to work under pressure, have great patience with being misunderstood, and have a high moral sense of responsibility. You will often get very frustrated working with people who waited too long to begin their career planning. You will feel helpless many times trying to constantly be creative in meeting the varied needs of your counselees and sifting through the mountains of literature that flood the field—it's horrendous trying to keep up with it and sift through career information for the valuable stuff. Then, you must struggle with your conscience when recruiters ask you to advise them which of your counselees are "hot prospects." It is a tremendous responsibility to be honest, fair, and accurate. And throughout it all you must fight against the expectations your counselees have for your services.

The name of your office, Career Planning and Placement, makes some people think you "find people jobs," but you don't "find people jobs." You must help them learn that they must find their own jobs. And you must continually help them learn exactly what you can do—career planning, not placement.

I worked hard to get this job, and I love it. But don't let anybody tell you in this kind of counseling that you "let the client do the work," because YOU do the work! You are actively involved with each counselee—listening hard and searching your mind for ideas and places to go for information. And you are actively involved in a variety of activities every day. If you can handle frustration, enjoy tough challenges, and are flexible, then you might make a pretty good career counselor.

—*A Career Planning and Placement Counselor*

---

surrounding testing. Other tests are designed to determine how well the taker will perform in some specifically defined future learning or performance situation. Such tests are called "aptitude tests." Finally there are achievement tests, tests developed to determine how much of some previously taught material the person who takes the test actually knows. Achievement tests are also used to verify the achievements of those who have learned in nontraditional ways by comparing the outcomes of such learning to that produced by conventional educational programs. For example, the widely used and accepted high school equivalency examinations are actually achievement tests that compare the performance of the equivalency candidate to that of high school graduates.

Because the range of interest and personality inventories is great, I am unable to provide you with any simple classification scheme. These instruments do not have right answers, and the meaning of a counselee's responses is determined by comparing those responses with those of some group. The particular meaning assigned to responses or groups of responses is sometimes determined by statistical procedures that produce groupings of similar items. The instrument's author typically assigns meanings to the statistically determined groups and designates scale names. The process of determining item groupings and assigning meanings to those groupings is called *homogeneous scaling*. Another procedure used in the development of inventories is *criterion-referenced scaling*. Criterion-referenced scaling requires that the responses of persons taking the inventory be compared with the responses of specifically defined groups (criterion groups) who have previously completed the inventory. Scale items are determined by the responses of criterion groups and scale names are based on the criterion group membership. I hope this sketch has convinced you that the counselor's understanding of how inventories are developed is vital for their appropriate use.

Other Assessment Devices

The types of instruments I have mentioned are standardized tests and inventories. There are other assessment devices that can have an important influence on counselees, and counselors should develop an appreciation of those. Assessments can range from anecdotal comments in a student's school record to evaluations of a candidate's performance in a simulated work situation at an assessment center. Despite the contention by a noted test critic that standardized tests are society's "gatekeeper" (Williams, 1975), we must recognize that most colleges and universities assign more weight to applicants' secondary school performance than to test scores and that graduate and professional schools likewise value grades.

School grades are a nonstandardized form of student assessment that has a major role in determining students' futures. Professional counselors must work with their teaching colleagues to bring the assignment of student grades under the same scrutiny and demand for fairness that we so rightly ask of standardized tests. Counselors should be familiar with the range and role of nonstandardized assessment devices as well as published standardized instruments.

I have continued to mention how the performance of test takers is compared with that of some defined group called a "norm group." One of the topics about which counselors must have knowledge is the concept of norm groups. To properly understand and evaluate a standardized test, counselors must be able to determine the adequacy and relevance of the norm group for their clients. Another major topic in tests-and-measurements courses is the derivation and types of scores used to report the results of standardized tests. If counselors are not comfortable with their understanding of the systems used to report scores and to compare the performance of their clients with that of the norm group, they cannot expect to facilitate the clients' understanding of the scores. Counselors will also use assessment instruments that do not rely on norm groups, and so they must be able to explain clearly and accurately the meaning of the scores from instruments they use.

School counselors will be exposed to the idea of competency tests. Such tests are used in some states to establish qualification for high school graduation and have been the subject of intense debate. Competency tests are typically criterion-referenced tests. The person who takes a criterion-referenced test does not compete against a norm group but is working to achieve an established performance standard. An example of a performance standard might be the ability to accurately multiply four-digit numbers by four-digit numbers or to type forty words a minute in a standard ten-minute test. Success or failure on such tests does not depend on the performance of a norm group or the performance of others taking the test. Potential employers might use criterion-referenced tests to determine whether an applicant had the minimum skills. For example, an employer may be interested only in knowing whether the applicant has the ability to read directions, not in the applicant's standing relative to others who have the ability to read directions necessary to the job.

Reliability and Validity

Counselors must also know about the various threats to the accuracy of the scores on assessment devices and the methods used to determine and report the accuracy of instruments. Such concerns fall under the general topic of test reliability and errors of measurement. Each person who takes a test is assumed to have a hypothetical score that represents the true performance on whatever is being measured. Owing to errors of measurement, the score actually obtained by the person is only an approximation of that true score. By studying the consistency of instrument content, the effect of time delays, and alternate forms and testing procedures, the test maker can provide users information about how much the scores obtained by those who take the test are likely to deviate from the true score. Unfortunately, not all test publishers make such information clearly available in a user-oriented form. Counselors must understand reliability and know how to gain the information necessary for their proper use of test data from the publisher's manual.

Important as the concept of reliability (a form of accuracy) is for counselors and their clients, it is secondary in importance to the concept of validity. The American Psychological Association manual (1974) states: "Validity refers to the appropriateness of inferences from test data or other forms of assessment" (p. 25). The manual reduces validity questions to two: (1) What is measured by the test? (2) What can be inferred from that about other behavior? Those questions are critical for counselor and their clients. Simply to tell a counselee "You rank high on a worry scale" tells the person little to help her with decisions she faces. Although we cannot be sure the information would be helpful, we can be sure that knowing what "worry" means and knowing what certain scores on the worry scale had meant in the behavior of others would be prerequisite to appropriate counselee action based on the information about the results.

Although they acknowledge the existence of numerous other terms, the APA *Standards* (1974) discuss three types of validity. *Criterion-related validity* is the relation of scores on the instrument to some other variable. Criterion-related validity estimates address the relation of the scores to some variable in the future and are called "predictive." Those that address present standing on the criterion are called "concurrent."

Content validity, the second type of validity discussed, is especially important for tests of skill and knowledge because it assesses how well the instrument samples the skills and/or knowledge it purports to measure. A good sample would be one that adequately represented the skill and/or knowledge claimed as a basis for the test.

The third type of validity, *construct validity*, is difficult to explain concisely and clearly and without resorting to circular definitions. Counselors and other psychological helping professionals often use constructs as terms to refer to complex concepts. Examples of such terms would be *interests* and *readiness*. Those terms obviously are subject to varied definitions and assessment approaches. Investigation of construct validity is a process of attempting to know and understand what is meant by the constructs on which the particular instrument is based.

Errors of Difference and Prediction

Finally, counselors who use tests properly must understand and know how to use the concepts of errors of difference and prediction in their work with clients. Since each assessment or measurement attempt is subject to error (unreliability), any consideration of two or more scores must take into account the fact that both the scores in question may have been influenced by test error. Even though we can feel confident in making statements about the amount of test error present in the assessment of groups, we cannot know for which individual members of the group errors are present. Nor can we know the amount and direction of the error for those individuals. We can, however, advise our counselees of the presence of errors and discourage them from assigning meaning to small differences between scores. Your study of the concept of errors of difference will provide the basis for your work with sets of scores.

Just as errors affect the interpretation of the meaning of differences between scores, errors are also present when scores are used to predict clients' future performance. Whether the prediction is future academic achievement in a college or the dollar volume of life insurance that a person will sell, reasonably accurate aggregate predictions can be made for large groups of people. The counselor's problem is that clients are *individual* and are interested in how well they might perform at some future time. Despite the sophistication of statistical techniques, counselors cannot escape the error inherent in individual predictions. We can, however, learn the concept of error of estimate (or prediction) and learn how to use that concept to make accurate statements to our clients. We can, for example, use errors-of-estimate information to construct experience tables, which will allow us to show our counselees what performances have actually been achieved by people like them who had similar records on the predictors.

A counselor who has a clearly developed rationale for the use of assessment devices in counseling, who is sensitive to the social and ethical issues surrounding assessment, and who gains an essential mastery of the concepts suggested above is prepared to use tests. Such counselors will not do harm with tests and will also have the potential to make assessment information a useful part of their counseling. But a word of caution: Given the variety of clients and settings in which counseling takes place, testing may be appropriate for few if any of a given counselor's clients. Moreover, mere concept mastery of assessment methods and techniques will not a competent counselor make. Counselors must acquire an appreciation of the social, ethical, and legal issues surrounding assessment. These are examined in the following section.

Social, Ethical, and Legal Issues

That numerous legitimate issues surround the use of assessment devices of various types and especially standardized tests is not news to those interested in the psychologically based helping professions. Likewise, there are numerous questions about the content and role of career information traditionally used by counselors as they help students make decisions that have far-reaching implications. If the decisions students make have far-reaching consequences, then so do the decisions made about students. To the extent that assessment information contributes to decisions about which curriculum or courses a student enters, to that extent are questions about the assessment process necessary and legitimate.

The controversy surrounding the use of standardized testing programs, though not new, is far from resolved. A survey of test use in secondary schools shows that tests are still widely used and that many schools would do more testing if funds were available (Engen, Lamb, & Prediger, 1982). The introduction to that report is a listing of the various groups that have called for the elimination of standardized testing from schools or for a moratorium on the use of standardized tests. Numerous special issues of professional journals (for example, *The American Psychologist, 36* (10), October 1981) and featured articles have presented the arguments of those involved in the testing controversy. The cover of the January 1980 *NEA Reporter* introduced the topic with the headline "Teachers and Citizens Protest the Testing Ripoff." On the other side, the Association for Measurement and Evaluation in Guidance has published a response to the "attacks" (Zytowski, 1981).

Because the current editions of tests-and-measurements texts as well as numerous articles present the basic issues in the standardized-test controversy, I have compressed the issues into those I consider essential for your present consideration. The first and major charge typically leveled at standardized tests is that they discriminate.

With the possible exception of a few critics who believe that we should not try to determine the differences among individuals, the discrimination concern is really one of unfair discrimination. That is, are the differences among test takers related to race, sex, socioeconomic status, and culture in ways that have no connection to what the test is actually trying to assess? I prefer to call this issue the issue of test fairness. Simply, the issue is "Are tests fair to those who take them?"

The issue of test fairness is not limited to the traditional disadvantaged groups in our society. If a White, upper-middle-class male is prevented by test scores from acquiring an education to which he aspires and is capable of, the tests have been unfair. At least the results of the testing have contributed to an unfair result. I believe that focusing on questions of tests and race, sex, age, and social class obscures the basic issue of test fairness. Numerous investigations have confirmed that results of national testing programs contribute something to the prediction of the performance of first-year college students (for example, Fincher, 1974). The social issue is whether the information gained is worth the cost in money and time and the potential for unfairness to many of those who take the tests.

Despite our legitimate concern about test fairness, we should not lose sight of the fact that differences among individuals do exist. When we compare individuals, some will excel and others will be at the bottom of the group, whether we are assessing physical talent, artistic talent, musical talent, or talent for schoolwork. If counselors attribute all differences among individuals to unfairness in the assessment procedures, they may contribute to faulty decision making. At some point in the decision-making process, counselees may need to, and in fact want to, make an accurate and fair comparison (to the extent such is possible) of the skills and achievements they possess with those necessary to achieve some goal.

Even if we have great faith in the potential of individuals to achieve far more than can reasonably be predicted for them, we must recognize that such achievements are typically the result of effort and sacrifice. Realistic planning should be based on an informed estimate of the *cost* of a decision, and counselors who withhold unfavorable data from their counselees do not contribute to informed planning. I suggest that we must consider the counselee's right to be given the best information we possess, at the same time that we consider the limits of assessment procedures and our desire to encourage our counselees to do more than could be reasonably predicted.

I believe that counselors should take a leading role in asking that tests be used only when the information gained is absolutely necessary for making a reasonable decision and is worth the cost and the potential for unfairness. To take the most pervasive national testing program as an example, most of the colleges that require the Scholastic Aptitude Test (SAT) might find their admissions equally valid if they relied on the applicant's school record and other data related to the applicant's past behavior and performance. This position is compatible with the recently announced recommendations of the Ford Foundation Commission on the Higher Education of Minorities ("Text of the Recommendations . . . ," 1982):

> The Committee on Ability Testing for the National Research Council (The council is an arm of the National Academy of Sciences.) has issued a report of a four year review of testing. Although the committee did not find ability tests biased against minority candidates, it questioned the expense and inconvenience of their use by other than selective schools. On that point the findings were similar to the Ford Foundation study of minority applicants.

I suggest an extension of the recommendations to benefit *all* students.

You may wonder, if standardized tests are unfair, why doesn't someone make them fair? Despite many sincere efforts to make the results of tests fair, the problem of unfairness remains. The reasons are too complex for our current purpose, except to say that tests rest on an assumption that those who take them have had backgrounds and experiences reasonably similar to those of the norm group for whom the instruments were designed. Even a cursory examination of the diversity in our society will show that this essential and fundamental assumption presents an obstacle for test makers that is almost impossible to surmount.

Another major grouping of criticisms of testing can be lumped under the concern for forced uniformity. Forced uniformity may occur in the school curriculum when all students are exposed to the same material so that they will score well on a standardized test. Or the uniformity may be imposed on ways of thinking so that the creative, divergent thinker is unable to perform well. These concerns are legitimate and valid, and I can only suggest that tests do not force undesirable uniformity but that such forced uniformity results from an unjustified use of the test results. Counselors must be in the vanguard of those who suggest that tests should not be used to define curriculum or define the desirable attributes of individuals.

A third major category of criticism of tests concerns labeling and stereotyping. The widely publicized California court case *Larry P. v. Wilson Riles* was really a court test of a broader issue—namely, the legitimacy of the use of standardized intelligence tests to place students in special classes. Such placements can result in the labeling or stereotyping of students. Although the test can contribute to such unfortunate outcomes, we must ask whether the issue is the test or the use of the test results. Again, in my opinion a far more important issue is whether the tests contribute to the fair assignment of students to special classes. Whatever our opinion on that issue, counselors must be leaders in the fight to avoid stereotyping and labeling on any basis.

Related to the issue of labeling and stereotyping has been the issue of access to information resulting from tests. The issue has actually had two aspects, the availability of information to students and parents and the ability of students and parents to control access to information in the student's file. Both concerns were addressed nationwide by the Family Educational Rights and Privacy Act of 1974 (the "Buckley-Pell Amendment"). Essentially, the act gives students and the parents of minor students the right of access to information in their educational records and gives them the right to limit access to that information.

The issues related to the information counselors use are related to those that surround testing. Occupational information has been criticized for showing women and minorities only in occupations that were traditional for those groups. The sex-specific language of interest inventories has been challenged. The issues raised grow out of the same social concerns that are related to testing. The social concerns are based in a belief that counselors' activities and the materials they use should encourage all groups to make choices based only on their personal characteristics and limitations, and independent of membership in any group.

In response to the social issues surrounding the use of assessment devices and information by counselors, the American Personnel and Guidance Association has published a policy statement, *Responsibilities of Users of Standardized Tests* (1980), as well as a position paper, "The Responsible Use of Tests" (1972). The Association for Measurement and Evaluation in Guidance, a division of the APGA, has published *Statement on Legislation Affecting Testing for Selection in Educational and Occupational Programs* (1980). These statements, like the sections of the APGA *Ethical Standards* relating to the use of test data and information, show the response of counselors' professional associations to the criticisms of testing programs, as do legislative proposals that have resulted in making the questions from some national testing programs available to those who take the tests. The National Vocational Guidance Association, another APGA division, has standards for career literature that recognize the legitimacy of many of the concerns about such publications.

Standardized tests and information sources are inanimate objects and can do no harm without the assistance of a willing human agent. Unfortunately, the willing human agents do not see themselves as doing harm. In most cases they are convinced they are acting correctly. Counselors must first ensure that their use of tests and information is based on sound counseling principles and recognizes the many limitations of the materials. They must also ensure that colleagues with whom they work use tests and information in a professionally appropriate and ethical manner.

The fact that counselors engage in activities other than the traditionally viewed individual and small-group sessions does not mean that counselors are only counselors part-time. Counselors are always counselors, and the attitudes and skills that we hope distinguish counselors from other helpers should always be present and observable in their behavior. Those important skills and attitudes are vital components of the counselor's work with assessment procedures and information giving.

Counselors are good listeners. A counselor working in an agency who has to disseminate information about the agency's policies and procedures to clients of that agency should communicate to the clients an attitude of willingness to really listen to their questions and concerns. By using the counseling techniques of feedback and clarification, the counselor can communicate respect, acceptance, and understanding of clients even though the counselor is working to facilitate an administrative procedure.

Counselors are concerned about individual differences. A counselor working in a publicly funded agency that seeks to move clients from public assistance rolls to full employment needs to constantly remind the control board that the information gathered about the agency's clients demonstrates a significant range of reasons for their current, un-, or underemployment. The assessment of the clients could be the basis for programs designed to accommodate individual differences.

Counselors are concerned about promoting opportunities for all their counselees. A school counselor serving on a committee charged with designing a school-system plan for identifying students who could benefit from a special program for academically talented students might need to remind the group that assessing the academic potential of students by means of traditional standardized ability and aptitude tests might be unfair to many talented students who had backgrounds markedly different from the background of the test norm group.

Counselors are concerned about counselee development. The goal of all information and training programs developed by counselors should be to make the counselee independent of any particular program or source of assistance. Because counselors are concerned about the *future* success of their counselees, they will perform those functions that will develop and enhance their counselees' skills. Competent, concerned counselors will perform all counselor functions in an ethical, professionally competent manner because counselors are concerned about each counselee's development.

Perspectives for the '80s

The socioeconomic changes occurring in our society will have a significant impact on the work of counselors in the 1980s. Certainly prediction is at best an inaccurate science, but we must recognize that certain changes we can now observe will influence the activities of counselors in the future.

The world of work is changing dramatically. Consider the automated office, in which telephones automatically dial numbers when the required lines are free, the internal messenger is a wheeled robot, and typewriters are computer-controlled word processors. Such offices exist today, as do assembly lines where robots controlled by computers assemble automobiles. These offices and factories are worthy of comment now but will be a commonplace fact in the world of work entered by those now served by school counselors. Those who are displaced by mechanical devices will also need the services of counselors as they make decisions about retraining and redirecting their lives. As job opportunities shift from manufacturing to service, so will ways of life.

The shift will be not only in the type of work available to the clients of counselors but in the location where work is available. The population shift to the Sunbelt has caused many families to be separated from relatives and familiar surroundings. The stress resulting from a national migration of workers will surely affect the types of assistance sought from counselors in many settings.

Not only the location of families but the concept of what is a family will continue to change during the '80s. There will be more single-parent families, and the economic necessity for all adult members of a family to be earners will increase. The single parent will be joined by the workers from conventional families who require day-care facilities. As the population becomes older, counseling services related to health issues will be in greater demand, as will counseling for retirement and preretirement planning.

Counselors who work with young people may find that basic value shifts have occurred in our society. Recent reports suggest that students have become more materialistic and see education as a means to financial success. Certainly, if this is true, counselors will face great demands for accurate educational and career information. Later, perhaps, counselors will serve counselees who discovered that education does not guarantee financial success or does not bring satisfaction.

The counselor of the '80s will work in a rapidly evolving society in which there are many needs for counselors' services and scarce public funds to pay those services. Counselors will be called on to defend the need for, and outcomes of, their programs. Counselors will deal with rapidly changing information management devices. The demands by numerous groups that assessment be fair and that it not limit the growth potential of those tested will increase. Counselees will see themselves as consumers and will want to know what kind of services they will receive. As active participants in the counseling process, counselees may choose to participate in assessment in order to gain what they consider to be useful information. They will be less willing to have counselors make decisions about or for them.

Counselors who work both in and out of school settings will be more directly involved in counselee education and the use of information. The information will be used directly with counselees or indirectly, as a part of the counselor's consulting function. Counselors will be expected to consult with teachers and parents, and the use of information will be one of the more critical ingredients in such consultative relationships. Likewise, counselors will be more directly involved in matters of curriculum and program review and design.

Counselors will be providing information to groups about a variety of topics. Counselors must have the information that people consider personally relevant and useful, and they will be called on to function as education consultants. Students in schools will want to know about sources of financial assistance for higher education, and their parents will also expect more systematically organized presentations of this information. Community counseling services will be providing group consultation sessions on job-seeking strategies for women seeking to enter or reenter the work world and men seeking reemployment. School counselors, as the only persons in a school with graduate-level training in tests and measurements, will be looked to as never before to provide administrators, teachers, parents, and students with the critically needed information about standardized tests. School counselors traditionally have been responsible for organizing and coordinating the many testing programs implemented during a school year. In addition to college entrance examinations, most secondary schools have regular programs of standardized testing to assess their students' aptitudes and achievements. Whether or not the students wanted or even needed the testing, the counselor might have been expected to administer the tests and provide students and parents with feedback on the results. In the '80s, counselors will be expected to perform all these functions, but they will be increasingly more involved in consultations with teachers and administrators about the meaning of the results for the school.

The results of standardized tests will have a major impact on the decisions made by pupil-services teams engaged in developing the educational plans required by the 1975 Education For All Handicapped Children Act (PL 94-142). This national law requires that handicapped students be placed in the least restrictive environment, or "mainstreamed," and have an appropriate educational plan developed for them.

It has caused counselors to be involved with school psychologists, special educators, school social workers, and school administrators as members of teams making placement decisions and developing individual educational plans for affected students. Counselors of the '80s will face new challenges as a result of this law. They must know and understand the language and limits of testing if they are going to be effective members of such teams. Some of the specific instruments used by such teams are not those traditionally used by counselors; nevertheless, counselors of the '80s must have familiarity with individually administered tests and a mastery of the basic concepts of assessment because they will be expected to be valued and contributing team members.

But school counselors are not the only counselors who will work with tests in the '80s. Counselors in agencies will be called on to demonstrate the effectiveness of their programs, and they will be doing so with assessment devices for their clients, their services, and so on. Counselors of the '80s will be more involved in a greater variety of research and evaluation activities, which will range from gathering simple demographic data on their counselees to using sophisticated and complex research designs for analyzing the data generated by their funded research projects. All these activities have always been a necessary part of the work of the counselor, but in the '80s they are critical to the work of the counselor if the knowledge base on which the counseling profession rests can be expected to expand.

Summary

Assessment and information are combined in this chapter because they present similar problems and opportunities in the work of the counselor. Assessment in all its forms ultimately produces information about the counselee. Whether that information is used by the counselee or to make decisions about the counselee is a major consideration in the work of the counselor. Counselors also collaborate with their clients in the use of occupational, educational, and personal/social information. The critical question is whether the counselor uses the information in a prescriptive, directive fashion to narrow the range of choices available to the counselee or whether it is used to help the counselee learn more about the available options. Equally important is the question of who is making the decisions on the basis of assessment data.

Although there are those who question the role of information in a counseling relationship, counseling theorists can be cited to demonstrate the compatibility of information and counseling. Assessment and information are important to, and are used by, those who argue that the provision of information has no place in the counseling process. Counseling is only one function in the role of the counselor.

There are issues and problems surrounding the areas of assessment and information giving. Many of the problems are the result of inappropriate actions by those who have made assessments and used information. The professional associations have addressed these issues and provided guidelines for counselors. Counselors who are following the guidelines suggested by their professional associations and who are acting within the ethical codes of their profession are at an appropriate starting point to use tests and information for the benefit of their clients. Maximum benefit for clients of counselors will come when those counselors base their actions on the concept that the information resulting from testing, like information about occupations, is provided by the counselor to give clients the best possible basis for determining their own courses of action.

Counselors should learn about the technical aspects of standardized testing so they can judge the adequacy of the instruments and translate technical information about those instruments into statements that are accurate and easily understood by their clients. As professionals who know and understand something about the proper uses of assessment, counselors should and must speak out about assessment abuses. Counselors must also recognize that there are situations in which test information, admittedly imperfect, is one uniform way, for those who must make decisions, to gain information about those for whom decisions must be made.

The '80s are likely to be a period of continuing reevaluation of the utility and adequacy of standardized test instruments. The number of instruments and devices involving the test taker as an active participant with the counselor will grow. Card sorts, self-scoring instruments, and interactive programs on microcomputers will be alternatives to current instruments that, when completed, must be processed at a distant location, to be returned two weeks later. Society will reject assessment methods and informational materials that unfairly restrict individual development. Rather, society will demand assessment methods and informational materials that will be used to expand and promote individual opportunity.

Now It's Your Turn

1. Ask your classmates about their experiences with standardized tests and testing programs. If they have criticisms and concerns, how could counselors have acted to eliminate them? Are there concerns beyond the immediate control of the counselors?
2. Ask a counselor working in the type of setting in which you would like to work how he or she uses assessment devices and information. Examine the tests and information sources the counselor suggests.
3. Find out whether the counseling or career-services center of your college has an automated or computerized career-information retrieval system. If so, visit it and try the system; if not, find out whether you might examine such a system at a nearby public school.

4. Examine some currently published interest inventories and occupational literature and note how the occupational titles have been made gender-free.
5. Get a copy of the materials the College Entrance Examination Board, through the Educational Testing Service, provides those who take any of their tests and note how the technical concepts of testing are explained in language understandable to those who take the tests. (The CEEB has been the subject of many recent attacks. I do believe counselors should acknowledge its attempts to publish model materials for counselors and those who take the tests.)
6. Read the section in any recently published tests-and-measurements text that covers the topic of testing and social issues—for example, Shertzer and Linden (1979, Chapter 6); Sax (1980, Chapter 2).
7. Divide into working groups. Assume that the group is the admissions committee of a medical college. The admissions staff has just reported that the applicant pool has been screened by the staff and that those who do not have superior grades in an appropriate premedical curriculum, glowing letters of reference, and a long history of school and community involvement have been eliminated. There are still three applicants for every open position. The admissions committee is charged with finding a way to determine who gets the available spaces. After a determined time period, groups should share their recommendations and discuss the reasons for them.

References

American Personnel and Guidance Association. *Standards for preparation in counselor education.* Falls Church, Va.: American Personnel and Guidance Association, 1979.

American Personnel and Guidance Association. *APGA policy statement: Responsibilities of users of standardized tests.* Falls Church, Va.: American Personnel and Guidance Association, 1980.

American Psychological Association. *Standards for educational and psychological tests.* Washington, D. C.: American Psychological Association, 1974.

Arbuckle, D. S. *Counseling and psychotherapy: An existential-humanist view* (3rd ed.). Boston: Allyn & Bacon, 1975.

Association for Measurement and Evaluation in Guidance. *Statement on legislation affecting testing for selection in educational and occupational programs.* Falls Church, Va.: American Personnel and Guidance Association, October, 1980.

Association for Measurement and Evaluation in Guidance, American Personnel and Guidance Association, and the National Council on Measurement in Education. The responsible use of tests: A position paper of AMEG, APGA, and NCME. *Measurement and Evaluation in Guidance,* 1972, 5(2), 385–388.

Burks, H. M., Jr., & Stefflre, B. (Eds.). *Theories of counseling* (3rd ed.). New York: McGraw-Hill, 1979.

Corey, G. *Theory and practice of counseling and psychotherapy* (2nd ed.). Monterey, Calif.: Brooks/Cole, 1982.

Cronbach, L. J. *Essentials of psychological testing* (3rd ed.). New York: Harper & Row, 1970.

Engen, H. B., Lamb, R. R., & Prediger, D. J. Are secondary schools still using standardized tests? *Personnel and Guidance Journal,* 1982, *60*(5), 287-290.

Fincher, C. Is the SAT worth its salt? *Review of Educational Research,* 1974, *44*(3), 293-305.

Goldman, L. Tests should make a difference. *Measurement and Evaluation in Guidance,* 1969, *2*(1), 53-60. (a)

Goldman, L. *Using tests in counseling* (2nd ed.). New York: Appleton-Century-Crofts, 1969. (b)

Goldman, L. It's time to put up or shut up. *Measurement and Evaluation in Guidance,* 1972, *5*(3), 420-423. (a)

Goldman, L. Tests and counseling: The marriage that failed. *Measurement and Evaluation in Guidance,* 1972, *4*(4), 213-220. (b)

Grummon, D. L. Client-centered theory. In H. M. Burks, Jr., & B. Stefflre, *Theories of counseling* (3rd ed.). New York: McGraw-Hill, 1979.

Holland, J. *The psychology of vocational choice.* Waltham, Mass.: Blaisdell, 1966.

Hoppock, R. *Occupational information* (4th ed.). New York: McGraw-Hill, 1976.

Keller, K. E., Biggs, D. A., & Gysbers, N. C. Career counseling from a cognitive perspective. *Personnel and Guidance Journal,* 1982, *60*(6), 367-371.

Maples, M. F. Humanism and testing: Are they compatible? *Humanist Educator,* 1977, *16*(1), 38-43.

Parsons, F. *Choosing a vocation.* Boston: Houghton Mifflin, 1909.

Patterson, C. H. *Relationship counseling and psychotherapy.* New York: Harper & Row, 1974.

Rogers, C. R. The necessary and sufficient conditions of therapeutic personality change. *Journal of Consulting Psychology,* 1957, *21*(2), 95-103.

Sax, G. *Principles of educational and psychological measurement and evaluation* (2nd ed.). Belmont, Calif.: Wadsworth, 1980.

Senour, M. N. How counselors influence clients. *Personnel and Guidance Journal,* 1982, *60*(6), 345-349.

Shertzer, B., & Linden, J. D. *Fundamentals of individual appraisal: Assessment techniques for counselors.* Boston: Houghton Mifflin, 1979.

Test of panel's conclusions and recommendations on testing. *Chronicle of Higher Education,* February 10, 1982, pp. 9-10.

Test of the recommendations of the Ford Foundation panel. *Chronicle of Higher Education,* February 3, 1982, pp. 10-14.

Williams, R. L. The politics of IQ, racism, and power: An editorial. *Journal of Afro-American Issues,* 1975, *3*(1), 1.

Williamson, E. G. *How to counsel students.* New York: McGraw-Hill, 1939.

Zytowski, D. G. Pro-test: A response from the Association for Measurement and Evaluation in Guidance. *AMEG Newsnotes,* 1981, *17*(1), 3-10.

CHAPTER **8**

Research and Evaluation

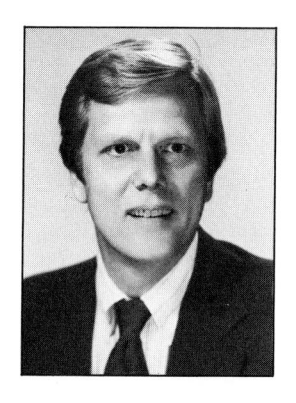

N. Kenneth LaFleur

N. Kenneth LaFleur is a University of Virginia counselor education faculty member. He is a graduate of Michigan State University and has held field leadership positions in the American Educational Research Association, Division E, and the American Psychological Association, Division 17. He is the coauthor of a research text and teaches counseling research.

The quest to understand events and know the "what," "when," "how," and "why" of phenomena is a basic component of the human experience. This desire to know and understand aids the process of building theories and paradigms that provide a map to guide current and future actions. The evaluation and research methods used by counselors are a natural outgrowth of the human endeavor to understand.

Counselors work with individual clients, groups of clients, the social systems in which clients live, and the environments in which the counseling activities occur. The counselor's effort in a process of evaluation and research is to understand these phenomena. Is the counseling technique being used of help to this client? What are the employment possibilities for rehabilitation counselors in the Southwest? Is the client's home environment conducive to helping the client achieve the counseling goals? What are the major types of counseling concerns brought by clients to the Center? What are the personal strengths of the members of this counseling group that could be used to foster a sense of cohesiveness in the group? These are the types of questions on which counselors focus their evaluation and research efforts in an attempt to know and understand their professional world. Often the questions are complex, and the processes used to find the answers are unique and designed to fit the specific question and situation.

The codes of ethics of professional organizations require counselors to carefully and continually examine their counseling activities. The codes of both the American Personnel and Guidance Association and the American Psychological Association advocate an examination of the efficacy of the helper's prevention and intervention efforts with clients. Such an evaluation and research activity is one of the hallmarks of the professional counselor. As a professional, the counselor must continually search for knowledge and understanding about counseling activities.

There is no one way of doing evaluation and research; it is a *process* with particular characteristics that separate it from other methods of knowing and understanding. The process has two major components: asking questions and seeking the answers to questions. As counselors engage in the evaluation and research process, they may identify new questions, reopen old questions, find the answers sought, and discover knowledge that was not the specific focus of the current research effort. In the research and evaluation process, the counselor becomes involved in consuming the evaluation and research production efforts of others *and* producing research activities to respond to the counselor's individual question. Both consuming and producing evaluation and research are integral parts of the professional counselor's work. Reading and listening to the work of other counselors is just as important a research and evaluation activity as producing evaluation and research.

This chapter is an introduction to evaluation and research in counseling. An overview of the process, an examination of the current issues, and a statement of future direction in the area of professional counseling research will be presented.

Ways of Knowing and Understanding

The process of evaluation and research used by counselors rests on the two basic sources of learning: authority and experience. These two sources are the major ways in which counselors learn about their professional work.

Authority

Authority is a technique used when counselors desire to learn items not possible or available from experience. Authoritative sources are identified, and information is sought from these sources. The reading and hearing of others' experiences, customs, and traditions are all examples of using authority as a source of learning. The use of authority as a major learning source was particularly prevalent during the Middle Ages. Plato and Aristotle were influential because they were viewed as important learning sources. The church, acting as an authoritative learning source, was able to influence what people believed and how they acted during the Middle Ages. In recent times, inexperienced counselors often ask veteran counselors for various types of information. Tradition and custom often form the foundation for the building of counseling programs.

Authority is most often used as a learning source when the evaluation and research venture involves the learning of facts. Authority would be more useful than experience in a counselor's attempts to identify employment opportunities for secondary school counselors in Arizona. A report by the Arizona State Department of Education would be a more efficient use of the counselor's energy than the application and interview with each secondary school in Arizona.

As a method of learning and understanding, authority has limitations. It is most reliable when focused mainly on facts rather than on understanding process. Another limitation occurs when two sources identified as possessing authority can disagree on a particular item. Authority is not necessarily infallible.

Experience

Experience as a way of knowing and understanding is most often used when the counselor's questions involve processes rather than a specific factual issue. As a learning source, experience is used when counselors observe phenomena associated with a question and then reach conclusions or answers based on their observations. Experience as a learning source places much trust in observational abilities and primary importance on the individual counselor's skill in interpreting the experiences. The major limitation of the experience category of learning is that some personal bias of the counselor may so distort the learning that it is not correct. Personal perceptions enter into the collecting of information and the conclusions reached when experience is used as a learning source.

Recently, in several sections of an introductory research-methods class, over 100 people completing a master's degree program in counseling were asked to identify something they knew about counseling and how they knew it. The group included students who had never acted as counselors with clients and those who had varying amounts of client contact in either training or employment activities. After dividing the responses to the first question (something known about counseling) into specific facts and process observations, it was possible to predict with 100% accuracy whether the source for the knowledge would be in the authority or experience category. Examples of authority were "I read it in the text used in the introductory course," "The professor said so," "A counselor in the Center told us that in a seminar course I took last semester," "The director informed me that that was the best program to help the parents they saw last year." Most of the experience-category statements pointed to knowing the item because "I saw three clients in the practicum who were helped that way," "I have been a paraprofessional counselor in a local agency for the past four months and I know it to be true." Using identified authority and experience categories, predictions of 93% accuracy were made of whether the person responding had counseling experience or was yet to act in a counseling situation with a client.

Authority and experience as ways of learning and understanding have individual advantages and limitations. Each is used to gain specific types of information, and each is used with varied degrees of reliance by inexperienced and experienced counselors. Both are valuable, and probably both should be used by the professional counselor in attempts to know and understand the facts and functions of counseling.

Methods of Reaching Conclusions

What counselors do with the knowledge gained through authority and experience will influence the conclusions they reach about counseling. The major methods employed to reach conclusions are deductive reasoning, inductive reasoning, and a scientific approach.

Deductive Reasoning

As a method of reaching conclusions, deductive reasoning uses a system of logic that enables the counselor to move from general to specific statements. The logic system involves a series of statements termed a syllogism, which contains a major premise, a minor premise, and a conclusion. An example of syllogistic reasoning is: (1) all counselors are self-actualized—major premise, (2) Sue is a counselor—minor premise, (3) Sue is self-actualized—conclusion. If the premises are true, then the process of deductive reasoning will lead to true conclusions. As an evaluation and research process, deductive reasoning can help the counselor organize existing knowledge and indicate new relations between known information. It can also help the counselor make links between theory and observations. Deductive reasoning has a major limitation in that the premises must be true if we are to reach a valid conclusion. Since it is often difficult to establish universal truths in the field of counseling, the deductive method is used mainly to organize existing information and provide questions and hypotheses to be examined by other methods.

Inductive Reasoning

The difficulties involved in establishing the truth of the premises used in the deductive method led to the development of the inductive reasoning method. Francis Bacon (1561-1626) called for knowledge not to be totally guided by an acceptance of authority as absolute truth. Bacon urged the inductive method of reasoning, which is based on taking observations of specific events and then making generalizations to entire groups. It is the reverse of the deductive method, which starts with a generalization (major premise) and works to a specific event.

In order to make valid generalizations using the inductive method, the counselor must examine or observe all of the specific events. Generalizations or conclusions that counselors make after completing observations on less than all of the specific events would be considered imperfect. Since it is often impractical or impossible to make observations on all events associated with the particular counseling question, evaluation and research activities completed by counselors using the inductive method are typically valid for limited groups or situations. This is a major limitation to use of the inductive method alone in evaluation and research activities. On the basis of limited observations, it was often thought that all "gifted children" were poor physical specimens. Such a generalization was based on the use of the inductive approach but was not valid for the entire group of all gifted children. Lewis Terman, a pioneer in the field of mental measurement, observed over 1000 gifted high school students and found them average in physical characteristics for their age. Even though the inductive method has limitations, it is of value in that it enables the counselor to gather reliable information about a limited group, which can be of use in making decisions about that group.

The Scientific Method

A method using both deductive and inductive reasoning was developed. Commonly labeled the scientific method, this inductive/deductive method uses observations from experience, and knowledge of authority gained from reading and listening to formulate hypotheses. These hypotheses, or best guesses about the answer to the counselor's research question, are then tested by gathering additional observations and coming to conclusions about the validity of the hypotheses. As such, the scientific approach involves both inductive and deductive reasoning methods. The main difference is in the use of hypotheses. Generalizations are made based on empirically testing the validity of the hypotheses by gathering data or observations designed to help test the hypotheses. Use of the scientific approach enables the research and evaluation efforts of the counselor to attend to the body of knowledge about counseling *and* to make decisions about the specific aspect of counseling under question.

Use of the scientific approach in counseling research and evaluation requires a methodology and attitude of knowing that are founded on the characteristic of objectivity. Both aspects of the research and evaluation process—asking and answering questions—are subjected to and based on the attribute of objectivity. The goal of the counselor in research is to ask and answer questions that are relevant for the counselor's work and are reliable. Such an endeavor demands that the procedure used to conduct the research be objective. The procedures and explanations are not based solely on common sense, reason, or authority; rather, the basis is empirical in that the foundation is objectively conceived, conducted, and explained research. The scientific method, therefore, requires a constant and conscious effort to proceed through the entire research and evaluation process in an objective manner. Such an effort by counselors is the only way to gain valid knowledge and understanding of the complex situations that are the work of the professional counselor.

Whatever method counselors use to learn about their work, several basic phases should be included. In some form, these major phases are the following: (1) get the involved parties to participate in the research process, (2) determine the goals of the activity to be studied and the research endeavor itself, (3) design the steps of the project, (4) gather the necessary information, (5) interpret the data, and (6) utilize the data interpretation. These six phases should be completed in the order presented. Utilizing results is determined by the method used to interpret the data collected. What data to collect depends on the goals of the research and evaluation activity, and the goals are best established by the parties involved in the venture to be studied. Research is a logical endeavor, and the skipping of a phase can provide counselors with erroneous or misleading answers to the research questions. A variety of procedures can be used to perform each of the major phases, and these are described in the following sections.

Methods of Research and Evaluation

A variety of research and evaluation types are available to counselors. Each method of research has its own strengths and limitations, and which method is used is determined by the particular research question.

Historical

The method of research that collects and examines existing information is historical research. Historical research examines past information in the form of documents or relics for the purpose of learning about the past. This method of research is not used often in counseling. An example of historical research was reported by Rockwell and Rothney (1961), who examined the writings of five pioneers of the guidance and counseling movement to discover ways in which the pioneers, and therefore the early guidance and counseling activities, were influenced by the social ideas of the late 19th and early 20th centuries. Other historical research activities have examined how federal and state government statutes have helped mold the practice of counseling. Use of the historical method of research is needed but is often neglected as an avenue to examine information because it does not have its major focus on current topics of interest in the counseling field.

Case Study

The earliest research and evaluation efforts in counseling were of the case-study method. The reports of this method of research typically are in the form of descriptions of counselor/client activities. Because the focus of the case study is on only one unit—one group, one client, one program—it provides the counselor with the opportunity to study the many facets of the research question. If counseling and the clients counselors serve involve complex interactions of many factors, the case-study method of research is an excellent choice for an intensive examination of one unit. The primary focus of the case study is to examine how the information collected on the one unit and its related factors changes over time. It is not designed to be used when the research question involves generalizability to other units, but it can be of importance in the development of questions and hypotheses or generalizations that can be investigated later using a different method. Anton (1978) has proposed several research designs that would be of aid to the counselor using a case-study procedure. Several of the designs permit the researcher not only to describe the changes of data over time but also to begin to make cause/effect statements about the relations of all the factors examined to one another.

The case study provides the professional counselor with a skill to constantly examine the practice of counseling. The use of the case study in the research and evaluation efforts of professional counselors requires more than just global descriptions of nonspecific counseling activities. Jayaratne and Levy (1979) suggest the following six-part summary of the orientation, knowledge, and skills of a counselor engaged in research:

1. An understanding of the treatment methods used.
2. Knowledge of the client system and its environment.
3. An empirical and objective orientation toward the process of counseling.
4. Ability to put research and evaluation designs into operation.
5. Ability to functionally use empirical feedback that is obtained during counseling.
6. Ability to evaluate, incorporate, and use the research of others.

The study by Ross (1979) summarized in the later section on participant-observer research is an example of a case study using the six items listed above.

Survey

The process of gathering information that is a response to selected questions is used in survey research and evaluation. Survey research is used frequently to collect data in an effort to gain factual knowledge. Recently, the Association of Mental Health Counselors completed a survey designed to discover age, sex, experience, placement, and training information about its members. The research was designed to gather the information in an effort to learn more about who were members of the association and solicit the members' thoughts about future association activities. Often organizations will conduct survey research to learn about the preferences, attitudes, and behaviors of a specified group of people. School counselors conduct survey research to determine whether the students think the counseling services provided are aimed at their needs. Rehabilitation counselors conduct survey research to identify whether the medical services provided by the regional office for spinal-cord-disability clients are effective. In most instances survey research is aimed at gathering facts selected to help the counselor plan and evaluate a variety of services.

Longitudinal

When the focus of the research and evaluation is on developmental concerns and the long-term effects of institutional or counseling activities, counselors often conduct longitudinal research. Longitudinal research is helpful not only in making conclusions about the long-term effects of a counseling activity but also in helping complete interim evaluations. The most important feature of longitudinal research and evaluation is the need to document all activities under examination. The major steps of longitudinal research are (1) statement of the research question, (2) development of the research and evaluation plan with a focus on the goals of the activity to be examined, (3) specifying the data of interest and the method for collecting them, (4) making use of a variety of data sources and types, (5) arranging for repeated collections of data, (6) continued review and possible revising of the research plan and activities, (7) determined efforts to gain 100% response from the data sources, and finally (8) analyses of both the gross data (those focused on the total activity goals) and the individual case data.

The most constant use of longitudinal research in counseling has been conducted in Wisconsin. Under the direction of John W. M. Rothney a series of longitudinal research projects were conducted to examine specified counseling activities in many secondary schools in Wisconsin. Similar research has been done at the University of Wisconsin to evaluate several student groups counseled by members of the university staff or counseling students. Currently, Marshall Sanborn, of the University of Wisconsin, is continuing the longitudinal research efforts started by

Rothney. Many of these efforts are conducted with clients who are provided services through the university's Research and Guidance Laboratory.

Participant Observer

It is possible for the counselor to conduct research and evaluation activities when the counselor is an actual participant in the counseling service. This is termed the participant-observer method of counseling research and is becoming used more frequently by counselors. Though used by sociologists and political scientists for a long time, participant-observer research has recently become the method of research practiced by professional counselors to evaluate ongoing counseling services. It is most useful to gain insight and understanding about how the individual client interacts in the client's particular environment. While a participant in the environment, the researcher must make and record observations of the events that occur. Patricia Ross (1979) has reported the use of a participant-observation research project with a group of troubled adolescents. Ross and a colleague used the research during a group counseling program to attempt an understanding of the adolescents and their environment as perceived by the young people. The establishment, conduct, and follow-up of the group counseling program provided the data for Ross and her colleague to examine the phenomena they were experiencing. It is an excellent example of the promise and problems of participant-observation research and also presents the method by which hypotheses and questions can be formed, tested, and revised during the research process.

Experimental

Counselors facing questions aimed at the discovery of cause-and-effect relations use the experimental method of research. This method can have as an interest one unit or an entire class or group of units. It is often designed to examine theory, as opposed to practice. The primary purpose of the research activity is not a decision about the counseling activity taking place but rather theoretical relations. Counseling research of the experimental type typically uses a series of statistical analysis procedures to examine collected data and makes conclusions based on the results of these analyses. The major limitations of experimental research lie in the need for control necessary to permit the counselor to make cause/effect conclusions about the data gathered. Anton's (1978) suggestions are helpful in that they enable the counselor to conduct experimental research with smaller units and make individual decisions focused on single cases. Therefore, conducting research aimed at cause/effect questions with single units is possible even though it has rarely been done in counseling research.

Data Sources in Research and Evaluation

What counselors know is based not only on the method used to conduct the research but also on the way information is collected. The information gathered is the data examined to find possible answers to the questions posited by the counselor. The value of the information collected is dependent on its validity and reliability as a source of data designed to provide needed facts focused on the research question.

Validity is a measure that attends to a determination whether the data collected are really what they were intended to be. As an index, validity responds to the issue of whether the data gathered are a true measure of the concept investigated. There are many types of validity and multiple methods to determine the validity of the data examined in a research or evaluation project. Most issues of validity begin with the question: "What should I examine to answer the question?"

Reliability is a concept aimed at the accuracy and consistency of the measures used to gather the data. As with validity, there are multiple types of reliability and multiple methods available to assess the reliability of the measures used. Methods of assessing reliability range from questions about the who, what, when, where, and how of observations to complex issues relating to the psychometric properties of questionnaires, inventories, and tests.

Observational Data

Countings or frequencies, responses or verbalizations, and ratings are examples of observational data used in counseling research and evaluation. The major item of interest in observational data collection is the need for controlled, systematic, and easily recorded information-gathering procedures. These items of interest require attention so that the researcher can make the necessary estimates of the reliability of the data. There are a variety of observational data types available. Frequency counts of negative and positive self-statements or thoughts have been used to examine the concept of self-esteem (Hannum, Thoresen, & Hubbard, 1974). Mayer and Butterworth (1979) used counts of the number of classroom disruptions and the amount of public money spent to repair school property damaged by vandals. Although a host of observational types of data can be gathered, the issue remains whether the data collected through observations are valid and reliable.

Questionnaires and Inventories

Much of the counseling research and evaluation literature provides descriptions of the use of questionnaires and inventories to measure items of interest. These data-gathering devices are structured to elicit specific information that will be helpful in answering the research question. Frequently the assessment instrument requires the person responding to identify levels of the response on a scale. Open-ended questionnaires are also used, and then the responses are reviewed, placed into categories, and evaluated. Most measures of vocational interest and vocational maturity are examples of inventory data. Questionnaires focused on demographic and attitudinal data are also examples of this type of data source.

Instruments for data collection that provide scores on one or more traits of the individual are often labeled *tests*. Tests have their most frequent use in diagnostic work but are used for theoretical evaluations and research as well. There are two basic approaches to tests in the field of counseling: impressionistic and psychometric approaches. The impressionistic approach examines any available cue in an attempt to understand client actions. A numerical estimate of the client's performance in terms of predetermined characteristic categories is the major method used by the psychometric approach. In an attempt to gather data about a client, the impressionistic approach may be to request that the client write an autobiographical sketch. The sketch would be used to identify what experiences the client viewed as important, why they were viewed as critical, and how different events interacted. A counselor using the psychometric approach to data collection with the same client would ask the client to complete a biographical checklist of experiences thought to be important events by others. The client would indicate which events had occurred in his or her life, and the counselor would "score" the checklist according to the number of items checked in predetermined categories of events.

The important consideration for the counselor is to use the data that are valid and reliable. Multiple sources can be used, and there are many possible methods to gather the data. The data collected, however, must be appropriate for the research question under study.

Standardized tests and inventories are also used in group situations to determine the characteristics of the group. Achievement tests are used as measures of educational efforts. Career-maturity inventories can be used to evaluate career group guidance efforts. Self-concept tests are used to measure counseling intervention activities in halfway houses within the justice system. Many research and evaluation activities use a variety of several standardized measures to answer the posited question. The first decision to be made in the use of a measure is what the question is. This information will provide direction toward choosing an appropriate measure.

Professional counselors may be asked to use standardized measures in group evaluation efforts as well as with individual clients. In each instance, knowledge of norming information, reliability, and validity for the measure is central and must be understood by the counselor if the instrument is to be used effectively.

A COUNSELOR IS A COUNSELOR?

I am a counselor and proud of it. My work setting is a United Way–funded Center for Child and Family Service. During a typical day I have between four and seven counseling sessions. Some sessions are family groups, and occasionally I have an adolescent group. Most of my counseling sessions last an hour, but some group sessions last longer. We usually meet with our clients weekly.

My counseling tends to be for several sessions because the problems dealt with typically concern friction in the client's interpersonal relationships. We do some short-term "concrete" counseling, which is basically information giving on the topics of sexuality, birth control, and abortion, and we often make referrals to other agencies after one session. If people want a divorce, we refer to the Legal Service Center. Many clients "walk in," but we get a lot of referrals from other professionals—lawyers and doctors, and from the courts and welfare agencies.

My primary job is counseling, but I do some other things. All the Center counselors do community relations work. We prepare and present programs to community groups. Some of our programs are to give the audience new interpersonal relations concepts and skills. Others are straight PR because we depend on community funding. Some of our programs do receive grant money, but we don't count on that. I also keep case records and follow up my clients. We must have evidence we are doing some good to get funds. I also do some coordination with other agencies so that we have a liaison with sources of help and of client referrals.

The biggest complaint I have is that we have no on-the-job time to read and keep up. Also, we don't get money for workshops and professional skill building. Unfortunately, our director is or was a counselor. I guess she got the job because she was a good counselor, so now we have lost a good counselor and gained a poor administrator. I don't think counselors should be administrators any more than administrators should counsel. We could do more if we had more time to do it, and more time would cost more money, but my agency is a great place for a person who really wants to be a counselor.

—*A Family Service Counselor*

Use of Statistics in Research and Evaluation

Statistics are often used by counselors to describe the data collected and to make judgments about the information gathered. It is important to remember that statistics are tools used to aid the counselor in a quest for knowledge. The foundation of counseling research and evaluation is the research and evaluation question, and the procedure to gather data—not the statistical procedures employed.

The work of professional counselors does require some facility with the use of statistical research tools. Both the consumption of others' research and the production of one's own research and evaluation require that the counselor be knowledgeable about a variety of statistical techniques.

One use of statistics is to summarize a description of the data collected. A counselor may desire to learn or report the "center place" or "middle point" of the data collected. Such a summary would be a measure of central tendency, and the counselor could use a statistic of the mean, mode, or median to determine the "middle point." Counselors often also wish to establish the variability of the data. In these instances the standard deviation, quartile deviation, and range are the statistical techniques used.

A second use of statistics in counseling research and evaluation is to make inferences from representative information (sample data) to the group (population) of interest. In these instances the counselor uses inferential statistical techniques that provide an estimate of the probability that the results of the research are accurate. Probabilities are also involved when counselors examine information from the entire group (population rather than sample data) and make decisions about whether the results of the research were due to chance.

The point is that some knowledge of statistics is necessary for the counselor to act in a professional manner. Statistical procedures are tools used to aid the building of a research and evaluation endeavor established on the firm foundation of appropriate question-formation and data-gathering procedures.

Perspectives for the '80s

The practice of doing counseling and the activity of research and evaluation in counseling traditionally were viewed as separate functions. So separate were the functions that the most common instance was that the two activities were performed by different people. However, for the professional counselor, the functions of the practice of counseling and the activity of research and evaluation often cannot be separated. If the professional counselor's work is meaningful, then the practice and research activities are combined. Conceptually, professional counseling requires a constant asking of, and seeking of answers to, questions about what is occurring in counseling.

The traditional separation of counseling practice and counseling research has caused severe limitations in both activities. Recently counseling research and evaluation has come under criticism for its lack of meaning to the practice of counseling. Goldman (1976) and Raush (1974), among others, have made three basic criticisms of the current state of counseling research: (1) Research has as its audience other researchers rather than people involved in the practice of counseling. (2) Research has as its focus topics that are not of major concern to the practice of counseling and are limited because the research employs designs requiring the use of averages rather than in-depth examination of individual changes in clients and/or counseling programs. (3) Research produced is often completed in settings that are not "real" in that they are laboratory environments or analogue studies.

These criticisms are valid and are due to the growth process of the field of professional counseling. As the profession emerged, the desire to gain stature led counselors completing research to identify with a view of science that promoted complex research designs and statistical analyses as the only method of arriving at answers. Such a view is parochial and fails to note that scientific inquiry is a process comprising both the formulation of questions and the seeking of answers. Failure to view scientific inquiry as having multiple methods of analysis and as being as much attitude as method was largely responsible for the loss by research efforts in counseling of their meaning for the practice of counseling. In its efforts to attain statistical significance, the counseling research of the past three decades has often lost practical significance. The errors of counseling research resulting from viewing scientific inquiry as being synonymous with statistical analysis and experimental controls have done much to make the research produced of little value to the actual practice of counseling. As a counseling activity, research and evaluation were methodologically cumbersome and complex and not relevant to the critical topics of the practice of counseling. The consumer function of research was also limited because the research produced was not on topics considered relevant and was reported in a fashion considered too complex for persons not deeply involved in research.

The call of the critics of counseling research is for evaluation and research efforts focused on relevant topics, conducted in "real" settings, reported in a manner meaningful to the practice of counseling, and using multiple research methods that are appropriate for the study of individuals and their environments. Such a mandate requires the professional counselor to be actively involved in the consumption and production of research. It also suggests that the research activities adhere to the attitude of scientific inquiry in that both the asking of questions and the attempts to attain answers to questions be included in the process of science and both be examined. To meet the mandate, the professional counselor will have to attend to the basic issues of research designs, methods of measurements, influences of personal perceptions, and the ethics of research activities.

Because the practice of counseling does not occur in a vacuum, the issue of the proper evaluation or research *design* to focus the research activity on the specific question is critical. In attempts to "be scientific," research in counseling adopted designs that focused on group procedures when the basic question being investigated was not a group issue. Anton (1978) and Oetting (1976) have presented an organized procedure and series of designs that would be appropriate for investigating questions focused on individual client or program changes. The procedures are examined within the process of scientific inquiry. The point is that the professional counselor must first adequately frame the research and evaluation question and then choose an appropriate design procedure. To complete the process of question and design choice in reverse would lead to answers not necessarily meaningful to the field of counseling practice and would not adhere to the process and attitude of scientific inquiry. Multiple designs are available, and the choice of a research design is determined by the question and setting.

The choice of a *measurement* procedure in counseling evaluation and research is often made on the basis of what is the easiest or most rigorous available. To make the choice of measurement on such a basis often results in a research activity that misses the target. Measurement is made in terms of "what makes sense" on the first hand and what is the most reliable and valid measurement procedure on the second hand. To reverse these items could lead to reliable and valid measures of data that are not relevant to the question. Again, the question determines the measurement procedure to be used in the evaluation or research effort. The call for counseling research to include examination of the interrelations between counseling clients and environmental variables dictates the need for creativity in the construction of measurement procedures. What happens in counseling is scientific subject matter, and the job of the professional counselor is to determine what the question is and then proceed to formulate a research design, measurement, and analysis procedure focused on helping find the answer to the question. Counseling involves complexities—complex clients, complex institutions, complex programs, complex environments, and complex interrelations between the clients, institutions, programs, and environments. This is no reason to conclude that the field of counseling is too complex to provide opportunities for research and evaluation. Rather, the mandate for the professional counselor is to constantly practice the attitude of asking questions and seeking answers in the world of counseling.

Personal *perceptions* influence many of the steps in the consumption and production of counseling research. The theories and paradigms held by the counselor influence what is examined and how it is investigated. Two counselors holding different theories may view the relevant questions differently, make different design and measurement choices, and come to different conclusions in the same research study. Mahoney (1976) has pointed to the many ways in which the researcher's belief system influences the formulation of research questions, choices of measurement and design procedures, and reasoning used to attain answers from the research data analyzed. If counseling research and evaluation were viewed as a process of exploration and investigation to improve the field of counseling rather than a constant contest to prove a point, then the researcher's perceptions would not be an important source of bias. The goal is not to eliminate the personal perceptions of the researcher but rather to recognize them and focus the research efforts on the research process, as opposed to a "who won" struggle.

Protection of the subjects in a research study is the major element in the *ethics* of counseling research. The guiding principle is that a subject should never leave a research project in worse condition as a result of the research than when the subject entered. The American Psychological Association has established an ethical code to be followed in research activities. The code provides a guide for ethical behavior in the formulation, execution, and result dissemination of research. Many of the ethical issues are also involved with the legal matters of client (research subject) privacy and the right of the subject to give "informed consent" in the research activity. Davidson and Stuart (1975) have provided a decision-making grid to aid counseling researchers in efforts to protect subjects' rights of privacy and informed consent. The scheme of their decision-making grid takes into account the levels of risk to the subject, of the subject's freedom to grant consent, of potential benefit to the subject for participation in the research, of benefit to society for the research activity, and of experimental nature of the procedures to be used in the research. For each of those various levels, varying activities are provided as suggestions to be used in gaining and protecting the subject's right to informed consent. It must be remembered that the major purpose of research in counseling is to help clients, and at all times the ethical guidelines should be followed. To do less would move counseling out of the realm of a profession.

Summary

Thoresen (1978) has suggested that as an aid to clients the professional counselor might attempt to teach a client the skills of research. Such a suggestion is well within the view of counseling research and evaluation provided in this chapter. The view of scientific inquiry as a process in which the goal is to ask meaningful questions and use multiple methods in attempts to discover the answers has been the focus of the discussion on counseling research. Helping clients learn this attitude and basic skills of data collection and examination may be of aid as they examine their individual actions. Counseling activity as a professional practice requires continual examination of the field. The experience and authority ways of knowing and learning, the deductive, inductive, and scientific methods of knowing, and the various types of research procedures (case study, longitudinal, historical, survey, participant observation, and experimental) provide the basic framework for the consumer and producer research activities of professional counselors. The focus on the reliability and validity demands of a variety of data sources enables the field of counseling to conduct research and evaluation that has acceptability across counseling professionals. Meaningful research intended to examine relevant questions, using appropriate design and analysis procedures in "real" settings, and reported in a manner understandable by the practicing counselor is needed.

Research and evaluation in counseling is not an appendage to the practice of counseling—it is a constant aspect of the practice. The professional counselor continually conducts research that is intended to bring together the activities of the theoretician, researcher, and clinical practitioner. What counselors deal with is subject matter for a scientific research process. It is amenable to investigation provided the proper research attitude presents itself in the behaviors of the professional counselor. The practicing counselor has an important place in the profession. Research and evaluation activities by practicing counselors can aid the profession in attempts to advance itself. The crucial issue is for the counselors to conduct research and to communicate the research to others. The professional counselor is a producer and a consumer of research—and both activities are continual.

Now It's Your Turn

1. Page through a journal in the field of counseling and select an article which is of topical interest to you *and* which involved the collection of data. Read the article and determine the following:
   a. What was the major question(s) of the research?
   b. What information (data) was collected to answer the question?
   c. What was the answer to the question?
   d. How will the information gained from the research affect counseling?
2. Identify a question you have about counseling. Determine what information you need to find the answer to your question and how you would gather that information.
3. Interview a practicing counselor and identify:
   a. What are three important questions the counselor has about the various counseling activities he or she is performing?
   b. What are some procedures that could be or are being used to find answers to each of the questions?
   c. How would answers to the questions alter the counselor's work?
4. Choose something you do or something that happens to you at least three or four times each day and is something you would like to change.
   a. Carefully define the chosen item in specific terms and for each of the next ten days record each occurrence, noting the time and situation and what happens after the occurrence.
   b. Examine the information recorded and identify any questions and/or

hypotheses you have about the information and possible relations between the chosen item and the events surrounding the occurrences.

References

Anton, J. L. Intensive experimental designs: A model for the counselor/researcher. *Personnel and Guidance Journal,* 1978, 56(5), 273–278.

Davidson, G. C., & Stuart, R. B. Behavior therapy and civil liberties. *American Psychologist,* 1975, 30, 755–763.

Goldman, L. A revolution in counseling research. *Journal of Counseling Psychology,* 1976, 23, 543–552.

Hannum, J. W., Thoresen, C. E., & Hubbard, D. R. A behavioral study of self-esteem with elementary teachers. In M. J. Mahoney & C. E. Thoresen, *Self-control: Power to the person.* Monterey, Calif.: Brooks/Cole, 1974.

Jayaratne, S., & Levy, R. L. *Empirical clinical practice.* New York: Columbia University Press, 1979.

Mahoney, M. J. *Scientist as subject: The psychological imperative.* Cambridge, Mass.: Ballinger, 1976.

Mayer, G. R., & Butterworth, T. W. A preventive approach to school violence and vandalism: An experimental study. *Personnel and Guidance Journal,* 1979, 57, 436–441.

Oetting, E. R. Planning and reporting evaluative research: Part II. *Personnel and Guidance Journal,* 1976, 55, 60–64.

Raush, H. L. Research, practice, and accountability. *American Psychologist,* 1974, 29, 678–681.

Rockwell, P. J., & Rothney, J. W. M. Some social ideas of pioneers in the guidance movement. *Personnel and Guidance Journal,* 1961, 40, 349–354.

Ross, P. *Trouble in school: A portrait of young adolescents.* New York: Avon Books, 1979.

Thoresen, C. E. Making better science, intensively. *Personnel and Guidance Journal,* 1978, 56, 279–282.

PART 3

The Clients of the Counselor

Counselors-in-training tend to favor one particular work setting over another. Some of you have projected your professional lives into community agencies or educational settings; others of you believe that the only meaningful work occurs in business and industry, private practice, or federal and state agencies. We would like you to reexamine this limited and limiting view of your professional training and your professional future. We ask you to do that by looking at your potential counselees, not at your work settings.

You should be reminded that APGA standards for the professional preparation of counselors stipulate a common core experience for all of you, regardless of your current and future career goals. Each of you will have certain training experiences that are identical to everyone else's training. As a matter of fact, only a few of your course experiences will be for a specific setting. For example, your classmates in this course include future rehabilitation counselors who want to work with alcoholics, battered wives, abused children, or mental-health patients. They also include future elementary or middle and high school counselors. Sitting next to you may be someone whose career goal is higher education and one of its several student personnel positions. Your class may also include people who want to be employed by business and industry, penal institutions, the military, or some other arm of the federal government.

The point is, a counselor is a counselor—not a setting. And the professional colleague group you are about to join planned it that way, for several reasons. Not the least of these has to do with your own needs. You need job flexibility and professional versatility. None of us can ever be certain we will wind up where we think we are going. As competent counselors, your future professional colleagues have helped you to examine a variety of alternatives for your future and to be equipped to explore them.

When you complete your program of professional preparation, you will be prepared to work as a counselor. A past APGA president used the term *counselor unadorned* to emphasize that a counselor is a counselor and that work-setting distinctions only indicate the place where counseling services are delivered. Your program should and will include courses and experiences that will help you to reinterpret your counseling skills and generalize them to particular work settings. Nevertheless, your desire or need to expand your career field beyond your current intentions can be accomplished only by building on a solid core of counselor competencies.

One more thought: Whatever you think you know about the work of a counselor in a particular setting may be distorted. For example, you have decided your completeness as a person and a professional rests in your becoming a marriage and family counselor, and so the only pertinent inclusions in your training should be those relating to *adult* behavior. Wrong! Married people often have children, and quite frequently they also have parents. If you have any illusions that marriage problems can be solved outside the family constellation, then let us dissuade you from such notions. To perform effectively as a marriage counselor, you must understand the behavior dynamics of adulthood, childhood, adolescence, and the senior years. Similarly, prospective elementary school counselors will fail if they are trained only in child development. These counselors must interact with older brothers and sisters, teachers, parents, grandparents, and a plethora of others. And if alcoholics are your mission in life, be reminded that they, too, come in all sizes. And so do their families.

This discussion is an attempt to remedy any myopic problems you may have been supporting and to suggest that shortsightedness will deter you in the pursuit of your professional identity. It is also an effort to convince you that your professional commitment requires you to learn as much as you can about as many things as you can, not only because you just might *not* know where you are going or how you will get there but also because a counselor is a counselor, not a setting.

The chapters in this section are designed to help you learn about, and become more able to understand, the dynamics of human behavior—all human behavior—so that you can become the kind of counselor your profession needs and will be proud to claim. We have used and defined the term *developmental counseling* to indicate that although there are unique developmental challenges at each life stage, our most important consideration is the *continuity* of human development. Counselors can ignore neither the past development of their counselees nor the future developmental challenges they face.

PART 3   THE CLIENTS OF THE COUNSELOR   193

Chapter 9, written by Joan C. Franks, is a discussion of childhood. It is a stage of development you may have many memories of but few understandings about. You may remember some of the things you did, but you might not know what influenced you to do them. Joan's discussion of how children behave, why they sort things out the way they do, and how they learn to interact productively with their environments provides not only an interesting excursion down Memory Lane but a fruitful one. It provides many useful insights into the abilities, interests, and motives of children who are trying to learn and/or circumvent the rules of adult society. Joan Franks suggests practical approaches to the perfectly normal abnormalities of children that counselors can use as they work with the children themselves, their parents, teachers, classmates, siblings, or others.

In Chapter 10, Barbara S. Fuhrmann reintroduces you to the most painful time of your life—for others. Or so the story goes. According to Barbara, this should not be the case, and if it is, then it is because all those others failed to understand adolescent behavior. The characteristics of adolescents, their needs, and their tentative strivings to achieve adult status are sympathetically and expertly described. Barbara Fuhrmann has dealt with this period of growth and development in a comprehensive and refreshing manner.

Chapter 11, written by Maureen R. Worth, explores that developmental stage labeled adulthood. The issues that adults must resolve and the sources of counseling open to them are discussed with reference to early and middle adulthood. Maureen identifies and explains the life-cycle concerns of men and women in terms of their similarities as well as their dissimilarities. If you find it difficult to envision yourself counseling someone of your own age group or older, then Maureen Worth's analysis of intervention strategies could assuage your fears. If you also believe you understand adulthood, then this comprehensive discussion of the topic may give you some surprises.

In Chapter 12, Paul Grobe introduces you to society's senior members. You may find several surprises in this chapter, too. Paul's presentation of the *measured* attributes of this age group indicates many discrepancies between the known characteristics of seniors and the myths that surround them. We are reminded also of our reluctance to accept the aging process in ourselves as a powerful influence on our attitudes toward seniors. When the only alternative is considered, we might discover that aging is a blessing. Paul Grobe's discussion of counseling approaches useful with seniors, together with his discussion of the attitudes, perceptions, and knowledge prerequisite to effective counselor interactions with seniors, is definitive, informative, and contemporary.

Chapter 13, written by Charles F. Gressard and Keith R. Hume, gives you an opportunity to increase your understanding of the diversity inherent in the counselees you may serve. Counselors have a proud heritage of concern for individual differences, but this discussion of special populations should increase your appreciation of the unique capabilities of these individuals. Your professional involvement with individuals can be disappointing and difficult, but it can also provide many rewards. In describing social deviances and physical handicaps, the authors also discuss the professional competencies needed by counselors who work with these populations. It is an informed and informative presentation.

While you are reviewing your work schedule in your office at a senior citizens' residence, a physically handicapped 9-year-old girl comes in. She is accompanied by her 15-year-old brother, who is out on parole, her alcoholic father, and her mother, who still displays the bruises inflicted by her husband. The little girl and her brother want to visit their grandfather. Their older sister was to meet them there, but she must have been late leaving the *unplanned*-parenthood center.

Have we persuaded you? A counselor is a counselor, not a setting. Professional counselors must be prepared to deal with a diversity of counselees and concerns, not just those stereotyped for a particular setting.

CHAPTER **9**

Children

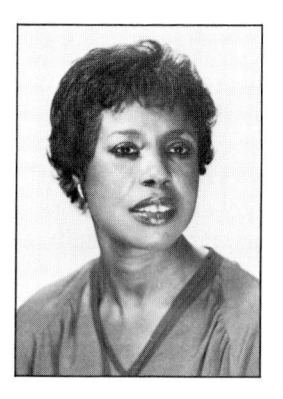

Joan C. Franks
Joan C. Franks is an associate professor of counselor education at the University of Virginia. Her area of specialty is elementary school counseling. Dr. Franks has presented numerous programs and workshops on the use of play in child counseling.

If counselors are to facilitate smooth and orderly development of the "whole" child, they need a clear understanding of the complex processes that govern the child's physical, social, emotional, and intellectual growth. Without these understandings, effective intervention and assistance cannot be provided. Therefore, the purpose of this chapter is to delineate some development stages of childhood and to discuss the implications of these theories for the counseling process. The chapter will include (1) a historical overview, (2) theories of human development, (3) implications for counseling, and (4) perspectives for the '80s.

A Historical Overview

It was during the 17th and 18th centuries that society showed a major interest in childhood. Before that time, childhood was viewed as a prologue to adulthood, and, therefore, adult standards were imposed on children.

During the Renaissance, childhood emerged as a distinct period of life. Rousseau was one of the first writers to stress the special needs of children. He wanted to understand children, not just to control them by physical force. He envisioned the goal of education as trying to help children exist as children. In his book *Émile* he emphasized the importance of childhood.

> Nature wants children to be children before they are men. If we deliberately pervert this order, we shall get premature fruits which are neither ripe nor well-flavored, and which soon decay. . . . Childhood has ways of seeing, thinking, and feeling peculiar to itself; nothing can be more foolish than to substitute our ways for them [Greenleaf, 1969, p. 64].

After society recognized childhood as a separate period of life, there was a growing interest in the plight and development of children. Much of this interest in children came from a new absorption in the biological and social sciences. Children suddenly attained new status as subjects of scientific inquiry. In the 20th century, scholars such as Hall (1957), Havighurst (1972), Gesell, Ilg, and Ames (1977), Erikson (1963), and Piaget (1965) conducted research studies on children and child development. For the past several decades, there has been a plethora of research about children, child development, and the education of children. According to Brophy (1977), this interest in the study of children can be attributed to a renewed interest in Piaget, a concern about the underprivileged, a shift from animal to human experiments, and an interest in the promotion of positive mental health.

Theories of Human Development

The works of such developmentalists as Piaget and Inhelder (1969), Erikson (1963), Kohlberg and Turiel (1971), and Havighurst (1972) are notable in the field of human development. Although each author has focused on a specific aspect of development during the early years, collectively these theorists have provided a solid basis for understanding the childhood years. In the sections that follow, these theories of child development are briefly summarized.

Piaget and Cognitive Development

The bulk of our knowledge of cognitive development in childhood comes from the works of Jean Piaget and individuals who were influenced by him. Piaget's research was based on systematic observations of children involved in cognitive and problem-solving tasks. He and his colleagues concluded that intellectual development appeared to take place in stages. Therefore, no stage can be eliminated, because each new stage is dependent on the preceding one. According to Piaget and Inhelder (1969), there are four stages of cognitive development: sensorimotor (or preoccupational), preoperational, concrete operations, and formal operations. These four stages are summarized below.

1. Sensorimotor stage (ages 0-2). During this stage the infant creates a world based on his desire for physical satisfaction. The infants realize people exist even when they cannot see them. They begin to engage in organized activities in which they manipulate objects. The child progresses from the reflexive stage to an exploratory stage. This period ends when the child can comprehend that concrete objects can be translated into words and concepts.

2. Preoperational stage (ages 2-7). During the *preconceptual subphase* (ages 2-4), children investigate their environment and their role in the environment. This phase includes a rapid increase in language. Even though the child and adult may use the same language, they do not necessarily have a common framework for communication.

During the *intuitive subphase* (ages 4-7), children become less egocentric and more social as individuals. They start to model adult behavior, and show the first sign of cognition. By the time children reach age 5 and are ready to enter school, their thinking is basically verbal. Usually children can deal with only one concept at a time.

3. Concrete operations (ages 7-12). Children in the concrete operations stage are capable of mental representations, conservation, relational terms, class inclusion, and serialization.

- *Mental representation.* The child is able to use symbols to carry out mental activities.
- *Conservation.* The child is now aware that length, mass, weight, and number remain the same despite a change in appearance.
- *Class inclusion.* A child can reason about the whole and parts simultaneously.
- *Serialization.* The child can now arrange objects according to quantified dimension—for example, weight, size, and ordinal scale.

4. Stage of formal operations (ages 12 and over). The final stage of cognitive development appears at approximately age 12, marking the end of childhood and the beginning of adolescence. Several important attributes distinguish this formal stage from the concrete operational stage. First, children examine all possible ways of solving a particular problem. Secondly, their thoughts are more deductive. Finally, they deal with the future rather than the here and now (Mussen, Conger, & Kagan, 1974, pp. 310-312).

Piaget's theory provides the counselor with a frame of reference for understanding the child's intellectual growth. However, counselors must be aware that this theory by itself is inadequate for understanding children and must be supplemented by other concepts. For example, emotional competence may be as important as cognitive competence in assuring adequate development.

Erikson and Emotional Development

According toe Erikson's theory (1963, p. 247), psychosocial development consists of eight stages. Each stage is related to the previous one, and each plays a significant role in the total scheme of development.

1. *Trust.* One of the most important characteristics a person can develop is a sense of trust. This stage dominates the first year of life. It is during this stage that children learn that they can trust the world and other people. Trust is considered one of the most important characteristics in personality development, and fortunately most infants acquire it without any problem.

2. *Autonomy.* During the second and third years of life, the child wants to be self-reliant. The child can now walk, can manipulate objects, and is capable of choosing and deciding. If children are to develop autonomy, their parents must give them opportunities to make choices within limits during these two years. During this stage parents need to be consistent in their discipline.

3. *Initiative.* This stage takes place during the fourth and fifth years of life. After children have been able to establish themselves as individuals, they seek to discover how much they are capable of achieving. During this time their conscience is in the process of developing, and their behavior is determined partly by their own concept of right or wrong. There is no other time in life when a person learns so willingly.

Erikson believes that if children are able to get through the first three stages without problems, they will have a foundation that will sustain them throughout life.

4. *Duty and Accomplishment.* During the years from 6 to 12, children become interested in activities that are socially acceptable. They are less self-centered and more interested in others, and they are interested in becoming workers and producers.

5. *Identity.* The problem of identity is central during adolescence, when rapid physiological changes contribute to inner turmoil. This is a period of life when youth examine their role in society in terms of who they are and what they are capable of becoming.

Erikson's adult developmental stages are intimacy, generativity, and integrity. These stages will be discussed in Chapter 11, on adults.

Erikson's work on emotional development can be extremely valuable to counselors trying to understand this aspect of child development.

Kohlberg and Moral Development

After a 12-year study of the moral development of 75 boys aged 10 to 16, Kohlberg and Turiel (1971, p. 415) developed a three-level, six-stage approach to moral development.

Level I: Premoral. Stage 1 is the punishment-and-obedience orientation. The individual adheres to the rules to avoid punishment, not because of respect or moral support for the rule.

Stage 2 is the instrumental-relativist orientation. The current action is determined by what satisfies one's own needs and occasionally the needs of others. Some elements of fairness and sharing are present, but they are always defined in a physical or practical manner—for example, "You do something for me and I will do something for you."

Level II: Conventional. Stage 3 is the "good boy" or "good girl" orientation. The individual is interested in maintaining good interpersonal relationships. Correct behavior is that which pleases or helps others and that which earns the approval of others.

Stage 4 is the law-and-order orientation. There is respect for authority, rules, and maintenance of the social order for its own sake. Good behavior includes doing one's duty, respecting authority, and maintaining the social order.

Level III: Postconventional, autonomous, or principle level. In Stage 5, the social-contract-legalistic orientation, right is interpreted by laws and regulations that have been scrutinized and agreed on by society. These laws and regulations take precedence over individual needs.

In Stage 6, the universal-ethical-principle orientation, the individual takes laws and regulations into consideration but bases his decisions on his own ethical principles, mutual respect, and trust.

Kohlberg's theory helps counselors realize that there is a moral element in behavior. These stages of moral development serve as a guide for people interested in moral education.

Havighurst and Developmental Tasks

In 1948 Robert Havighurst presented a theory of human development based on the concept of developmental tasks. He defined *developmental task* as "a task which arises at or about a certain period in the life of the individual, successful achievement of which leads to his happiness and to success with later tasks, while failure leads to unhappiness in the individual, disapproval by the society, and difficulty with later tasks" (Havighurst, 1972, p. 2). These tasks encompass the behavioral, cognitive, and social/personal skills that a person must master. Havighurst (1972, pp. 9–16) identifies these tasks and classifies them by age. The developmental tasks of children are listed below:

Developmental tasks of infancy and early childhood.
1. Learning to take solid foods.
2. Learning to walk.
3. Learning to talk.
4. Learning to control the elimination of body wastes.
5. Learning sex differences and sexual modesty.
6. Forming concepts and learning language to describe social and physical reality.
7. Getting ready to read.
8. Learning to distinguish right and wrong and beginning to develop a conscience.

Developmental tasks of middle childhood. Middle childhood is the period from 6 to 12 years of age. According to Havighurst (1972), during this period the child must deal with three major thrusts: (1) the thrust out of the home and into the peer group, (2) the physical thrust into the world of games and work requiring neuromuscular skills, and (3) the mental thrust into the world of adult concepts, logic, symbolism, and communication. The developmental tasks of middle childhood that originate from these three thrusts of growth in the child are as follows:

1. Learning physical skills necessary for ordinary games.
2. Building wholesome attitudes toward oneself as an organism.
3. Learning to get along with age mates.
4. Learning an appropriate masculine or feminine social role.
5. Developing fundamental skills in reading, writing, and calculating.
6. Developing concepts necessary for everyday living.
7. Developing conscience, morality, and a scale for values.
8. Achieving personal independence.
9. Developing attitudes toward social groups and institutions (Havighurst, 1972, pp. 19–31).

Basically, the developmental stages of Piaget, Erikson, Kohlberg, and Havighurst describe the capabilities of the child at various stages in his or her development. The profile of any child will indicate highs in some areas and lows in others. Moreover, differences will exist among children of the same age.

Implications for Counseling

Counselors who study the works of Piaget, Erikson, Kohlberg, and Havighurst will have a better understanding of the total development of children. These concepts give the counselor some useful guidelines for understanding the major task of each stage of life and some valuable information on the cognitive and psychosocial aspects of child development. Thus, the works of these theorists are most helpful in determining the needs of each child and in planning approaches that will contribute to his or her development.

Counselors can assist children with the developmental process by providing them with the following services: individual counseling, group guidance and counseling, classroom guidance, consultation, and referral services. These services are delineated below.

Individual Counseling

Individual counseling is a relationship in which a counselor seeks to help children understand and accept themselves. It provides an opportunity for children to explore their feelings, abilities, and interests so that they can make maximum use of their potential. This increased knowledge of the self that the child attains through individual counseling can benefit emotional, intellectual, and moral development.

Group Counseling

Group work provides the child an opportunity to share ideas and experiences with others. In a group the child is able to interact with peers, observe behaviors, and examine alternative behaviors. Counselors may form groups to deal with such concerns as self-concept, social skills, interpersonal relationships, problem solving, academic skills, communication skills, and values. Group counseling contributes to the development of healthy personalities because it provides opportunities for children to learn how to interact effectively with one another.

Classroom Group Guidance

Counselors employed in schools will find classroom guidance a very helpful technique. Classroom guidance can be used to merge career and human development into the learning process. In classroom guidance, the teacher and counselor work together in conducting the guidance activity. The counselor also serves as a resource person for the teacher by providing the teacher with follow-up activities. Some of the areas the counselor may focus on are values, attitudes and beliefs, personal and social development, and career development. Classroom guidance activities can improve the classroom environment, thus enhancing the intellectual, emotional, social, and moral development of children.

Consultation

Consultation is a means of providing information, sharing information and ideas, clarifying problems, or developing strategies for helping the child.

TIRED BUT HAPPY

It's the most exciting work in the whole world. Everything you do seems to make a difference because everybody you try to do it for—children, teachers, parents, school specialists, everybody—is coming and going with a great big smile. Who could be unhappy in a job like that? What's hard about my job? The workload. Elementary schools are very busy places. Children are trying to learn their lessons. But they are also trying to learn how to get along with one another and all those adults in their lives. Parents are trying to learn how they can help their children grow up as painlessly as possible, and teachers are trying not to lose their patience and still live with the disappointments they face every day. It's a boiling pot of energy and anxiety, and sometimes it's tough to keep the lid on and not let things boil over.

But it's terrific to know that you can. That's what it's all about. You've got to help keep everything together and running smoothly so crises won't erupt all over the school. You've got to know who needs what almost before they do, and you've got to get it to them before they find other ways of trying to get it for themselves. So you work with everybody and try to understand what it takes to keep them happy. Parsons was right: happy workers are productive workers.

How do you do it? By counseling with the kids and leading group guidance sessions for them. By consulting with groups of their parents and teachers. And by consulting with other school specialists and community agencies—not just every now and then but all the time. You can't keep everything coordinated unless you've got an organized program and work through teachers and parents.

Would I advise counselors-in-training to think about my kind of work as their career choice? Not unless they've got a lot of energy and know how to get a job done without getting constant direction and recognition, and not unless they get a kick out of being where the action is. When you help an elementary school child, you're getting in early enough to really make a difference. And when you help the adults who can really make a difference in the child's life, you may find, like me, that it really makes a difference in your own life.

—An Elementary School Counselor

Teachers, parents, and significant others may seek the counselor's help regarding a child's behavior or academic progress, or the counselor may request information from the teacher or other adults about a counselee. The counselor works individually or in groups with parents, teachers, and significant others to help them understand and facilitate the total development of children.

In summary, if the counselor is to provide meaningful services for children, it is essential that the counselor understand the intellectual, emotional, and moral development of children. The above paragraphs provide some guidelines that may be helpful throughout the counseling process.

Referral Services

In an effort to meet the needs of children, counselors make referrals to other specialists. These specialists may be available in the school system or in the community. For example, within the school system, counselors may refer children to school psychologists, school social workers, reading teachers, speech therapists, and other specialists. In the community, counselors may refer children to such services as mental-health clinics, child guidance clinics, and family services and drug-abuse centers.

Perspectives for the '80s

Because of the changes in family structure and emphasis on the rights of children and the needs of exceptional children, the '80s will bring about many challenges for counselors.

Changes in Family Structure

The American family has undergone tremendous changes during the past decade. Much of the change in family structure can be attributed to the high divorce rate. The U.S. Department of Commerce (1977) reports that between 1960 and 1970 the divorce rate was 34% and from 1970 to 1977 it increased to 79%. Changes in family structure may create problems for children. The counselors of the '80s may be asked to provide additional services for children to help them cope with these changes.

Rights of Children

The rights of children will be an important issue in the 1980s. Rodham (1979) lists four areas of basic rights for children: (1) the rights of children with families, (2) the rights of children without families, (3) the rights of children in institutions, and (4) the rights of children in society. Children are dependent on adults to assist them in achieving these rights. Therefore, counselors who will serve as advocates for children need to understand the role they will play in helping children attain their rights.

Needs of Exceptional Children

The passage in 1975 of PL 94-142, which requires that services available to "normal" children be available to exceptional children, presents a challenge for counselors. A study by Lebsock and DeBlassie (1975) of school counselors in the Southwest revealed that 43% of the counselors did not feel adequately trained to work with exceptional children. This feeling of inadequacy was also expressed in a study by Huber and Westling (1978); they reported that only 34% of the school counselors in Florida felt adequately trained to work with exceptional children. The training of counselors to work with exceptional children and the role that counselors will play in the implementation of this law will be a challenge for counselors in the '80s as they strive to meet the needs of all children.

The counselor, in her effort to meet the developmental needs of children, may become discouraged and frustrated. When this happens, the counselor needs to recall the statement made by Abraham Lincoln on behalf of children.

> A child is a person who is going to carry on what you have started. He is going to sit where you are sitting, and when you are gone, attend to those things which you think are important. You may adopt all the policies you please; but how they are carried out depends on him. He will assume control of your cities, states and nations. He is going to move in and take over your churches, schools, universities and corporations. All your books are going to be judged, praised or condemned by him. The fate of humanity is in his hands [Burgess, 1979, p. 126].

Summary

In this chapter I have depended on the theories of Piaget, Erikson, Kohlberg, and Havighurst for an explanation of child development and behavior. Even though the four theories discussed are based on different groups of assumptions, they are in many respects compatible. These theories supplement one another and provide the counselor with a foundation for understanding total development.

Piaget, Erikson, Kohlberg, and Havighurst emphasize that human life develops in an orderly manner and in predictable ways. Each theorist describes the individual child as having the potential for independent decision making and problem solving.

The emphasis in this chapter has been on normal, healthy development. However, it is recognized that some children, because of physical, emotional, or social impairments, may not develop normally.

Now It's Your Turn

1. Explain the rationale for counselors' studying the developmental stages of children.
2. Discuss the theories of Piaget, Erikson, and Kohlberg. How are they alike? How are they different?

3. List the services a counselor can provide for children. Discuss how these services can aid in meeting children's developmental needs.
4. Compare and contrast Erikson's psychosocial stages of development and Havighurst's developmental tasks.
5. Observe a 5-year-old child and a 9-year-old child. Compare their cognitive, psychosocial, and moral development.

References and Suggested Readings

Beard, R. M. *An outline of Piaget's developmental psychology for students and teachers.* London: Routledge & Kegan Paul, 1970.

Brophy, J. E. *Child development and socialization.* Chicago: Science Research Associates, 1977.

Burgess, D. S. An international perspective on children's rights. In P. A. Vardin & I. Brody (Eds.), *Children's rights: Contemporary perspectives.* New York: Teachers College Press, Columbia University, 1979.

Dimick, K. M., & Huff, V. W. *Child counseling.* Dubuque, Iowa: William C. Brown, 1970.

Erikson, E. H. *Childhood and society* (2nd ed.). New York: W. W. Norton, 1963.

Gesell, A., Ilg, F., & Ames, L. B. *The child from five to ten.* New York: Harper & Row, 1977.

Gowan, J. C., Coole, D., & McDonald, P. The impact of Piaget on guidance. *Elementary School Guidance and Counseling,* June 1967, *1* pp. 212-213.

Graham, R. Moral education: A child's right to a just community. *Elementary School Guidance and Counseling,* May 1975, *9* pp. 229-308.

Greenleaf, B. K. *Children through the ages.* New York: McGraw-Hill, 1978.

Hall, C., & Lindzey, G. *Theories of personality.* New York: Wiley, 1957.

Havighurst, R. J. *Developmental tasks and education.* New York: David McKay, 1972.

Huber, C. H., & Westling, D. L. School guidance counselors and the mildly retarded: Roles and preparation. *Mental Retardation,* 1978, *16,* 174-177.

Kameen, M. C., & Huber, C. H. Counselors and disabled children: The special educator's viewpoint. *School Counselor,* 1979, *27,* 24-27.

Kohlberg, L., & Turiel, E. Moral development and moral education. In G. S. Lesser, *Psychology and educational practice.* Glenview, Ill.: Scott, Foresman, 1971. pp. 415-416.

Lebsock, M. S., & DeBlassie, R. R. The school counselor's role in special education. *Counselor Education and Supervision,* 1975, *15,* 128-134.

Maier, H. W. *Three theories of child development.* New York: Harper & Row, 1969.

Muro, J. J., & Dinkmeyer, D. C. *Counseling in the elementary and middle schools: A pragmatic approach.* Dubuque, Iowa: William C. Brown, 1977.

Mussen, P. H., Conger, J. J., & Kagan, J. *Child development and personality.* New York: Harper & Row, 1974.

Papalia, D. E., & Olds, S. W. *A child's world: Infancy through adolescence.* New York: McGraw-Hill, 1975.

Piaget, J. *The moral judgment of children.* Glencoe, Ill.: Free Press, 1965.

Piaget, J., & Inhelder, B. *The psychology of the child.* New York: Basic Books, 1969.

Rodham, H. Children's rights. In P. Vardin & I. Brody (Eds.), *Children's rights: Contemporary perspectives*. New York: Teachers College Press, Columbia University, 1979.

Rousseau, J. J. *Émile*. New York: E. P. Dutton, 1969.

Singer, R. D., & Singer, A. *Psychological development in children*. Philadelphia: Saunders, 1969.

Smart, M. S., & Smart, R. C. *Children, development and relationships*. New York: Macmillan, 1977.

U.S. Department of Commerce, Bureau of the Census. *Marriage, divorce, widowhood and remarriage by family characteristics* (Table K). Current Population Reports (Series P-20, No. 312). Washington, D.C.: U.S. Government Printing Office, 1976.

U.S. Department of Commerce, Bureau of the Census. *Marital status and living arrangements*. Current Population Reports (Series P-20, No. 323). Washington, D.C.: U.S. Government Printing Office, 1977.

Williams, J. W., & Stith, M. *Middle childhood behavior and development*. New York: Macmillan, 1974.

CHAPTER **10**

Adolescents

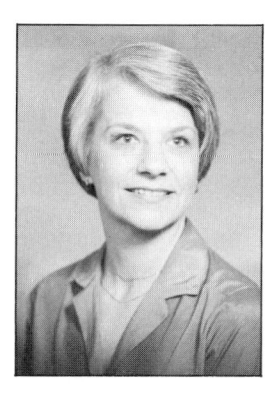

Barbara S. Fuhrmann
Barbara S. Fuhrmann is an associate professor in the Department of Educational Services at Virginia Commonwealth University. Dr. Fuhrmann's teaching responsibilities include adolescent growth and development courses. She also has a private practice specializing in the counseling of adolescents and their parents. Barbara S. Fuhrmann is the editor of the Virginia Counselor Journal.

I don't even know what people mean by adolescent. It seems to me people nowadays jump from being children to being adults.

You may not know that's what's happening, but it does . . .

I don't think I'm so special. Lots of kids I know, they feel all of a sudden they can't be kids anymore . . .

You can tell by looking at them too; their bodies aren't kids' bodies either. It's hard to guess people's age nowadays because everybody looks older; even if they don't, they act older. Everybody's acting one way or another. If you don't act you get lost; the world passes by without you [Cottle, 1979, p. 40].

The 16-year-old who made the statement above expresses clearly the major dilemma of the adolescent years, years which young people must "get through" on their way to adulthood and which they must also experience day by day, "making it" *as* adolescents. Unfortunately, for some the dual task is difficult at best, for they belong neither in the world of children nor in the world of adults. They are, Lewin (1939) said, "marginal" people who aren't accepted by either group. For others, the task is not so problematic; for some, it is joyful.

There are many definitions of the young we call adolescent. Perhaps this definition by Ambron (1975) says it most clearly:

> Adolescence is the bridge between childhood and adulthood. It is a time of rapid development: of growing to sexual maturity, discovering one's real self, defining personal values, and finding one's vocational and social directions. It is also a time of testing: of pushing against one's capabilities and the limitations as posed by adults [p. 393].

The issues that surface during these years are varied and complex and are dealt with by counselors in many settings—schools, social agencies, community organizations, courts, churches, group homes for specialized populations such as foster children, runaways, drug and alcohol abusers, unwed mothers, and emotionally disturbed or intellectually or physically handicapped youngsters. Counselors become involved with adolescent behavior,

> most of which appeared in childhood in less developed forms. The most common of these patterns of behavior include interest in heterosexual activities; marked conformity to peer-group ideals, standards, principles, and behavior patterns; a strong desire for social approval and attention; resistance to adult authority; a desire to help others; prejudice and discrimination; and social competency, or a facility in dealing with people and social situations [Hurlock, 1973, p. 90].

Adolescence: A Cultural Phenomenon

Both the personal comment and the definition that open this chapter come from the experience of adolescence as it exists in 20th-century America, a culture that has, in fact, developed the notion of adolescence as a necessary sociological and economic phenomenon. Adolescence is a modern Western invention arising from the economic need to delay the entry of young people into the marketplace and to train them for detailed, technological work. Although most Western nations have some form of adolescence, only in the United States is it typical for adolescence to extend from the onset of puberty until the early (or even late) twenties, when people leave school and assume the full economic responsibilities of adulthood. In many parts of the world adolescence as we know it does not exist—and in many more it didn't until relatively recent years (Ralston & Thomas, 1974).

For example, among the Cheyenne Indians, adolescence was virtually nonexistent. Adult status was granted to growing individuals as soon as they were capable of adult tasks; children became adults without fanfare, almost without notice, as their adultlike contributions were accepted and rewarded (Hoebel, 1960). In our own history, one can picture the typical agrarian extended family of the mid-19th century. As soon as they were able, children were given meaningful and appropriate tasks, tasks which contributed to the family's welfare and which were rewarded accordingly. As children became increasingly capable, their tasks changed, so that by the time their bodies matured to adulthood, they were also sociologically capable of adulthood. Although our great-grandparents did not experience the formal puberty rites practiced by some tribal cultures, their passage from child to adult was noted by a change in the clothing they wore. The transition from short to long pants was a clear indication that a boy had become a man, and his acquaintances treated him accordingly.

But today long pants do not an adult make. (It is now common to see miniature versions of adult styles in size 2.) In an ever more technological and complex world, we have developed ever greater dependence on a long educational process. Whether more years of schooling do or do not increase competence, our society is geared to paper credentials, and paper credentials are accumulated only through long years of directed schooling. Until people can support themselves both financially and psychologically, they are not considered full-fledged adults, and in this society, economic and psychologic independence is almost never achieved before 18 years and often not until the mid-twenties. Thus, the adolescent period extends from the general onset of puberty, around 12 years, to the time when a person achieves full adult responsibility—physically, socially, legally, and economically. Physical adulthood obviously comes first, girls reaching it by age 14 or 15, boys by 15 or 16. Legal and social adulthood come next, as defined by compulsory education laws (the end of which come at 16 in most places, child-labor legislation (16 or 18, depending on the work), juvenile justice codes (15 to 18, depending on the law and the crime), and ages required to drive a car, buy alcohol, and marry without parental consent. Although these legal adult-reaching ages vary from about 13 to 21, depending on specific circumstances and local legislation, everyone has achieved all of them by age 21. But not everyone has achieved financial independence from parents by age 21. Thus, our extended educational system, in which people rely on parental support for ever-increasing lengths of time, can be seen as the primary factor in the extended adolescence that is common today.

Development in Adolescence

As young people pass through adolescence on their way to full adulthood, they experience a number of significant changes. First is the change in body and resulting adaptations to a new body and body image. In the

YOU'VE ONLY JUST BEGUN

The things you must learn to be good "on the job" aren't in any textbooks. They are right there in your work setting, and so you've got to get out of your office and go learn them. You can't sit behind your desk and wait for the world to come to you. You must be an active and viable part of your school, and there is only one way. Counselors must be seen, and they must see what's going on.

You must be thoroughly familiar with all phases of the school operation. You've got to understand the curriculum offerings, extracurricular activities, school philosophy, faculty, and administration—really understand, not just be familiar with. If you don't know the difference between one kind of math and the dozen other kinds of math, and this teacher's expectations and another teacher's requirements, then you will be creating problems instead of helping to solve them—for everybody, not just your counselees. You must understand the world of work—its opportunities, demands, trends, and so on—because your counselees need your help in planning their futures. You must not let your shortcomings become their burdens, and so you've got to learn all you can about the world of work and the world of higher education. They are related, you know.

You must also understand that you will be working with a wide range of ages and personalities: students, teachers, parents, administrators, blue-collar workers, professionals, and community representatives. And it is imperative that you be able to communicate with these persons in a positive and cooperative manner. You must earn their respect and confidence. You need their help in order to help your counselees.

You must be able to evaluate situations and offer knowledgeable solutions and alternatives. Every situation will be different and unique, and your best resource for answers will be your ingenuity. Counselors have many responsibilities, but their greatest responsibility is professional affiliation. You need professional association membership—local, state, regional, and national. And your professional associations need your active involvement.

—A High School Counselor

approximately four years that it takes for the body of a child to become the body of an adult (the time known as puberty), the person must become accustomed to a new body size, changes in body proportions, the development of primary sex characteristics (the sex organs), and the development of secondary sex characteristics (all those physical features—breasts, musculature, body hair, voice, shape—that differentiate male from female).

As adolescents test this new body and mind, they wander farther and farther from the familiar surroundings of home and neighborhood and develop new groups with whom to interact and new situations with which to cope.

We are brought, then, to the problem of the new adolescent attempting to maintain himself as a unique individual (that is, to hang on to the personality that he has developed as a child) in situations where it is not altogther appropriate still to be a child. At the same time we are expecting him still to be himself, to be the Joe, Tom, Sally, or Meg that he or she has always been and we are expecting; but he is trying to fit in, to belong, in these new groups with his new body and his new thoughts [Manaster, 1977, p. 128].[1]

If there is one fundamental assumption underlying our conceptions, not only of adolescent development, but of development in general, it is that an individual becomes the kind of person he is as a result of continuing and continuous interaction between a growing, changing biological organism and its physical, psychological, and social environment [Conger, 1973, p. 33].

Current Cultural Effects

We exist in a period of extremely rapid social change—of "future shock" in which change is occurring so fast as to leave today's problems and today's solutions already outdated. The views, attitudes, and experiences of one generation are not appropriate for the next, and differences in knowledge itself separate generations. Adults cannot rely on their own experiences as adolescents to relate to the new adolescents, but rather new social situations must be faced together, with no one having a corner on the right or most appropriate way to think, feel, or behave. Whereas at one time in history children learned from adults, we now live in a time when children learn some things from adults, adults and children learn some things together, and adults learn some things from their more knowledgeable, more experienced children.

In addition to dealing with pubescence at earlier ages (the average age of menarche is now 12 1/2, in contrast to 16 or 17 a hundred years ago), adolescents must also accept the social fact that they will not be ready to utilize their physical maturity for procreational purposes until many years have passed. Yet we provide them with adult-styled clothing (much of which is sexually provocative), encourage their heterosexual interactions, and introduce them to perfume and beauty-care products while simultaneously requiring that they deny their newly developed sexual impulses.

[1] From *Adolescent Development and the Life Tasks,* by G. J. Manaster. Copyright © 1977 by Allyn & Bacon, Inc. Reprinted by permission.

And all this takes place in a society that espouses ever more liberal attitudes. Subjects that once were discussed only behind closed doors are now out in the open. Controversial issues are discussed in the media and in the classroom, and people who were once considered deviant are now on the lecture circuit. In sum, children are exposed to significantly more than their parents were, and at significantly earlier ages. Pre- and extra-marital sex, abortion, contraception, homosexuality, bisexuality, group marriage, open marriage, transsexualism, pollution, nuclear energy, fuel shortages, space exploration, diet, and drug use are concepts that average 14-year-olds have already been exposed to. They must learn to deal with them.

As recently as 50 years ago, adolescents made few decisions about how they would live their lives. Most were prepared to take on responsibilities much like those of their parents and to live similarly. Almost all married and raised children. But today children often don't know how their parents earn a living; most know (either through personal experience or through a close friend) what single-parent families encounter; many live far from adults other than parents and teachers. They are exposed through less personal means to a wide variety of life-styles and are told to choose—single or married, heterosexual or homosexual or both? children? career? work patterns? education? military service? religion? place to live? The choices are endless, and they continue throughout life. Decisions are not as binding as they once were, as newspapers report that people now make a major occupational change three to five times, and more than half change marriage partners at least once.

Alternate life-styles, the possibility of frequent change, liberalized attitudes, availability of adult material goods, increased mobility and affluence, knowledge explosions, and increased technology make for a highly unpredictable society. Tomorrow will surely not mirror today; adolescents have a huge challenge to face and numerous tasks to accomplish.

Tasks of Adolescence

Manaster (1977) has combined the life tasks as proposed by Adler (1932) with the developmental tasks of adolescence as proposed by Havighurst (1972). The life tasks encompass those areas of life that demand attention and must be contended and coped with at all times, from infancy through old age. Adler's life tasks include *love and sex, work and school, friends and community* (society), *self,* and *the meaning of life* (the existential task). The developmental tasks are those accomplishments necessary at one stage of development in order to permit successful movement to the next stage. A developmental task is "a task which arises at or about a certain period in the life of an individual, successful achievement of which leads to his happiness and to success with later tasks, while failure leads to unhappiness in the individual, disapproval by the society, and difficulty with later tasks" (Havighurst, 1972, p. 2).

The relationships proposed by Manaster (1977) for developmental tasks and life tasks are identified in Figure 10-1.

FIGURE 10-1. Developmental tasks and the life tasks with which they are associated

	Developmental Tasks	Life Tasks
1.	Achieving new and more mature relations with age mates of both sexes	Friends and community (love and sex)
2.	Achieving a masculine or feminine social role	Self (friends and community): Love and sex
3.	Accepting one's physique and using the body effectively	Self, love and sex
4.	Achieving emotional independence of parents and other adults	Self, friends and community (love and sex)
5.	Preparing for marriage and family life	Love and sex
6.	Preparing for an economic career	Work and school, self
7.	Acquiring a set of values and an ethical system as a guide to behavior—developing an ideology	Existential (friends and community)
8.	Desiring and achieving socially responsible behavior	Friends and community, work and school, existential

From *Adolescent Development and the Life Tasks*, by G. J. Manaster. Copyright © 1977 by Allyn & Bacon, Inc. Reprinted by permission.

To master the developmental tasks that will allow the adolescent to attain adulthood while dealing with the here and now of the life tasks as they interplay in daily existence: that is the challenge of adolescence. Development itself is varied, changeable, and complex. In the following pages, I will highlight the most popular of the theories of adolescent development that accompany physical maturation, including cognitive development, psychological development, and moral development.

Cognitive Development: Jean Piaget

Adolescents have been described as both sensitive and callous, considerate and inconsiderate, conservative and liberal, optimistic and pessimistic, materialistic and idealistic. They are often thought of as impulsive, introspective, impetuous, and intense. Although none of these descriptors apply to all adolescents, many apply to at least some and are possible to apply only because of a qualitative and quantitative change in the thinking processes of the adolescent.

Jean Piaget, a Swiss psychologist, has done extensive work in studying the development of thinking processes through childhood and into adulthood. His theory includes a series of invariant stages through which people pass. The childhood stages are universal, and although they can be influenced by teaching, everyone of normal intelligence achieves and passes through them. These stages are discussed in depth in Chapter 9 of this text. It should be reemphasized that "each stage of development is characterized much less by a fixed thought content than by a certain power, a certain potential activity, capable of achieving such and such a result according to the environment in which the child lives" (Piaget, 1970, pp. 171–172). In early adolescence the person moves into the stage that Piaget calls "formal operations." "The adolescent, unlike the child, is an individual who thinks beyond the present and forms theories about everything, delighting especially in consideration of that which is not" (Piaget, 1973, p. 148).

Although the concrete and tangible basis for thought attained during childhood is still present and reliable, the adolescent just beginning to develop formal-operational potential discovers new ways of thinking. These new ways, operating from propositions and hypotheses, open vast new vistas, openings that may be both intensely invigorating and somewhat frightening. New adventures invariably involve both excitement and risk.

Three specific thinking processes characterize the formal-operational stage. Instead of being locked into the tangible, the formal-operational thinker begins to think instead about possibility and is therefore able to entertain realistically improbable ideas. Second, the formal-operational thinker is able to use the hypothetico-deductive method to deduce from hypotheses (which may or may not be true) the logical consequences of the hypotheses as if they were true. Third, the formal-operational thinker can manipulate ideas, juggling intellectual relations among thoughts that have no basis in fact. These new skills allow the adolescent who achieves them the ability to think in the abstract, to weigh alternative possibilities, and to imagine a variety of futures.

Many adolescents never progress into formal-operational thinking. Certainly those with limited intelligence do not. But most do, earlier or later depending on intelligence, family and social environment, and direct teaching. And for those that do, there are tremendous implications. The new social environments open to youth can be seen not only as they are but also as they potentially could be, as they might be at their best.

Formal-operational thought creates the possibility of a wide range of emotional responses to the new cognitive challenges of adolescence. Whereas at one time adolescents may delight in thinking about the unlimited possibilities they face, at other times they may despair in the overwhelming difficulty of achieving their ideals. Thus cognitive development contributes to the adolescent potential for vast mood swings.

The challenge of formal operations manifests itself in several ways. Thought often becomes focused on self, forcing youth to reestablish their personal identities to accommodate new information and new ways of

IF YOU HAVEN'T TRIED, DON'T KNOCK IT

I'm really glad you asked me for my reactions to counseling as a career, but you may not be happy to hear what I have to say. As a residential-preparatory-school counselor, I am responsible for helping students select and get admitted to college. I like what I do, and I think it's important work to do, so why do counselor educators try to put it down? Last year the professors and the other students in my classes tried to make me feel second-rate for wanting to do this kind of counseling—that it wasn't counseling at all, but at best just advising.

That attitude really disturbs me. It is narrow-minded, and it should be corrected. More than half of all high school students want to attend college, and if you look at the data on their lack of success, you would know that what is needed is more and better, not less, college counseling. Sure, I do a lot of information giving, and so do all other good counselors. But I also do counseling. What do you think happens when the students have to look at themselves and their plans? Deal with the pain of being denied admission? Making choices and developing decision-making skills? And what kind of problems do you think the need for financial aid can create? Because my school is small, I have the time to give to each student that is needed for a life-planning process. Choosing a college is one of the most important parts of that process, but students also come to me with a lot of other problems.

One thing about residential-school counseling is that you are never off. Anyone considering my kind of work should consider this part of it very carefully. And, if you can't meet deadlines and you don't know how to get things organized and stay on top of them, then you won't last very long in counseling jobs like mine—or any other that I can think of.

I guess you can tell I like what I do and I am proud of my work. I am not proud of some of my colleagues' rhetoric about serving all students and refusing to see that one of the best ways to do it is as a good secondary school college-placement counselor.

—*A Residential-Preparatory-School Counselor*

---

thinking. This inward focusing creates an egocentrism in which each youth is convinced that everyone is as focused on him or her as he or she is. Egocentric youths are always self-conscious and virtually unable to really pay attention to anyone other than themselves. Hence the small tragedies of adolescent "loves"—in which each person focuses so exclusively on self that each only worries that the other is accepting or judging, and neither is able to pay attention to the other.

Another effect of formal operations is to create a climate ripe for experimentation. Formal-operational adolescents are on the brink of examining their potentials and are to be expected to experiment with going beyond the limits they have known. Consequently, they may appear foolhardy, full of fantastic notions of who they might become, totally unaccepting of their own mortality. Potential and reality have yet to reach a compromise.

> The onset and growth in formal operations for many adolescents open new vistas for thought and behavior. Almost as a form of reality testing, adolescents try out their new thoughts and behaviors with friends, parents, and others to assess their reactions, as well as the adolescent's own reactions. In addition to the "reality-testing" function, the trying out of new hypotheses and potentials in thought and action can be very stimulating and just plain fun. In toto, as reality testing and an enjoyable facet of being an adolescent, this has been referred to . . . as an "experimenting" effect of the development of formal operations in adolescence [Manaster, 1977, p. 91].[2]

Adolescent thought, feeling, and behavior may therefore appear inconsistent. "Much of what is considered typically adolescent in the way of emotionality can only be fully understood in the context of formal-operational thought" (Elkind, 1968, p. 152).

Psychological Development: Erik Erikson

Erik H. Erikson trained as a psychoanalyst with the Freudian Society in Vienna in the late 1920s. He then moved to Boston, where he worked as a child analyst and developed his monumental stage theory of personality development.

According to Erikson, personality develops in an invariant sequence of stages, which he called "normative crises." Unlike traumatic crises, these crises are normative in that they are normal, healthy tasks of development that everyone must experience and master. Erikson's stages roughly approximate the stages identified by Sigmund Freud, but Erikson rejected Freud's mechanistic theory, which emphasized drives and predestination, in favor of a more developmental, more controllable, more humane emphasis. Erikson saw the ego as adaptive, constructive, positive. As we mature, we have a series of eight tasks to accomplish, and although we approach these tasks primarily in sequence, all eight are really present at all times, and we may well regress to an earlier stage when a life crisis occurs, especially if an earlier task was not completely satisfactorily resolved. Each task has both a positive and a negative outcome. Healthy development occurs when we integrate the positive and negative valences so as to achieve a preponderance of the positive. Table 10-1 outlines these eight tasks, normative crises, or "Ages of Man."

---

[2]From *Adolescent Development and the Life Tasks,* by G. J. Manaster. Copyright © 1977 by Allyn & Bacon, Inc. Reprinted by permission.

TABLE 10-1. Erikson's eight ages of man

Approximate age	Task to achieve	Danger in not achieving	Examples of Circumstances of learning
Birth–2	Trust	Mistrust	Parental care
2–4	Autonomy	Doubt/shame	Toilet training, dressing, eating
4–6	Initiative	Guilt	Trying things alone
6–12	Industry	Inferiority	Making things, school
12–18	Identity	Confusion	Self-exploration, peer relationships
18–25	Intimacy	Isolation	Love relationships, deep friendships
25–50	Generativity	Stagnation	Childrearing, community service
50+	Integrity	Despair	Retirement, facing death

Since Chapter 9 has discussed Erikson's early stages already, our discussion here will be limited to those stages associated with adolescence. The first task in adolescence is to discover an identity, a sense of uniqueness from others and a projection of who the individual might become. The individual's identity, her separateness, emanates from her own personal history, from the success or lack of success she has achieved in preceding stages, and from her anticipation of who she might be in the near and more distant future. She must examine herself and her similarities to and differences from her family and peers and must determine for herself how to live her life. Life-style decisions, including sex role, career choice, and avocational pursuits, take on paramount importance. With the chronological extension of adolescence into the twenties, Erikson's next stage, that of intimacy, may also be included in our discussion of adolescence. Although the beginnings of intimacy frequently occur during the teen years, it is only after a person has achieved a sense of who he or she is in relation to others that the task of achieving intimacy can be successfully accomplished. Intimacy, the give and take of committed relationships, is possible only between individuals who have a solid sense of who they are and where they might be going.

Erikson was especially interested in the psychology of adolescence. Unlike Freud, Erikson saw youth as an adaptive time both personally for the individual and socially. Recognizing the importance of these years to future psychological health, the society, said Erikson, grants youth a "psychosocial moratorium," a kind of way station or reprieve from social responsibility and an encouragement to experiment in the attempt to discover an identity.

> The integration now taking place in the form of ego identity is . . . more than the sum of the childhood identification. It is the accrued experience of the ego's ability to integrate all identification with the vicissitudes of the libido, with the aptitudes developed out of endowment, and with the opportunities offered in social roles. The

sense of ego identity, then, is the accrued confidence that the inner sameness and continuity prepared in the past are matched by the sameness and continuity of one's meaning for others, as evidenced in the tangible promise of a "career" [Erikson, 1963, pp. 261–262].

In order to be introspective, to come "face to face" with self and develop this sense of uniqueness, at least two conditions seem necessary. First is the mental ability to weigh alternatives, to evaluate strengths and weaknesses, and to perceive both self and environment accurately; in other words, the ability to think in formal operations may be a necessary condition for experiencing an "identity crisis." Second, the society must grant the psychosocial moratorium necessary for such personal and intense self-confrontation. The implications of these conditions are significant: if people do not achieve formal operations, they will probably not have the identity crisis that Erikson describes. Since a significant minority of adults apparently have not achieved formal operations, many young people will likely become adults without the introspection characteristic of the identity-gain task. In addition, the longer the psychosocial moratorium, the longer the identity crisis. It may be convenient to roughly equate the psychosocial moratorium with the educational years, as Manaster (1977) does:

> It may be that dwelling on issues of personal identity is a luxury that comes with an extended psychosocial moratorium. Adolescents who are not pressed into the adult social and occupational world, most probably because they are pursuing courses of higher education, are granted the time, and to some degree are expected to look closely at themselves and their future [p. 123].[3]

But many adolescents finish high school, get jobs, marry, and set up housekeeping without the luxury of time for self-examination. It is interesting to speculate on whether these young people experience an identity crisis and even whether there is any necessity for them to do so.

But regardless of when or whether an identity crisis occurs, all adolescents must wrestle with identity-related questions—Who am I? What will I become? How do I want to spend my life? How will I earn a living? For some the answers may come easily and early; others may weigh the alternatives and change directions throughout their lives. For all, identity formation is a central issue, one that will occupy a significant place in their lives.

Moral Development: Lawrence Kohlberg

As young people mature physically, cognitively, and psychologically, they are continually faced with questions of right and wrong, good and bad.

---

[3]From *Adolescent Development and the Life Tasks*, by G. J. Manaster. Copyright © 1977 by Allyn & Bacon, Inc. Reprinted by permission.

Their responses to these questions and, even more important, the reasoning behind the responses constitute the moral development of the individual. It too can be viewed as progressing in identifiable and sequential stages. Jean Piaget (1932/1965) studied moral reasoning by examining the marble-playing behavior, and the reasons they gave for their behavior, of children between 2 and 12 years old. He discovered that moral reasoning is directly related to cognitive reasoning; that is, a person at the concrete-operations stage can reason morally only at a stage that does not require the thinking processes of formal operations. John Dewey identified three levels of moral development: the *premoral,* or *preconventional,* level, in which behavior is motivated by physical and social consequences ("I'll do it because I'll get a reward if I do"), the *conventional* level, in which behavior is motivated by uncritical acceptance of the standards of the group ("I'll do it because it's the law"), and the *autonomous,* or *postconventional,* level, in which conduct is guided by the individual's personal judgment following reflection (I'll do it because I believe it's right, regardless of what others think") (Blatt & Kohlberg, 1973). In over 20 years of research, Lawrence Kohlberg has both validated and expanded these three stages:

Preconventional (premoral): Based on meeting personal needs
Stage 1: Punishment and obedience orientation ("I'll do it so I don't get punished").
Stage 2: Instrumental-relativist orientation ("I'll do it if you also do something for me").
Conventional: Based on meeting group norms
Stage 3: Good-boy orientation ("I'll do it to please you").
Stage 4: Law-and-order orientation ("I'll do it because it's my duty").
Postconventional (autonomous): Based on moral principle
Stage 5: Social-contract orientation ("I'll do it because it's best for the majority").
Stage 6: Universal ethical orientation ("I'll do it because my conscience tells me it's right").

Kohlberg's theory is a fully developed one, complete with an instrument for measuring moral reasoning, many activities that teachers and counselors can use to stimulate development of moral reasoning, and years of action research into the processes that help people reason morally at increasingly higher stages. Kohlberg's research shows that any one person generally reasons more than half the time at one level, with the rest of his or her reasoning at adjacent levels. Furthermore, people generally do not regress, but rather remain where they are or slowly move to the next higher stage. In a moral discussion, people understand argument from the levels below their own but do not accept them. They also understand arguments one stage above their own but do not understand arguments more than one level higher. It is futile, therefore, to use level 5 reasoning (for example, "I have the right to engage in peaceful protest!") with a person whose moral reasoning is at stage 1 (for example, "Take down that protest sign or I'll knock your block off!"). Most important, people prefer the reasoning at the highest level they can understand. The implications for teaching and counseling are great: it is only through extensive and intensive discussion of moral issues, in which all views are freely exchanged, that young people will be consistently exposed to moral reasoning that leads them to reevaluate their own thought processes and advance up the moral-reasoning ladder.

Moral reasoning is obviously dependent on intellectual development. The concrete-operational child or adult is capable of moral reasoning at stages 1, 2, 3, and 4, but formal operations are required for stages 5 and 6 moral reasoning. And although cognitive development sets limits to moral reasoning, it is not sufficient for it. Most people are at a cognitive level that is higher than their moral-reasoning level. Further, mature moral reasoning is necessary for principled moral behavior, but being able to reason at a high moral level does not ensure concomitant moral behavior. For example, I can reason that driving at 55 mph or less on the highway is right because it conserves fuel and lowers the highway death toll (level 5), but I may well drive faster when I think I won't be caught—or maintain the speed limit only out of fear of the consequences (level 1).

It can therefore be seen that cognitive development is a necessary but not sufficient condition for mature moral judgment, and mature moral judgment is a necessary but not sufficient condition for mature moral action. In order to develop mature moral judgment and action, adolescents need not be told what to do, but need instead to experience an environment that gives them freedom and power to wrestle with moral issues, argue positions, make decisions, act on those decisions, and assume responsibility for the consequences of those decisions. In fact, some of the problems of adolescence may be attributed to the adolescent's ability to think maturely while not being encouraged, or even allowed, to act maturely. In all high schools, for example, the values of democracy and individual rights and responsibilities are held in high regard and taught as the best form of government. Yet few high schools *practice* democracy in any form, and fewer still afford students equal rights with the adults in the school. The students are encouraged to think democratically, but their ability to act in democratic fashion is severely restricted.

Just as cognitive and moral development are interdependent, so too are cognitive and psychological development. The reflection necessary for an examination of identity has already been shown to be dependent on the attainment of formal operations. Therefore, formal-operational thinkers who reason morally only at the conventional levels of stages 3 and 4 will probably never experience an identity crisis. Although they can think in hypotheses, propositions, and possibilities, their conventional acceptance of group norms will prevent them from questioning conventional morality or conventional expectations of them.

In summary, then, adolescents develop physically, cognitively, psychologically, and morally. Their bodies change, and they must adapt to and accept the changes. For most, the very quality of their thinking changes too, and they can feel both the excitement and the confusion of new thought. This new thought can even turn inward, leading to extreme self-consciousness and the adventure of self-discovery. As this happens, all the old constructs and rules, along with everything that was once so sure, are questioned. And all this takes place in a society that suddenly places new and often conflicting demands on its young, with whom it doesn't know how to deal. For some adolescents, this may indeed be a time of tumult, of wild extremes in thought and behavior, of unpredictability and confusion. But for others it may be reasonably stress-free, full of good experiences. And for some the changes may hardly be noticeable. Reactions on the part of the young are as varied as everything else about them.

Adolescent Concerns: The Counselor's Role

Manaster (1977) identifies three general types of adolescent problems. First are those that might be called primarily educational in nature. These problems, like facing a new situation, trying out a new behavior, or making a decision, may be addressed through experience, in discussion with peers, or with the help of a professional. Most of the work of secondary school counselors, as well as counselors in colleges, community organizations, social service agencies, and church groups, involves these kinds of problems.

Counselors in these settings help youth with problems of sex-role adjustment, sexual behavior, vocational and leisure-time choices, social concerns, developing and keeping friends of both sexes, school-related problems, family adjustments related to adolescent development, educational choices, life-style choices, religious and moral issues, and any other concern that arises primarily because the body, mind, feelings, and social world of the adolescent are so rapidly changing. These are issues that, though vitally important, will eventually be solved by time alone. It is the quality of the solutions and the immediate experience of support in this time that can be positively affected by counselors who understand and support the young people who are experiencing these normal life and developmental tasks.

Second, those adolescents who achieve formal-operational thought and mature moral judgment are likely to experience some degree of confusion over who they are and who they want to be. Some experience the identity crisis most acutely. In Erikson's (1968) words, the adolescent is searching for "a new sense of continuity and sameness" (p. 128) and, in so doing, may experiment, try on alternate roles, feel elated and/or depressed, and most certainly question self as well as everything and everyone else. Counselors can assist these young people, many of whom experience this crisis during college rather than high school, by longer-term counseling, during which the young person is made to feel the warm, understanding support of the counselor and is given permission to freely reflect and experiment within the counseling relationship. For some, knowing that they are not alone in their search for themselves is the main support that they need to get through the crisis. The greatest danger of the search for identity is the potential for self-rejection.

Because self-rejection leads to poor personal and social adjustments, it is important to recognize and correct the common danger signals of maladjustment: excessive irresponsibility, feelings of inadequacy and inferiority, expressions of unsocial behavior, use of defense and retreat mechanisms, hypersensitivity to real or imagined slights, anxiety and worry, perfectionist attitudes, over- or under-concern about appearance, and hostility toward authority (Hurlock, 1973, p. 344).

For those who are beginning to feel some self-rejection, long-term counseling may be essential. With these problems, counselors must be able to help adolescents more accurately assess themselves and their worlds. With realistic concepts of both their personal characteristics and the facts of their existence, young people will be able to adjust their views and plan realistically and assertively.

The third and least common kind of adolescent problems are those that are neurotic. Neurotic adolescents are in distress because "the way of acting or thinking which they have employed as children is not amenable to functioning as an adolescent and then adult" (Manaster, 1977, p. 120). Their behavior is not acceptable, but they don't understand why not. They perceive the world and themselves inaccurately, and their problems encompass all life and developmental-task areas.

Anyone who works with adolescents encounters all three kinds of problems, and all can be compounded by situational factors—the home, school, neighborhood, social contacts, money, and immediate traumas. Some teachers and friends can deal effectively with problems of an educational nature, and counselors spend most of their time with these too. Problems of an identity nature are more encompassing, are more time-consuming, and often require greater counseling skill than a teacher normally has. These, then, are definitely within the realm of the counselor. In addition to educational and identity issues, counselors of adolescents often spend considerable time and energy consulting with parents, teachers, and community resources in the attempt to educate them about adolescent needs and to improve the external environment in which the adolescent lives. Young people with neurotic problems will certainly also be seen by counselors, but for the most part, these adolescents are experiencing conflicts that are usually referred to professionals trained to work with them. Therapy, not counseling, is indicated.

In the settings in which counselors work, flexibility is a primary requirement. Although a particular day may be set aside for specific activities and tasks, a spontaneous issue may take precedence, and the counselor must be able to respond, to adapt to the new situation.

Along with flexibility is required the ability to stay current with situational issues of society, the neighborhood, the profession, the school district, interpersonal relations, and the myriad of other concerns and topics that pass through the counselor's office. In no situation does a counselor have the luxury of attending to just one thing; the counselor must be an expert juggler, with juggling pins of various sizes, shapes, and weights. Although most counselors work in institutions and therefore have to keep regular office hours, never are the scheduled hours sufficient. Paperwork is taken home, simply because it is often the least immediate of daily demands, and home visits and community consultation are done at the convenience of the parents or agency, often "after hours." The demands of others also interfere. Administration, even the "system" itself, demands the completion of tasks (often quasi-administrative) by counselors, tasks that frequently interfere with what the counselor would prefer to do. In sum, the counselor must be a highly skilled professional, competent in human relations and counseling with adolescents and adults, knowledgeable in developmental psychology, organized and efficient, flexible, spontaneous, adaptable, willing to work long hours, deeply committed, and, to balance, must possess a sense of humor that will allow laughter and fun.

Given the requirements and the demands, the rewards are also great. Wealth is certainly not the end point of a career in counseling adolescents, but the personal satisfaction of significantly affecting positive lifetime decision making is enormous. In many instances, the effects can be readily seen—in good decisions, accomplishments, and positive attitudes—and the kids are not shy about letting their counselors know how they helped. Most counselor's offices are filled with the important tokens of affection presented by the adolescents with whom the counselor worked.

Perspectives for the '80s

During the 1980s, adolescence will continue to encompass anywhere from five to ten or more years of every person's life, and during these transitional years, the young people will face situations that will likely separate them from all previous generations.

The role of the counselor of adolescents undoubtedly will evolve in reaction to rapidly changing societal needs, but it will continue to be focused on assisting maturing individuals in their acceptance of adult tasks.

Among the several societal changes will be certain changes in institutions that employ counselors and in the differential emphasis to be placed on various adolescent needs. Several panels of educators, including the Panel on Youth of the President's Science Advisory Committee (Coleman, 1972) and the Carnegie Council on Policy Studies in Higher Education (1980), have proposed significant educational changes, the implications of which include the following:

1. *Vocational education.* More attention must be paid to the needs of youth who are not bound for college. For many years, counselors have concentrated their efforts on the few students who were college-bound. With the development of a society in which a college degree is no longer a ticket to success, the needs of the non-college-bound are more prevalent. Counselors will have to work with youth in all areas of career development, from first-time and part-time employment to entrance into complicated technical programs. The counselor will have to be familiar with an ever-increasing specialization of careers.

2. *Nontraditional students.* The traditional comprehensive high school, with its programs for full-time students between ages 14 and 18, may be on its way out. Instead, youth may be alternating school and work, attending school while on a work-study program, or developing work skills in technical settings or in on-the-job training. Educational institutions will thus be called on to serve a wider population in both age and interests. The counselor must be prepared to work with these nontraditional students. New skills will include job development, job placement, work-study coordination, and development of new ways of measuring competencies and recording accomplishments.

3. *Specialized studies.* There will likely be more attention to alternative forms of education. Some students may have the interest and opportunity to specialize early. It is entirely conceivable that with the possible demise of the traditional high school will come the development of specialized studies previously unavailable to most adolescents—computer technology, aviation, specialized business studies, for example. Counselors will be called on not only to help young people make decisions about such alternatives but also to assist in the design of the alternatives themselves.

4. *Basic skills.* There will continue to be more emphasis on basic skills in secondary programs. People who didn't master the basic skills in elementary school *used to* drop out and go to work. But today, and in the future, there are and will continue to be very few jobs for the nonliterate and unskilled. As a result, those who once would have dropped out are remaining in school, and the secondary schools are now required to provide effective remediation. Basic-skills programs will be combined with alternative training and educational programs, and counselors will be required to help adolescents make appropriate choices.

5. *Study skills.* Consistent with the above demands for appropriate career education and training programs, there will likely be more attention to the development of effective study skills and positive work habits. Because both attitudes and behaviors are so vitally important in this development, counselors will be the likely leaders in this area.

6. *National youth service.* For many people who do not want further education (at least immediately after high school) and do not yet have employment, the development of some form of national youth service (like VISTA, for example) is probable. Counselors may well assist in its development and will certainly be involved in its implementation.

7. *Coordination.* With alternative programs, alternation of work and school, and the possibility of a national youth service, counselors will have to develop sophisticated coordination techniques, for it is unlikely that any one institution or agency will serve all the needs of any one person. Thus, the counselor will be called on to coordinate business activities, agencies, industry involvement, transportation requirements, school demands, and individual needs. Computerized records and information retrieval systems will be mandatory, and counselors will have to be as proficient with them as they are with people.

8. *Consultation and humanistic education.* With increased emphasis on choices, acknowledgment of student rights, and a concern for the total well-being of each person, the guidance functions in any institution must be spread beyond the counselor's office. Thus, the counselor will likely be increasingly involved in teaching—of human relations skills, decision-making skills, problem-solving skills, communication, values clarification, and so on—to other staff members, teachers, parents, and adolescents. These skills will not remain within the sole domain of the counselor, but the counselor may instead become the human relations "consultant," who systematically helps others learn the skills that will provide them with the means for handling most situations and problems themselves. Counselors may truly become the persons who most effectively "give away" their skills.

9. *Special education.* There will continue to be increased attention to the special needs of handicapped adolescents. With the societal recognition of the rights of the handicapped has come the long-overdue need to both understand and work with the physically and mentally handicapped. Counselors must be both more knowledgeable about handicapping conditions and more competent in advocating for the handicapped.

10. *Life-style choices.* With an ever more open society, counselors must become comfortable working in previously taboo (or at least touchy) areas. Human sexuality, nontraditional career choices, possibilities for life-style choices other than the nuclear family, drugs, and alcohol need to be dealt with fairly and openly. Counselors must first examine their own learning and attitudes in these areas and must learn to accept views that differ from theirs. Only then can they be objective and fair in working with adolescents.

11. *Youth participation.* There will need to be more attention to youth-participation projects designed to provide meaningful activity and to reduce the segregation of young people from both those older and those younger than themselves. Included are likely to be projects in the community, projects of a business nature, projects in meaningful problem

solving (for example, energy conservation), and projects designed for youth to assist other youth. Many such projects already exist. As youth feel an ever-increasing need for meaningful involvement, such projects will continue to grow. Counselors will be called on to assist in their design and implementation. For example, a counselor might work with a local social service agency to develop experiential placements for youths who will deliver day-care services to children or to the elderly; another counselor might help a young person interested in architecture to "apprentice" herself as a volunteer in an architectural firm; still another might place a promising adolescent as a student member of a local governing board or committee.

12. *Counselor specialization.* Finally, given the vast array of responsibilities outlined above, counselors themselves are likely to become increasingly specialized. Instead of the traditional high school guidance-staff structure in which each counselor is considered a generalist who can deal with everybody in a particular class or section of the alphabet, it is likely that the counselors will develop specific areas of expertise. Specialty areas might include career development, college placement, vocational training, remediation, work-study, drug education, family-life education, special education, special programming, community liaison, study skills, computer technology and information systems, humanistic education, discipline, and staff development. Most likely, counselors of adolescents will maintain a generalist *attitude* but will develop one or two specialties as well.

While the demands on the counselor of adolescents in the '80s will be both varied and extensive, seeing individuals mature into the responsible and responsive adults of the next century will be the reward of those who meet the challenge.

Summary

This chapter has highlighted the unique developmental concerns of adolescents, especially as explained by the developmental theories of Jean Piaget, Erik Erikson, and Lawrence Kohlberg and viewed in the context of the society of the 1980s. It was emphasized that adolescence has a biological beginning but a societal ending and that counselors must be aware of the tremendous impact of society on the experience of adolescence.

During this period, people develop cognitively, psychologically, and morally as they attempt to master the tasks that are appropriate. They begin to think abstractly rather than concretely, to be concerned with their present and future roles, and to wrestle with increasingly complex moral dilemmas. At the same time, physical and hormonal development are as overwhelming as they were during the first year of life. The period of adolescence thus becomes filled with the *potential* for upset—physical, cognitive, and psychological—and is a period when counselors can play tremendously important roles in helping youth both experience adolescence positively and prepare effectively for adulthood.

Now It's Your Turn

Although a single sample never provides a valid picture of a group, each of us has one adolescence about which we are expert—our own. It is helpful to examine our experiences as adolescents and to compare those experiences with others' as we try to understand the developmental issues of this important period of life. To do so, imagine yourself in each of the scenes described below. Answer the questions and compare your answers with those of your classmates.

1. *Fantasies of the future*

    You are in the sixth grade, and a favorite but distant relative has come for a visit. (It often helps to recall a photo of yourself at this age and to try to remember a favorite outfit, your hairstyle, and what your home looked like, inside and out.) While visiting, this relative asks you "What do you want to be when you grow up?" What would you have answered? What would have been the reasons for your answer? Is there something else you thought about but wouldn't say? How realistic was your answer?

2. *Body acceptance*

    You are in the eighth grade. Imagine yourself at school, surrounded by the others in your class. Recall the popular clothing styles and note what you are wearing. Remember the grooming ritual you would go through each morning. Imagine yourself standing in front of a full-length mirror. How did you like your body? What about it did you like? Dislike? How did it compare with the bodies of your friends? How did your feelings about your body affect you?

3. *Social relationships*

    You are a sophomore in high school. Remember your school, your friends, your after-school activities. Who was your best friend? What qualities attracted you to him or her? When the two of you were alone, what did you talk about? What was your circle of friends like? What did you do together? What friendship or social issues were you most concerned about?

4. *Love/sex*

    Recall your first romance. Describe yourself and your boyfriend/girlfriend. What attracted you to that person? How did he or she make you feel? Was your interest directed mainly toward that person or toward yourself? Explain. What new issues were raised for you as a result of this romance?

5. *Cognitive development*

Recall a moment during your adolescence when an idea that had previously seemed exceedingly difficult suddenly made sense. Describe what happened. Or recall a philosophical argument or discussion that you became involved in. What thinking processes were you using?

6. *Parental relationships/moral thinking*

Think back to the first time during your adolescence that you had a significant philosophical (moral, religious) disagreement with your parents. Describe the situation, their point of view, your point of view, and the resolution of the disagreement.

7. *Experimental behavior*

Most adolescents at one time or another do something that is against the law. Describe a time when you did something for which you could have been arrested. What were the motivations behind your action?

References

Adelson, J. Adolescence and the generalization gap. *Psychology Today,* February 1979, pp. 33–37.

Adler, A. *What life should mean to you.* London: Allen & Unwin, 1932.

Allport, G. W. Crises in normal personality development. *Teachers College Record,* 1964, *66,* 235–241.

Ambron, S. R. *Child development.* San Francisco: Rinehart Press, 1975.

Blatt, M. & Kohlberg, L. The effects of classroom discussion on children's level of moral judgment. In L. Kohlberg, *Collected papers on moral development and moral education.* Cambridge, Ma.: Center for Moral Education, 1973.

Carnegie Council on Policy Studies in Higher Education. *Giving Youth a Better Chance: Options for Education and Work.* San Francisco: Jossey-Bass, 1980.

Coleman, J. S. *Youth: Transition to Adulthood.* Chicago: University of Chicago Press, 1972.

Conger, J. J. *Adolescence and youth: Psychological development in a changing world.* New York: Harper & Row, 1973.

Cottle, T. J. Adolescent voices. *Psychology Today,* February 1979, pp. 40–44.

Elkind, D. Adolescent cognitive development. In J. F. Adams (Ed.), *Understanding adolescents.* Boston: Allyn & Bacon, 1968.

Elkind, D. Growing up faster. *Psychology Today,* February 1979, pp. 38–45.

Erikson, E. H. *Childhood and society* (2nd ed.). New York: W. W. Norton, 1963.

Erikson, E. H. Identity and the life cycle. *Psychological Issues,* 1959, *1*(1).

Erikson, E. H. *Identity, youth and crisis.* New York: W. W. Norton, 1968.

Havighurst, R. J. *Developmental tasks and education.* New York: David McKay, 1972.

Hoebel, E. A. *The Cheyennes: Indians of the great plains.* New York: Holt, 1960.
Hurlock, E. B. *Adolescent development.* New York: McGraw-Hill, 1973.
Lewin, K. Field theory and experiment in social psychology: Concepts and methods. *American Journal of Sociology,* 1939, *44,* 868–897.
Manaster, G. J. *Adolescent development and the life tasks.* Boston: Allyn & Bacon, 1977.
Muson, H. Moral thinking: Can it be taught? *Psychology Today,* February 1979, pp. 48–68, 92.
Piaget, J. *The moral judgment of the child.* Glencoe, Ill.: Free Press, 1965. (Originally published, 1932.)
Piaget, J. *The psychology of intelligence.* Totowa, N. J.: Littlefield, Adams & Co., 1973.
Piaget, J. *Science of education and the psychology of the child.* New York: Onion Press, 1970.
Piaget, J., & Inhelder, B. *The psychology of the child.* New York: Basic Books, 1969.
Ralston, N. C., & Thomas, G. P. *The adolescent: Case studies for analysis.* New York: Chandler, 1974.
Seidman, J. *The adolescent.* New York: Dryden Press, 1953.

CHAPTER **11**

Adults

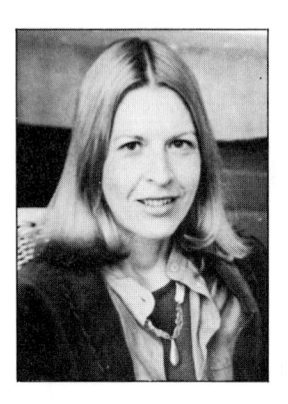

Maureen R. Worth
Maureen R. Worth is an instructor of psychology at Southern Seminary Junior College. Dr. Worth has coauthored texts on adult counseling and adult development. She is also a licensed professional counselor and has a private counseling practice.

    External circumstances as well as internal reappraisals are continually reshaping the lives of adults, and stability and certainty do not always persevere. Adults experience emotional pain, react to loss, reevaluate earlier decisions, and embark on new life experiences. Change is omnipresent. With it comes the need to cope with new situations, reconsider past decisions, and alter some goals or expectations. Thus, time and new experiences often alter the meaning and context of one's present life course. Stability and maturity do not always suffice to insulate adults from evolving internal and external circumstances.
    Today adult counseling is emerging in order to meet the specific

Note: Parts of this chapter are adapted from the following: *Counseling Adults: A Developmental Approach,* by William H. Van Hoose and Maureen Rousset Worth. Published by Brooks/Cole Publishing Company, Monterey, California, 1982.

developmental needs of this age group. Counselors who work with adults are unique in that their area of expertise is grounded in their in-depth study of the issues and needs of people in the adult years. With this knowledge they can intervene with an awareness of relevant concerns during particular periods in the adult life cycle. They can also address themselves to circumstances that cause people to question the course of their lives, such as divorce, death, job or career changes, and physical illness. Adult counselors are thus specialists in concerns of adults. They understand fully, for example, the meaning of a "midlife crisis" or the process of grieving for a loss. They can help adults evaluate their present needs and view these issues within the context of developmental theory of adulthood.

Intertwined with developmental concerns are social changes that have also altered the life course of many people and have created a need for adult counselors. Kimmel (1976) enumerates several of these factors that have created some unique circumstances for adults. First, people are living longer. This increased life span has produced more older adults, in number and proportion. Second, there is more leisure time. In some instances early retirement offers new challenges and changes for adults. Third, today adults are better educated and are privileged to have better health care services, including counseling. Fourth, our society is becoming more service-oriented, and there is a greater emphasis on the quality of life. Last, adults have more opportunities to experience a variety of life-styles. With these changes adults need to examine their values and goals in order to choose the style of life most appropriate for them.

Counselors who have specialized in adult development are needed to help people through these periods when questions are raised about life commitments and about the direction of one's life. These changes are "normal" and inevitable. For example, Jan, a woman in her late thirties, has decided that she wants more from life than being "just a housewife." She seeks counseling to make a career choice and to consider the impact of this choice on her family. A different decision is facing Jack. Shirley, his wife, has disclosed that she has fallen in love with someone else and wants a divorce. Jack knew that their marriage had lost some of its zest, but he never dreamed this would happen. It is often in such periods of transition and self-doubt that people seek counseling.

Because these periods are part of normal adult development, the client need not be defined as "mentally ill." These people need counselors whose skills are not in treating psychopathology but in helping adults make transitions in life-styles, careers, and interpersonal relationships as well as aiding them in a better understanding of themselves.

Adults are continually reconsidering past decisions and discovering new aspects of themselves. Kimmel (1974, pp. 526–527) believes that the biggest challenge during the adult years is self-renewal. One must continue to face new challenges, find new meaning to life, and learn new concepts and tasks. Without the flexibility to grow, change, and perform new roles, the person finds it difficult to live fully in the present. One who is bound up in the past cannot cope effectively with current demands. Adulthood is not a static period of life but a time of much change. This chapter will describe some specific developmental stages of adult life and then consider the role that counselors play in their professional involvement with adults in a variety of counseling settings.

Developmental Issues

Theories of adult development are helpful guidelines for specifying issues and concerns of adults at different periods or stages of adult life. Stage theory in development implies that at certain periods in their lives adults will encounter similar experiences. Each stage has a specific crisis, or period of time when certain issues must be resolved. When we speak of crisis in this context, we are not usually referring to trauma. Although a death, divorce, or job loss will cause depression and intense upheaval, for many adults a crisis may imply a less dramatic disturbance of one's life.

Simply put, a crisis can be conceived of as a period of doubt and decision making (Erikson, 1963). "Have I chosen the best career for me?" "Is my relationship with my spouse as rewarding as I would like it to be?" or "How can I improve my relationship with my adolescent child?" It is a period of concern for intimate relationships, careers, and personal aspirations. These concerns are often expressed, and most adults don't quit a job in the city and start over on a farm; they don't wait until their spouses move out or until their adolescent children are having drug problems before *they* begin problem solving.

The crisis period is usually a period of disequilibrium, a time of questioning one's values and reconsidering the course of one's life. Stage theory also suggests that each stage of development is more complex than, and qualitatively different from, the previous stage as the person progresses to greater maturity. Periods of crisis are usually followed by periods of relative calm.

When adults enter counseling, Bocknek (1976) notes, viewing them as having a *developmental crisis* is useful. The problems presented may have accumulated over the years, or they may be precipitated by current circumstances. In either event, Bocknek states "the client requests assistance *now* because somehow his/her present day life circumstances are unacceptable" (p. 38). More specifically, Bocknek enumerates several categories of developmental crises: (1) fear of an impending life stage; (2) reluctance to leave a gratifying stage; (3) trauma of unexpected developmental demands; (4) unresolved earlier issues; (5) a cumulative erosion of energies from seemingly overwhelming responsibilities, and (6) a desire to grow and live more fully.

Adults enter counseling for current concerns. These concerns are most likely to occur during periods of transition. Counselors who can recognize these transition points will be better equipped to help adults gain insight into their present concerns. Although research on the adult years is relatively recent, we are able to document some trends. Since the major works of Levinson et al. (1978) and Gould (1972) used only males as their subjects, caution must be exercised in generalizing the research findings to women. Based on the works of Levinson, the sequence of development outlined in Figure 11-1 and elaborated in the following pages is evident in the early to middle adult years.

Early Adulthood

The previous chapter focused on adolescence and the struggle to establish an identity as a separate individual. Although this issue is never completely laid to rest, the focus in the adult years is that of attaining intimacy with others without losing one's sense of self. Most adults at this time make initial decisions about a career and whether to marry (Havighurst, 1972). The person is expected to make these decisions with a minimum of help from others. Although, as we will see, previous decisions are often reconsidered in later years, the young adult views them as being permanent. Certainly, these decisions will have a major influence on later development. For example, the choice of a marital partner is a relatively large investment in the life of another person, and the birth of children will further obligate the individual to make a long-term commitment to their care.

During early adulthood one is expected to behave more *autonomously,* or independently. One must take responsibility for one's actions. One must also meet *intimacy* needs through relationships with other adults.

The transition from adolescence to young adulthood is not an abrupt or clear-cut change. As Havighurst notes, this period is often filled with stress and self-doubt as the person moves from an age-graded reference point to a social-status-graded structure. For many young adults, college or the military is a social vehicle for making this transition (Levinson et al., 1976). Gould (1972, 1975) and Vaillant and McArthur (1972) concur that this transition is not only gradual but sometimes precarious. For example, Vaillant and McArthur report that a number of men in their study were in their mid-adult years and still struggling with maternal dominance. Gould also found that although there is a strong need for peer relationships, these relationships tend to be "instantaneous and unstable" and are typically followed by "a temporary rebound back to parents."

By early adulthood the individual should have progressed in establishing an identity that is separate from others. This autonomy is facilitated by realistically examining specific strengths, weaknesses, attributes, and values. As discussed in the previous chapter, adolescence is viewed as a time of narcissism. The person becomes more introspective and questions

FIGURE 11-1. Phases of early and middle adulthood

Transition Period	Leaving the Family		Getting into the Adult World	Age 30s Transition	Settling Down		Midlife Transition		Middle Age
Stable Period	18-20s		20s	Late 20s to Early 30s	30s		Late 30s to Mid-40s		35-55
	Ambivalence between being autonomous or dependent on family. Conceptualization of a "dream" or "vision" for future. Development toward greater psychological and physical distance from family. Greater dependence on peer relationships		Creation of a lifestyle. Commitments to marriage and career. (Above choices viewed as permanent)	Questioning of initial commitments. Making necessary changes in job commitments and relationships	Intensification of career to pursue long-range goals. Time of deepening commitments to family life. Making of social commitments. Strong need for achievement and societal approval		Time of introspection. Identification of all aspects of oneself and incorporation of previously ignored parts of oneself. Realization that life is half over. This time viewed as the last chance to make changes		For those who have questioned lives and made changes this is often a period of productivity and creativity

abilities or desires to be a particular way. Through relationships with others, or the achievement of intimacy, and through developing a sense of autonomy, or separateness as a unique individual, young people begin to define themselves as adults.

Achieving Intimacy

The work of Erikson (1963) describes the psychosocial issues of individuals over the life cycle. In young adulthood the major developmental task is *intimacy and solidarity* versus *isolation*. Erikson identifies this polarity as a crisis, described previously as a period when the outcome of an issue is in doubt. The crisis for the young adult is whether or not one is able to sustain an intimate and caring relationship with at least one other person. One's failure in the interpersonal realm will result in withdrawal or isolation from others. A healthy resolution encompasses the ability to be intimate with another—to trust, to disclose, to give and receive. Yet the person does not become so fused to the other that a separate sense of selfhood is forfeited or subsumed by the other; and at the other extreme, the person does not move away or fail to share in intimate relationships because of a fear to trust or disclose personal beliefs and emotions.

To attain an intimate relationship with another, one must be mature enough to relate to the other in a trusting and reciprocal way. In contrast to the narcissism of earlier years, one must now be cognizant of the desires and individual needs of the other. When one cannot share with another in an intimate way, the relationship remains superficial and will not meet some basic needs of each person.

Counselors of young adults will verify that many a counseling session focuses on how one can meet this intimacy need. People who are dating are concerned about why a relationship ended as it did; married couples may come to counselors because they can't communicate their wants and needs. In both situations sexuality is often an issue.

Although intimacy is a major task in early adulthood, issues of intimacy continue over the life span. Not all people attain or sustain an intimate relationship during early adulthood. For example, Lowenthal and Weiss (1976) refute Erikson's supposition that intimacy is always attained in early adulthood. They contend that for developmental reasons or unique circumstances some adults are well past early adulthood before true intimacy is achieved. The young couple who married for the wrong reasons (parental pressure or rebellion against parental dominance) may divorce and later in life meet new partners when both possess the maturity necessary to attain intimacy. Lowenthal and Weiss further note that not only is intimacy an ongoing process but "the salience of intimacy waxes, wanes, and waxes again across the life course and . . . the rhythms vary between the sexes, often with disruptive consequences" (p. 14). From their perspective, intimacy, then, is a complex process and a lifelong pursuit.

Although marriage is the major social vehicle for attempts at meeting intimacy needs, there are alternative life-styles for meeting intimacy needs as well. Tools that can help meet intimacy needs include good communication skills, self-knowledge, and sensitivity to the needs of others. People must also learn to tolerate differences and to express their wants and needs to others when appropriate.

It is evident, then, that during the early adult years the person focuses on ways to form intimate relationships that are mutually rewarding. Most young adults consider marriage or some alternative intimate life-style. They also make initial career choices, and most become working, productive members of our society. Tolstoy and then Freud defined the healthy adult as one who can both love and work.

As both Freud and Erikson suggest, sexuality is important in attaining intimacy. The decision to counsel a client about sexual concerns should, of course, be based on the counselor's skill in sex counseling. At present many counselors lack adequate training (Kirkpatrick, 1980) and should therefore refer clients with sexual concerns.

Becoming Autonomous

Independence from the family of origin increases the young adult's autonomy. Levinson et al. (1976, 1978) suggest that becoming separate from one's family is a major developmental task. Gould (1972) also notes that negative and ambivalent feelings toward one's parents may emerge. The feeling of a need to break away from the family is strong, and the young adult looks to peers to help make this transition.

Counselors need to be aware of these inner conflicts. The urge for independence and a separate identity is strong. Parental intervention in attaining autonomy will cause intense conflict. One client, a college senior, was deeply troubled when his father offered him an excellent job with his business firm at a high salary. The young man was torn between wanting the good position (realizing that he could never land as desirable or high-paying a job on his own) and wanting to be out from under his father's jurisdiction. When a client must make such a decision, many questions emerge concerning independence, self-esteem, achievement, and loyalty to and respect for parents. Counselors will need to help clarify values and examine the alternatives.

Yet, as we have noted, not all adults make the transition to being psychologically independent during the early adult years. Autonomy issues are thus prevalent in early adulthood. For instance, some young women, instead of becoming autonomous, will become dependent on their husbands just as they were dependent on their parents. When a husband is willing to accept this role as protector and provider, this lack of autonomy may seemingly pose no problems. However, should the relationship dissolve through separation, divorce, or death, the woman may seek counseling in order to develop her independence. In a developmental context it is easier for people to make such transitions "on schedule" in early adulthood. However, particularly with women, autonomy is not always achieved early. Young women may be particularly ambivalent about investing energy in a career. At this period of life women are most intent on appearing "feminine." Some fear that aggressive and independent behavior may cause them to be unattractive to men. The young woman client who is struggling with these issues may have strong career aspirations but may fear competing with males in order to achieve her career needs. Counseling should help her understand the existence of these conflicting needs. Research on counseling women has provided valuable insight and techniques for counselors in helping women attain greater autonomy and independence. Tiedt (1972) suggests that counselors be aware of this literature. For example, counselors may be able to provide female role models who have successfully dealt with specific issues of autonomy. They can recommend books about sex equality and in general help to educate women about new alternatives. Evans (1978) further suggests that one of the most difficult therapeutic tasks is coping with women's hostilities when they discover that they have been duped by being sex-role-stereotyped. However, this anger must be confronted and constructively dealt with in counseling.

The assumption of adult roles will cause some young women to question their values, their socialization process, and their future goals. Counseling can help women explore all avenues of growth. Berry (1972) suggests that counselors redefine what it means to be a woman. Through this redefinition young women clients will be aware of their potential and see new alternatives and possibilities. Because women are more apt to be socialized to remain dependent, some young women may forgo experiences that would enable them to become more independent during this period. Counselors who are aware of this developmental course will be able to actively seek ways to help their young-adult women clients develop a fuller sense of self.

For most young adults the twenties are a period of making choices about adult roles. I have given examples of some ambivalent feelings that women and men may experience which deal with self-esteem, identity, achievement, and autonomy. Although decisions may come only after much introspection and examination of values, most young adults do make at least a tentative commitment to careers and adult relationships. Counseling issues may revolve around career choice or inability to make a choice, relationships with others, and feelings about undertaking particular responsibilities. It is not uncommon during this period for young adults to try out various jobs and commitments or to drift aimlessly for a time. However, if one has not attained some degree of commitment and purpose by around age 30, one may have a strong sense of urgency to attain more stability and order. Our society is tolerant of some delay in

THE STATE OF THE UNION

What's it like to be an assistant director of student-union activities? You're asking me what it's like to be responsible for a fully functioning building that serves thousands of students from 8:00 in the morning to 1:00 the next morning. How can anyone describe the management and organizational details associated with a program of activities that range from disco dancing and lost and found to food services and bookstore and "hot lines"? Add to that the crises of student club, fraternity, sorority members when each one is certain the calamity of the century has just been imposed on him or her. And these are members of the university community. Imagine what it's like when all those "nonresidents" move onto the campus for their annual conferences. Are they patient when they can't locate, or don't find vacant, their assigned conference rooms, or living accommodations, or eating arrangements?

It's like no other work in the world. Where else would students bring you a pizza as an excuse for being able to discuss a roommate, academic, lover, parental, or loneliness problem? Who else can pack into one day up-to-date information on course work, professors' idiosyncrasies, rape, suicide, the pill, abortion clinics, financial aid, housing, parking tickets, social events, grade-point averages, registration policies, and lost property? Who else gets asked all these questions while keeping records, counting money, selling tickets, and being on call 24 hours a day?

The hours are a transgression against human dignity, and the pay is an additional indignity. But constant interaction with people who need and want help means you can get pretty tired of keeping someone else's spirits up and smiling all the time.

Would I like to do something else? Not on your life! What work has such variability or permits such versatility? What other work assigns so much responsibility or permits so much freedom? What other work provides so many opportunities to learn so much, do so much, or add so much to so many lives? Each and every budding young professional counselor interested in higher education should give careful thought to student-union involvement.

*—Assistant Director
    Student Union (Information Services)*

---

making adult commitments, but those adults who have not been able to do so may experience social pressures to find their niche. George, age 30, is experiencing this pressure. George has attended four colleges but still does not have a degree. His pattern is to "start well" the first semester; however, after a period of time interest will decline and grades will suffer, whereupon he will drop out of school and find a menial job. None of the jobs is satisfying, since George is bright. He was also reared in a professional family with high achievement expectations. After a while he will lose interest in the job, declare a new major, and return to school. Although George has had several close friends over the years, he has never married, since the type of woman who interests him has so far not been interested in marrying a man with such indefinite career plans. As the years pass, his father has become increasingly more critical of his lack of attainment of a career and other adult roles. His mother, however, makes excuses for his behavior and subtly undermines his confidence in himself by giving him money or by protecting him from his father. George must eventually confront who he is as an adult, and he feels that time is running out for making these decisions.

The Thirties Transition

Between the ages of 29 and 34, most adults are married, have begun a career, and are parents. Gould (1972) observes that at this time some inner doubts may emerge. During this period people may question the present course of their life. They begin to question the meaning of their life and may make some changes. For some adults these changes will be minor; for others the changes will be more drastic. For example, Sandy is 29 and single. Although she enjoyed being single in her twenties, she always thought that by 30 she would be married. She had rejected marriage proposals in the past; now she wishes the "right" man would enter her life. Lately she has become increasingly pessimistic about meeting this person and is considering continuing her education in the event that she will always have to provide for herself. Fred is facing a different decision. On receiving his degree in law he went to work for a prominent law firm, where he is supervised by a very ambitious man. Fred has modeled himself after this person and often works a 12-hour day. His wife complains about his absence, and he feels he can never relax because of the pressures of his job. He feels depressed at the thought of spending the rest of his life with so much stress. He has begun to ask himself what he really wants out of a career instead of what he feels he "should" do. Thus, as Gould (1972) notes, motivation during this period changes from "should" to "want." In order to answer this question, Fred will need to examine his values, goals, and relationships.

Settling Down

Once choices of the twenties have been reconsidered, and some changes made, most adults move into a period of settling down. Levinson notes that men begin to pursue long-range goals. Having made decisions about what is truly important, they are free to act on these choices. Family life is usually emphasized, along with community and occupational activities. This is usually a period of high productivity and ascension in careers. During the middle to late thirties, men may feel a need to be independent of authority and control. If a man has a "mentor"—an older person whom he has turned to for advice—he may reject him during this time.

Thus, during the thirties men are involved in establishing careers. Many men also have families. Because of changing sex roles, men may be asked to become more involved with their children. Moreland (1979) suggests that some men may feel that their wives' and children's demands for nurturance, support, and spontaneity may cause them to examine the meaning of masculinity.

During their thirties some women become aware of their need for independence. Frieze, Parsons, Johnson, Ruble, and Zellman (1978) point out that the increased autonomy during this period may cause feelings of guilt about rejecting children and husband. Some women may be attempting to reestablish careers or pursue further education. Counseling issues may center on vocational aspirations, study skills, financial problems, self-confidence, role definitions, child care, scheduling of classes if in school, and time pressures.

Moreland (1979) also points out that questioning the satisfaction of the wife and mother role is prevalent at this time. This questioning may result in feelings of low self-worth and self-directed anger. He suggests that the developmental counselor help the woman client reappraise her commitments and values and help her deal with her guilt and anger. He notes that women may need to be taught to accept their angry feelings, which many women have been taught to deny.

The expansion of women's roles beyond homemaker creates new opportunities for women to explore new and challenging aspects of life. In previous times larger family size and a short life expectancy made motherhood a full-time life experience. Today, with fewer children to rear, modern birth-control methods, and greater longevity, women have many productive years left to pursue other goals and ambitions. Yet, the new roles for women have created new issues as well. How does a woman manage a career, children, and household responsibilities? How does a woman get her husband to cooperate? How does she resolve personal feelings of guilt about leaving her children's care to others? How does she find time for personal interests outside of career and home responsibilities?

The Midlife Transition

In the late thirties or early forties most adults experience a midlife transition. As they realize that life is half over and that death is a reality, they feel a sense of urgency to make adjustments "before it's too late." Typical responses to the midlife transition are a questioning of values and goals, self-examination, and embracing new activities or relationships. Moreland (1979) observes that this transition is often more intense than earlier ones. He suggests that counselors recognize that abrupt and radical changes during this period still are within the normal range of human development and are not a sign of deep emotional disturbance or pathology.

Part of the midlife transition entails ownership of parts of the self that have been previously suppressed or rejected. Part of one's personality has been denied expression because of initial adult choices. Now people who are reflecting on their lives feel a need to express some of these dormant traits. Neugarten (1968) has noted that during this period men become more aware of the "feminine," or nurturant and emotional, aspects of their personality, whereas women express suppressed "masculine" attributes and have a stronger need for autonomy and achievement.

Individual responses to the midlife crisis vary. Scarf (1972), in a review of Levinson's research, notes that some men may divorce their wives, move to a new location, and start a radically different life-style. Others may perform poorly at work and have several extramarital affairs. Still others may feel upset and depressed but do nothing. For others midlife is a time of greater personal growth whereby bonds of intimacy are strengthened, relationships with children become more meaningful, and work offers a means of enhancing oneself.

Women, during the midlife transition, become more aware of their needs for achievement. It is now common for women to return to school to gain the skills necessary for a career. This growth toward greater independence often places strains on marriages. Coupled with the husband's questioning of appropriate life goals, it is not uncommon for marital issues to emerge, since the growth needs of both suggest that the marital relationship must change to meet new needs. Couples at midlife often describe their marriage and sex life as dull, boring, and routine. The very security for which the couples were striving in their thirties now becomes stifling to some.

As men reach midlife, feelings of depression, anger, anxiety, and apathy intensify, and the realization that certain goals have not been attained may cause what developmental experts call the midlife crisis. Counseling issues at this time will center on men's expectations of financial success, their concerns about physical decline, their role as a parent and a spouse, and the values on which they have based their lives. Levinson (1977) notes that at this time a man may wish his wife were more of a companion and less of a mother figure. This is the time when some men attempt to break out of their past molds by changing careers, spouses, and ways of living.

Men at this time, because of their nurturant and emotional needs, may wish to have closer relationships with family members. One dilemma some men may face is the fact that now that they wish to have a more intense relationship with their children, the children, who are now adolescents, are beginning to move away from their family and establish their own independence.

At the midlife transition women too are questioning their current life-style. Counselors in higher education settings are discovering more "reentry" women on campus. These women are approaching middle age and are making the transition from being a homemaker to being a career woman. For some the decision to pursue a career was a joint family decision; for others marital discord, including divorce or widowhood, was a catalyst for this change. Some women may have expected to always be homemakers and are shocked, outraged, and frightened about the new demands on them to be independent and autonomous. Their self-confidence may be low, they may lack self-esteem, and they may sometimes be overwhelmed by new role demands. If they are the sole provider for their family, they must find the strength and support to care for children, achieve in a career, and still have time for personal growth and relationships with other adults. Others, because of their mounting need to express their independence and autonomy, may have instigated the change themselves. Nevertheless, they too may need support in creating a workable daily routine that now includes not only child care and home responsibilities but skills for success in college. Newman (1979) stresses the need for counselors to recognize three areas of life that need to be balanced in order for women to plan their lives. First, the individual self needs to be explored. Attitudes about being a woman and acceptance of one's personal needs and desires must be clarified. Second, the self in life work should be examined. This includes career plans and aspirations outside the family. Third, whether married or single, the woman needs to be aware of her need for relationships with others. Communication skills and issues in relating to friends, children, spouses, and other family members need to be explored.

Middle Adulthood

The resolution of the midlife crisis brings about a period of greater calm and self-assurance. Studies show that those marriages that have survived the midlife reevaluation are higher in satisfaction. Sheehy (1976) observes that by their fifties couples have learned that respecting each other's privacy and still sharing many interests do not have to be exclusive. In contrast to the uncertainty of the early forties, at this period couples expect to grow old together.

As a result of the midlife reevaluation, some people also find that their newly found inner resources and strengths bring about a period of intense creativity coupled with a greater self-acceptance. A recent survey indicates that happiness increases dramatically beginning in the fifties through old age (Sheehy, 1979).

During middle age, roughly from 35 to 55, men and women reach the peak of productivity and exert their greatest influence on society. At the same time society makes the greatest demands on people during this period of life. For most people the middle years are quite busy, which may explain why some arrive at the end of this period with surprise that the journey is finished so quickly. Some specific issues and circumstances of middle-aged adults are enumerated below.

Biological Changes

Biological changes, which have been going on mostly unnoticed since early adulthood, become more pronounced between ages 35 and 55. For women, the greatest biological change is the menopause, which typically occurs over a period of years during the forties or fifties. For men, physical change may take the form of slowing down on strenuous forms of physical activity and some loss of physical skill. Sexual activity may decrease slightly after age 50 or 55, but both men and women may remain sexually active far into old age.

Achieving Generativity

During early adulthood maintaining a sense of intimacy was a major issue. Although one never ceases to explore interpersonal relationships, the early adult years should have provided opportunities for the person to discover his or her unique capacity for intimacy. This achievement of a sense of intimacy paves the way for the next stage of adult development: generativity versus stagnation. *Generativity* refers not only to procreating but to the course the individual pursues in making the world a better place in which to live. The adult who is achieving generativity hopes to make a personal impact in this life through her or his own productivity and creativity.

Each adult accepts or rejects this task of assisting future generations in attaining a more fulfilling life. If this task is rejected or if the person fails to achieve this sense of generativity altogether, "regression to an obsessive need for pseudo-intimacy takes place, often with a sense of stagnation and personal impoverishment" (Erikson, 1963, p. 167).

Other Issues of Middle Adulthood

Kimmel (1976) has identified three other crisis points in middle adult lives where counselors may intervene. These include late parenthood, coping with aging parents, and bereavement. He notes that near the end of parenthood several developmental issues converge at once. The mother may be in menopause. Further, she may be questioning how she will spend her remaining years now that her child-rearing responsibilities are ending. Issues of identity, wills, life plans, and goals must be resolved by both men and women. At this age health concerns may bring the realization that life left to live is decreasing. Moreover, job changes at this time are not readily or easily made. Kimmel further notes that people in the generativity period may be asking "What am I producing that will outlive me?" The generativity issue may cause parents to look for validation in their role as parents. If the adolescent children are having problems, the parents may feel a sense of failure. A major theme of this period is "Where did we go wrong?"

Coping with aging parents will bring on concerns of one's own fears and anxieties of death, infirmity, and inability to care for oneself. Kimmel suggests that the theme "I hate putting mother in there" may be voiced by adults who must make the difficult choice of caring for their parents in their own home or placing them in a nursing home. Counselors must help these clients deal with their feelings of anger, fear, and guilt.

The final counseling concern Kimmel describes is helping people deal with the discomfort and anxiety of the death of a close relative or friend. Kimmel notes that this developmental issue is so common that many bereaved persons do not seek counseling, and yet many benefits are derived from this experience.

This brief discussion of some specific counseling issues of adults should clarify how adult developmental issues may be the focus of counseling sessions. The counselor's awareness of these concerns, based on an in-depth understanding of the nature of adult development, will enable the counselor to assist the client at a particular stage of life. The adult client must be viewed in a developmental framework in order to understand specific issues and concerns.

Women and Men as Clients

Because of the socialization process and the differential treatment of men and women in our society, the sex of one's client is a most significant variable. Identity, self-esteem, achievement, self-expression, and autonomy will be differentially perceived by men and women. We have already seen how women may have ambivalent feelings about career achievement in early adulthood and how they are often middle-aged before they pursue a career outside the home. Men likewise have often been socialized to invest heavily in careers, even at the expense of their emotional and physical needs. Attitudes about being a client thus depend on one's sex.

The Male Client

In counseling males, perhaps the biggest hurdle is getting men to ask for help. Wong, Davey, and Conroe (1976) suggest that revealing weakness is something that males are taught not to do. Many men avoid counseling because they see asking for help as an admission of vulnerability. Indeed, counseling statistics show that more women seek counseling than men. It is essential that counselors educate men about the specific ways that men can benefit from counseling. In this manner, they can help men realize that seeking help when needed is a strength, not a weakness. The developmental view that counseling is for normal people who wish to understand the developmental process more fully can provide a framework in which seeking help is an opportunity to more fully realize one's potential as a human being.

Male clients also are believed to have some valuable attributes that the counselor can rely on in the counseling interview. Some of these qualities are identified by Scher (1979), who suggests that men tend to be emotionally clear. He suggests that a male client who cries is usually sincere, since males have not been socialized to use crying as a manipulative device. Because his seeking counseling may be viewed as a weakness, questions of pride and self-esteem should be explored. Further, since males are more apt to be achievement-oriented, the counselor can expect, in general, that the male client will have a need to have a productive session. Masculine needs for power, competition, and control must be addressed in the counseling interview. Finally, the exploration of the affective realm should make the client aware that his emotions are the cause of the difficulty, not his thoughts and cognitions.

Effective counseling will allow clients to explore all avenues of awareness. Wong et al. (1976) emphasize that counselors should loosen and open the constraints of the typical male stereotype by "expanding masculinity" or defining appropriate masculine behaviors more broadly. They observe that men have been conditioned to avoid making a 180-degree turn toward values previously labeled as feminine, but by defining the masculine role more flexibly, men will be able to take on values heretofore considered feminine. This endorsement is consistent with the earlier-described ability to be androgynous and thus able to live a fuller, richer life.

Yet, because men have learned to function in the cognitive domain (Marino, 1979), they are often defensive against being steered to the affective realm. Men preserve their self-image by ignoring their emotions, since this domain is frightening and anxiety-producing. Techniques to overcome this fear suggested by Marino include, first and foremost, the necessity for the counselor to stay out of the cognitive realm. Asking questions that promote giving explanations for behaviors only circumvents the therapeutic process, since the male client may give a very cogent, rational diagnosis of the issues and appear to have gained insight into his problem. Marino suggests that terminating counseling at this point will not allow men to explore their feelings, because thus far counseling has centered on the cognitive aspects of the issue. How does one get men in touch with feelings? By confronting men when they use an angry tone of voice when they feel hurt, discouraged, or rejected; by looking for other inconsistencies in behavior and feelings, such as becoming stiff and tight-faced when feeling frightened; by exploring the polarities of the need to be hard and in control versus feeling soft and unsure. Since in these explorations the counselor is asking male clients to show their vulnerabilities, any sign of discomfort in the counselor—either male or female—will stop this process of exploration. Another issue concerning women counselors is that of nurturing male clients to the extent that the counselor is too much involved in "helping" the client, so that he becomes dependent on her to solve his problem. Although initially this may be comforting, the client will resent it later. Women counselors should be aware of a female issue—that of "feeling worthwhile by taking care of males."

Women as Clients

As with men, sex-role stereotyping limits women's exploration of their full potential. Marecek and Kravetz (1977) observe that it is not uncommon for women to have a lower self-concept and self-esteem as a result of this traditional perspective. Institutional sexism may also create role conflicts for women. Another concern is the professional orientation of the counselor or therapist. Therapists who embrace the psychoanalytic viewpoint may do women a disservice. Marecek and Kravetz write: "Psychoanalysis is the major theoretical substrate for current clinical practice. Psychoanalytic theory specifies women's 'innate' nature as passive, dependent, and morally inferior to men's. Motherhood is seen as a universal requirement for female fulfillment, and the desire to bear a child is taken as a sign of mental health. Psychoanalytic theory is devaluating to females."

Counselors need to address these issues both as individuals who intervene into the lives of others and as members of a profession that promotes practices of helping people expand their awareness. We are being asked to question not only societal values but the very nature of our theoretical underpinnings, which have contributed much to our theories of personality and counseling.

Concern over the effect that therapists have on their women clients has compelled the American Psychological Association to form a task force to study sexism in therapy. A survey of women clients revealed four categories of sexist behaviors by therapists: (1) therapists foster traditional sex roles, or the belief that "woman's place is in the home;" (2) women clients are devalued by therapists, and therapists limit their expectations of women's potential; (3) therapists adhere to sexist use of psychoanalytic concepts; and (4) therapists respond to women as sex objects. Seduction of female clients is included in this category (Brodsky, Holroyd, Payton, Rubinstein, Rosenkrantz, Sherman, & Zell, 1978).

In a similar vein the American Personnel and Guidance Association has responded to this concern by producing a booklet to help counselors examine their attitudes, *For Women and for Men: Sex Equality in Counselor Education and Supervision*. These guidelines give counselors a clear outline of specific practices that are unhealthy for women and men as well. The developmental counselor will thus have as a tool a basic understanding of men's and women's development and particular issues that they are addressing.

Work Settings

Intervention strategies for adult counseling can be adapted to a variety of community agencies and higher educational settings. A brief description of these work settings is outlined.

Higher Education

The new emphasis on continuing education has expanded the age of the college population. Not only do young adults in their early twenties seek counseling, but in just as much demand are counselors for middle-aged adults. College counselors must be equipped to handle a wide variety of counseling concerns. These issues include problems with sexual identity, forming intimate relationships, career changes, crisis intervention, drug and alcohol problems, marital problems, and sexual dysfunction, as well as academically related topics of study skills, test anxiety, and strategies that enhance classroom performance. Counselors in college settings and agencies that serve young adults will encounter many sessions with themes concerning their struggle for independence. For example, Susan, a college junior having difficulty studying, came to counseling to improve her grades. An exploration of her choice of nursing as a career revealed that her parents had encouraged her to make this choice. She had decided that she would rather study commercial art, but her parents felt that she would be better able to support herself in a nursing career: "Nurses can always get jobs, but commercial art is so competitive, you might not be able to find a good job."

Scott had a different dilemma. He was shy but wanted to date. He felt uncomfortable in the presence of women but longed to be able to have a "normal" dating relationship. When he did ask a woman out, he spent the several days from the time he made the date feeling intense anxiety about the impending date. His attitudes about women and his sense of selfhood would require a number of counseling sessions.

The issues of older college students will often revolve around the integration of the study role with other adult roles. Older students may have fears about competition with younger students, whom they perceive as having more recent practice with study skills and effective learning.

Doris was 43 when she decided to return to school. Her choice was prompted by her recent divorce and her realization that her minimal job skills were not adequate to attain a job that would support herself and her two children. Before marriage Doris had completed two years of college with above-average grades. Yet, at her age, she wasn't sure how successful she would be in school; homemaking and child care had left little time for reading or other intellectual pursuits. She was terrified at the thought of how she would ever manage child care, classes, and the home.

Community Agencies

A wide variety of community mental-health agencies exist to meet various and specific needs of adults. Many communities have comprehensive community mental-health agencies that deliver a range of services. Although traditionally these agencies employed psychologists, social workers, and psychiatrists, the newer emphasis on developmental needs has created jobs for agency counselors. A new division of the American Personnel and Guidance Association has recently been added out of the need for agency counselors to have a professional milieu in which to organize and explore common concerns and interests.

The employment of agency counselors is still an emerging phenomenon. At this point it is necessary to prepare counselors who are cognizant of their unique contribution to the field of community mental health. In this vein the emphasis on training for intervention into the wide array of adult needs as outlined in this chapter is necessary. Some agency counselors may further wish to specialize in one aspect of adult concerns, such as marriage and family counseling, drug and alcohol abuse, rehabilitation counseling, employment counseling, or sex counseling. It is evident that this specialization will be undertaken within the framework of the spectrum of needs of adults, since specific concerns of adults also relate to their overall pattern of development.

Perspectives for the '80s

In this chapter I have explored the emerging field of developmental counseling for adults. As I have indicated, this area of knowledge is relatively new but rapidly expanding. Several factors in our society suggest that we are just on the threshold of a new and exciting specialty in counseling. Rapid changes in careers, the status of women, and the intense interest among the American population in self-fulfillment will certainly enhance this area of specialization.

The American public is eager to explore various means of attaining greater self-awareness and personal growth, as evident in the popularity of numerous group experiences designed to promote self-understanding, and through local community service programs. Parents want to know how to be effective with their children. Married couples want to learn better communication skills through enrichment programs. Women who have been out of the job market for years hope to have a career. These people seek counseling to make a better life for themselves. Professionals can help, and adults are ready to avail themselves of these services.

For the professional, a coming trend for the '80s is to specialize. Some counselors specialize in concerns of women, such as family planning, rape, or abused wives. Others focus on the college population and a broader range of problems. College counselors may also specialize in concerns of reentry women or career planning.

Whatever population the counselor of adults chooses, she or he must be familiar with the underlying developmental issues of adults at different ages. The counselor must certainly be cognizant of the issues of a particular population. One must therefore keep abreast of social changes. These developmental and social issues have an intense impact on the final decisions that adults make.

The emphasis on counseling for the attainment of better coping skills will be a major thrust of the '80s. People do not want to be labeled "mentally ill" when they have problems or when they desire to explore new facets of living, and consequently they will not want counselors or therapists who adhere to such a model. They will want competent counselors who can help them reach out, explore, and discover new meaning in their lives.

So where should counselors look for jobs counseling adults in the '80s? Certainly in higher educational settings. In addition, community service agencies will be expanding to include more needs of the adult population. Programs that sharpen adults' skills in communication and coping with daily issues will continue to thrive. Counselors who receive training in presenting such programs may find many opportunities to do so for businesses, for educational employees, and through community resources.

The concerns of adults are being recognized by organized institutions such as educational institutions, businesses, community agencies, and churches. They are now requesting counselors to give their patrons better skills for daily interactions. Our society is complex, and adults want to comprehend how all facets of their lives mesh with their evolving sense of self. Adults strive for mastery and competence, and counselors of adults have the tools to help people live fuller, more rewarding lives.

Summary

Adults seek counseling for help with adult role performance, to find or clarify values and meaning in their lives, and for the ability to relate in more intimate and meaningful ways with others. Counselors offer the means and structure for helping people develop their fullest capacities. The adult population is becoming more aware of the services that counselors offer, not to sick or mentally ill people, but to all who wish to live a more productive life.

The early and middle adult years are distinguished by a series of developmental issues. This period is a time of questioning previously made commitments, as well as exercising adult roles and responsibilities. The fact that people are living longer is causing them to reflect on the most productive or meaningful ways in which to spend the remainder of their lives. This process brings them to old age with a greater sense of self and confidence in their ability to cope with everyday living and to strive toward a productive life.

This chapter reviewed some specific developmental concerns of adults in early and middle adult life. It was noted that counselors who have a thorough understanding of these stages are better equipped to gain a perspective on appropriate intervention strategies. Also cited were some specific concerns of adult clients. It is hoped that this brief overview will give students a focus on the needs of this counseling population and will direct them toward the type of skills they need to attain to become an adult counselor.

Now It's Your Turn

1. *Identity and autonomy development*

    Describe the transition from adolescence to adulthood. How are the developmental issues of identity and autonomy experienced by the young adult? Give an example of an identity issue; an autonomy issue.

    How might males and females differ in their attainment of autonomy? Give examples.

2. *Age thirties transition*

    Describe the age thirties transition. What are some possible counseling issues at this time?

3. *Midlife transition*

    What are some dynamics of, or the impetus for, the midlife reevaluation? Why might some counselors who are unfamiliar with adult-development theory consider this time "pathological?"

4. *Adult development*

    Explain and give examples of how adulthood is more than living out the choices of an earlier time. How does social change affect people in their adult years? Give examples.

5. Choose one of the brief vignettes in this chapter. Describe the developmental issues of the person and indicate what counseling strategies and techniques you would use in this counseling session.

References

Berry, J. B. The new womanhood: Counselor alert. *Personnel and Guidance Journal,* 1972, *51*(2), 105-108.

Bocknek, G. A developmental approach to counseling adults. *Counseling Psychologist,* 1976, *6*(1), 37-40.

Brodsky, A. M., Holroyd, J., Payton, C. R., Rubinstein, E. A., Rosenkrantz, P., Sherman, J., & Zell, F. Guidelines for therapy with women: Task force on sex bias and sex role stereotyping in psychotherapeutic practice. *American Psychologist,* 1978, *33*(12), 1112-1113.

Erikson, E. H. *Childhood and society* (2nd ed.). New York: W. W. Norton, 1963.

Evans, D. A. Emerging truths on the psychology of women, as through a glass darkly. In L. Harmon, J. Birk, L. Fitzgerald, & M. Tanney (Eds.), *Counseling women.* Monterey, Calif.: Brooks/Cole, 1978.

Farrell, W. *The liberated man; beyond masculinity: Freeing men and their relationships with women.* New York: Random House, 1974.

Frieze, I. H., Parsons, J. E., Johnson, P. B., Ruble, D. N., & Zellman, G. L. *Women and sex roles: A social psychological perspective.* New York: W. W. Norton, 1978.

Gould, R. L. Adult life stages: Growth toward self tolerance. *Psychology Today,* 1975, *8*(9), 74-78.

Gould, R. L. The phase of adult life: A study in developmental psychology. *American Journal of Psychiatry,* 1972, *129*(5), 33-43.

Havighurst, R. J. *Developmental tasks and education.* New York: David McKay, 1972.

Hunt, M. *Sexual behavior in the 1970s.* New York: Dell, 1974.

Kaplan, H. S. *The new sex therapy.* New York: Brunner/Mazel, 1974.

Kimmel, D. C. Early and middle adulthood. In J. O. Lugo & G. L. Hershey (Eds.), *Human development: A multidisciplinary approach to the psychology of individual growth.* New York: Macmillan, 1974.

Kimmel, D. C. Adult development: Challenges for counseling. *Personnel and Guidance Journal,* 1976, *55*(3), 103-105.

Kirkpatrick, J. S. Human sexuality: A survey of what counselors need to know. *Counselor Education and Supervision,* 1980, *19*(4), 276-282.

Levinson, D. J. The mid-life transition: A period in adult psychosocial development. *Psychiatry,* 1977, *40*(2), 99-112.

Levinson, D. J., Darrow, C., Klein, E., Levinson, M., & McKee, B. Periods in the adult development of men: Ages 18-45. *Counseling Psychologist,* 1976, *6*, 21-25.

Levinson, D. J., Darrow, C., Klein, E., Levinson, M., & McKee, B. *The seasons of a man's life.* New York: Knopf, 1978.

Lowenthal, M. F., & Weiss, L. Intimacy and crisis in adulthood. *Counseling Psychologist,* 1976, *6*(1), 10-15.

Marecek, J., & Kravetz, D. Women and mental health: A review of feminist change efforts. *Psychiatry,* 1977, *40*(3), 323-328.

Marino, T. M. Resensitizing men: A male perspective. *Personnel and Guidance Journal,* 1979, *58*(2), 102-105.

Masters, W. H., & Johnson, V. E. *Human sexual inadequacy.* Boston: Little, Brown, 1970.

Moreland, J. R. Some implications of life-span development for counseling psychology. *Personnel and Guidance Journal,* 1979, *57*(6), 229-303.

Neugarten, B. L. (Ed.). *Middle age and aging.* Chicago: University of Chicago Press, 1968.

Newman, B. Beyond the total woman: Creative life planning to meet women's needs. *Personnel and Guidance Journal,* 1979, 57(7), 259–361.

Scarf, M. Husbands in crisis. *McCall's,* June, 1972, pp. 22–31.

Scher, M. On counseling men. *Personnel and Guidance Journal,* 1979, 57, 252–255.

Sheehy, G. *Passages: Predictable crises of adult life.* New York: E. P. Dutton, 1976.

Sheehy, G. The happiness report. *Redbook,* July, 1979, pp. 54–59; 210+.

Tiedt, S. M. Realistic counseling for high school girls. *School Counselor,* 1972, *19,* 354–356.

Vaillant, G. E., & McArthur, C. C. Natural history of male psychologic health: I. The adult life cycle from 18–50. *Seminars in Psychiatry,* 1972, 4(4), 415–427.

Williams, J. H. *Psychology of women.* New York: W. W. Norton, 1977.

Wong, M. R., Davey, J., & Conroe, R. Expanding masculinity: Counseling the male in transition. *Counseling Psychologist,* 1976, 6(3), 58–61.

Note: A good teaching aid for the early and middle adult years is a kit that includes two sound filmstrips, a teaching guide, and a game for exploration of the adult years. This kit is available from The Learning Seed Company, 145 Brentwood Drive, Palatine, Illinois 60067. Title: *Life Passages: Personal Growth beyond Adolescence.*

CHAPTER **12**

The Elderly

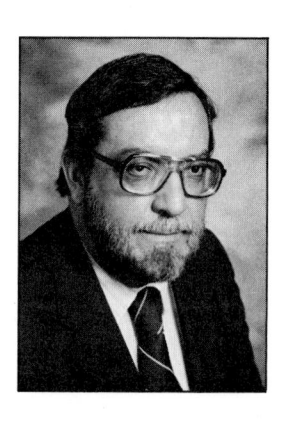

Paul Grobe
Paul Grobe is a rabbi in Asheville, North Carolina, and consultant to special projects in aging. He was a counselor educator and Community Health Professions faculty member at Old Dominion University. He had postdoctoral training in gerontology at the University of Michigan Institute of Gerontology and at the E. P. Andrus Center on Aging at the University of Southern California.

Widespread attention is currently being focused on the elderly throughout the United States. Much interest has been generated because of the increasing awareness of this most rapidly growing segment of the population (Butler, 1975). Numbering more than 23 million, the 65+ age group now forms about 11% of the population.

Because of concomitant biomedical, psychosocial, and economic concerns confronting the older person, it is inevitable that members of the counseling profession should be called upon to help the elderly, their families, and other health care providers. Yet, counselors currently find themselves inadequately prepared to offer appropriate assistance and hence are uncomfortable with, and tend to avoid, older persons in need as a potential client group.

Most established professional helpers share these concerns, perhaps because they, too, were educated at a time when formal training in gerontology was not available. Despite enrollment in colleges with established gerontology programs, they failed to see themselves as professionals who might someday be engaged in providing for the biomedical and pscyhosocial needs of the elderly. Yet, medical and psychosocial health care providers continue to report increasing numbers of older persons among their caseloads and patient loads.

Much has been done to eliminate or significantly reduce infantile mortality and the effects of early childhood diseases, thereby extending the quantity of life. However, a great deal more remains to be achieved in order to provide professional helpers with the knowledge base and the set of experiences required to enhance the quality of life for those extended years.

It is the purpose of this chapter to provide counselors and other health care professionals with an explanation of the effects of stereotyping, expectancy phenomena, and the associated myths of aging both on the professionals who work with the elderly and on the elderly themselves. The special concerns and needs of the aged will also be examined, as will training implications for those who prepare to offer counseling to them. It seems clear that, for the 1980s and beyond, emphasis in gerontological research will have to shift its focus from adding years to life to adding life to the remaining years.

Stereotyping, Expectancy, and Learned Helplessness

Because of detectable losses and decline in function related to old age, the expectancy phenomenon and the related concept of learned helplessness exert a powerful influence on the behavior of the elderly, who are viewed by society and themselves as less autonomous and hence as less worthy.

Stereotyping

Social stereotyping occurs when the mind casts about for a strategy to deal with the unfamiliar. An unfamiliar person with characteristics similar to those of a known group will come to be regarded as if he were indeed a group member. The quality of universality and/or homogeneity is a myth attributed to all groups who are targets of prejudice, and the elderly are no exception. Prejudice against the elderly may be referred to as ageism.

Senescence as a developmental stage contains the widest range (that is, ages 60–100) by far of all developmental age groupings. In addition to their varying ages, older people differ by sex, race, religion, national origin, socioeconomics, level of education, and level of well-being. And although the vast majority of older persons have had the opportunity to achieve certain common developmental tasks and to share common experiences (for example, marriage, employment, parenthood, grandparenthood, retirement, divorce, death of spouse), many have accomplished these at varying ages and locations. Thus, even if the experiences of individuals are similar to those of the group, the net effect of those experiences is different for each individual.

The critical point in social stereotyping is that the bias of categorizing persons into one group or another is not found only in the selectively prejudiced; rather, it is said to be universal and often involuntary and to be due to the very nature of the perceptual process. Krech, Crutchfield & Egerton (1962) described stereotyping as a sort of concept formation: "The properties of an object (person) are determined in large measure by the properties of the system of which it is a part (p. 32)." The expectancy phenomenon is a significant aspect of stereotyping.

The Expectancy Phenomenon

In addition to the "mind set" associated with stereotyping are the concomitant preconceived notions or related expectancies. The concept of expectancy effect or phenomenon as a determinant of educational outcomes has received much attention since Rosenthal and Jacobson's studies (1968a, 1968b) became known. Rosenthal and Jacobson postulated that teachers' biases about the abilities of students resulted in differential treatment, which influenced student achievement. By anticipating that the evaluated person will behave congruently with the held expectancy (the preconceived or biased assessment), the evaluator not only predicts but engages in behavior to ensure the fulfillment of the prediction (Finn, 1974), thus establishing a "self-fulfilling prophecy."

More pertinent to the older client populations are the findings of three separate but related studies in which patients' reports of symptom reduction in psychotherapeutic settings were significantly related to their expectations of improvement (Goldstein & Shipman, 1961; Goldstein, 1960; Friedman, 1963). The persuasive and contributing influences of stereotyping and its major component, expectancy, to the self-concept of the person have been documented (Finn, 1970). It is said that often certain aspects of the held expectancy tend to be incorporated into the self-concept and function as self-regulating mechanisms biasing the person's behavior in the direction of the preconceived assessment. Because of impending losses in autonomy due to declines in health, meaningful roles, economics, and so on, the effects of negative stereotyping on the aging are regarded as even more potent contributors to declines in self-esteem and related behaviors than for younger groups.

Learned Helplessness

Perhaps one of the most significant derivatives of negative stereotyping and expectancy as it relates to the elderly is the phenomenon of learned helplessness. As reviewed and discussed by Seligman (1975), "learned helplessness" postulates that as a person undergoes a series of events of which he has no control over the outcome (that is, he sees no relation between effort and desired change in surroundings or goal attainment), his behavior becomes debilitated, curtailed, and passive. Persistence is reduced, and performance deficits occur even for tasks at which the person was initially competent.

This is essentially what is observed among the institutionalized elderly. The increasing declines in health, memory, and meaningful roles experienced by older persons are often regarded by them and their counselors as predictive of incompetence leading to helplessness. The fact that, for more than 80% of the elderly, impairments do not restrict performance of the daily tasks of living is often ignored. Decompetence, or a decline in competence, is regarded as incompetence, and this negative expectation is projected. Especially in institutions and agencies, and often in the community at large, the elderly come to believe that they cannot produce desirable outcomes by their actions.

Real or perceived loss of autonomy propels the cycle of regression. In essence, older persons are taught to become helpless by the expectancy that they should. Because stereotyping and its derivative phenomena, expectancy and learned helplessness, are almost unavoidable and exert significantly more potent influence on those most vulnerable (for example, the aging, the handicapped), it is crucial for counselors to maintain a consistent level of alertness to, and awarenss of, the effects of stereotyping to which even the most well-intentioned are susceptible.

Arriving at old age has allowed the elderly an opportunity to accumulate many and varying experiences; hence, gerontologists have identified the elderly as the group with the most variance or heterogeneity (Birren & Woodruff, 1975). Biomedical, psychosocial, and socioeconomic stereotypes attributing negative characteristics to the elderly as a group abound. Selected illustrative examples are presented below.

Biomedical Myths

The most prominent among the biological and medical myths of aging are poor health and sexual incompetence. These two characteristics will be discussed from the perspective of the myth attributed to all target groups of prejudice, that of homogeneity.

The Myth of Poor Health

The elderly as a group are noted for more frequent physician visits, for longer durations of hospitalization, and for spending a larger percentage of their income on medications, but it would not be valid to assume they are in poor health. Although almost all the elderly have some chronic or degenerative disease (for example, cardiovascular-renal, cancer, diabetes, arthritis), 80% or more remain relatively free of restriction in performing their daily activities. An additional 10% require some assistance, and only 10% are either institutionalized or homebound and significantly impeded and dependent with regard to their daily activities (Weg, 1976).

Unless the elderly possess what Burnside (1975) has characterized as the "accoutrements of age" (for example, being crippled, having cataracts, wearing glasses), they will most often be ignored as elderly and "pass" as members of the middle-aged group. It is estimated that, before death occurs, 20 to 30% of the aged will have spent some time in an institution, such as a nursing home or residence for the mentally impaired. But despite their impairments, the vast majority of the elderly are active, alert, and able to function independently.

The Myth of Sexual Incompetence

Contrary to widely held opinions, it is untrue that all elderly persons are sexually incompetent. This myth of sexual incompetence may have derived from the fact that some of the elderly (for example, male diabetics and women experiencing senile vaginitis) are either impotent or too discomforted to engage in sexual intercourse. In addition, the attitudes held by a society glorifying youth and denigrating the old may contribute to the psychological decompetence associated with sexual behavior. Many elderly people have incorporated the societal view that gratifications associated with sexual fulfillment are primarily for the young, but research indicates that, barring illness or trauma, and with adequate nutrition and appropriate self-esteem, sexual interest and activity may extend for many well into the eighth decade of life (Masters & Johnson, 1966).

Refractory periods for males are extended with age, and men require more time and stimulation to achieve erection and ejaculation, but they remain quite capable of experiencing coitus, albeit less frequently than in earlier years. Women remain potentially capable of multiple orgasmic activity into old age and, except for irritation resulting from reduced lubrication, could continue to enjoy coitus indefinitely if partners were available. Unfortunately, there are more than one-third more women than men at age 65 and even more than two-thirds more women than men at age 75. It is reported that in the absence of the traditional partner there is an increased tendency to masturbate or engage in homosexual relationships. It needs to be stressed that, despite the incompetence of some elderly people to engage in sexual intercourse, very few are impeded from engaging in related sexual, sensual, and gratifying behaviors, which include touching, stroking, and caressing, as well as expressions of loving, caring, cherishing, and valuing.

Psychosocial Myths

Within the psychological domain, the two stereotypes most generally held are associated with the intellectual capacity of the elderly. It is generally believed not only that intellectual deterioration is inevitable but also that learning ability declines with age. Sociologically, the remarriage of the elderly is frowned on. All three of these are the subject of the following discussion.

Myth: Intellectual Deterioration Is Inevitable

Although the actual numbers of neurons (neurological cells) in a brain have not been determined, Busse (1977) estimated that as many as 20 billion neurons can be found in the central nervous system (CNS) at age 30. The concept of reserve is nowhere demonstrated more dramatically than in the CNS, for while neurons, which do not regenerate, are lost at the rate of .8% per year after age 30, our capacity to function intellectually is not impaired. Empirical evidence on intellectual decline is at best quite complex and contradictory and can be summarized in the words of Eisdorfer (1977): "Long term longitudinal investigations of middle aged and aged persons raise doubts about validity of any simple hypothesis that there is progressive, generalized loss of intellectual and training ability in all older persons" [p. 237].

Major problems in relating intelligence to aging include the following. (1) Comparing an individual's level of intellectual ability with herself over time (that is, longitudinal studies) may yield different results than comparing old persons with those younger (that is, cohort studies or cross-sectional research). (2) The role of physical or emotional illness in affecting cognitive behavior must be considered. (3) Present concepts of the nature of intelligence need to be clarified. Data suggest that the intelligence of most persons remains constant until at least age 70, except for those who show what Riegel, Riegel, and Meyer (1968) have called "terminal drops" signaling significant decline in physiologic integrity or imminent death.

Some worthwhile cautions to be observed are these: (1) Analysis based on superior as well as low-scoring subjects cannot be generalized to the average older person. (2) In studying the performance of older people on intelligence tests, it must be remembered that more than 2 million elderly are functionally illiterate, 12% had less than five years of schooling, and 32% completed only secondary school. Hence, the elderly received predictably lower scores on group tests of intelligence, which are more oriented toward younger persons at higher levels of education. It would seem likely that, in comparing the average older person with himself over time, crystallized intelligence (including such abilities as verbal meaning, numerical skill, and habits of logical reasoning) does not decline until the seventh decade and then only modestly. Fluid abilities of intelligence—

such as logical reasoning, association memory, and figural relations—reveal more decline with age (Cattell & Horn, 1967).

Myth: Learning Ability Declines

"You can't teach an old dog new tricks" is the folkloristic philosophy that pervades the attitudes not only of the young but also of many elderly people themselves. Botwinick (1967) defined learning as the acquisition of information or skills measured by an improvement in some overt response. Gerontological research has not yet elaborated a formal theory to account for age-related differences in learning. Although some research indicates that learning ability seems to decline in later life (Arenberg & Robertson-Tachabo, 1977), there is no conclusive evidence to suggest a great deal of change in that capacity. Though learning less rapidly than younger subjects, older adults can learn effectively and show little change in their ability to carry out cognitively demanding tasks. Knowles (1970) characterized adult learning as andragogy (as opposed to pedagogy) and mentioned motivation, self-management, relevancy, goal perception, and comfortable learning environments as conditions vital to the enhancement of lifelong learning. The andragogic approach to learning implies the continued capacity for the older person to continue to learn. Further, it emphasizes the capability of the older learner to design and control his own educational experience. The instructor is regarded more as a helping or resource person rather than as a dispenser of information. Adult education continues as the fastest-growing sector of the educational enterprise. With research indicating that the older person retains his potential and ability to learn and relearn, the pursuit of learning throughout one's life is becoming a more valid and valued lifelong activity.

Myth: Remarriage Is a Mistake

The basic family unit in old age is the marital pair; among persons 65 and older, 53% are married (Riley & Foner, 1968). One of the major role changes affecting husband/wife relations is the death of a spouse. Because women tend to outlive men by more than eight years, the role of widow is much more likely to occur than that of widower. A related trend is the emergence of more retirement marriages. The vast majority of these later marriages follow widowhood rather than divorce. In studying more than 100 retirement marriages, McKain (1969) suggested factors that predisposed toward the more successful remarriage. He found that persons who knew each other well, had the approval of their adult children, had coped with disengagement, had a stable income, and particularly were homeowners were more likely to have successful marriages. McKain also identified personality as crucial and predictive of remarriage success.

The myth of mistaken remarriage is often derived from the rigidity of expectations of the elderly person's adult offspring. Some children of the elderly announced they were shocked at their parents' remarriage plans, while in other cases fear of losing an inheritance was a factor. Some children's disapproval related more to a distorted notion that remarriage was an act of disloyalty or an insult to the memory of the deceased parent. Adult children who had assumed the role of caregiver to their parent also expressed realistic concerns about providing for the health care and related support services for yet another old person, the new spouse. McKain concluded that the negative attitudes of adult offspring probably inhibit the success of remarriage and further prevent a large number of retirement marriages.

Socioeconomic Myths

Perhaps the most tragic of the myths associated with the elderly are those stereotypes that influence their socioeconomic status and well-being. As a consequence of aging, people are believed to (1) be unproductive, (2) be in their golden years, and (3) have few needs. The following discussion examines these myths.

The Myth of Nonproductivity

A society that arbitrarily mandates retirement or economic unproductivity based on age and then proceeds to stereotype that age group as unproductive could be viewed as cynical or at best confused. In addition, retirement usually means eligibility for Social Security income, which is penalized if a retiree chooses to be more than allowably productive. Despite only scant research to support assumptions about emotional, cognitive, and temperamental declines in capacities related to job performance, many negative stereotypes serve to create resistant hiring attitudes among employers, in addition to undermining the confidence of the older worker. The Bureau of Labor Statistics research findings have consistently challenged the notion that older workers are less consistent or accurate than their younger colleagues. Older workers are not only more likely to remain on the job and experience lower absenteeism, they are also less likely to incur job-related injuries (Hendricks & Hendricks, 1977).

Despite discouragement and penalty, the Bureau of Labor Statistics reported in 1977 that more than 3 million persons over 65 were in the labor force in full- or part-time employment. Of this number almost 2 million were men, with more than 1 million women also employed (Hendricks & Hendricks, 1977). It has been speculated that the actual number of employed elderly people is at least double the reported number. Those failing to report are seeking to avoid the financial penalty imposed on allowable earnings with Social Security.

In addition to the reportedly employed elderly, who constitute almost 15% of the 65+ group, vast numbers of older persons are engaged in voluntary or contributive services to the community or the family. Retired Senior Volunteer Programs, Service Corps of Retired Executives, Green Thumb, and Foster Grandparents are some examples of federally sponsored programs through which the elderly express their contributive productivity. Further, many elderly people contribute services to churches, family agencies, and public schools. And it is not unusual for the 65+ to accept the responsibility of caring for octogenarian parents while still contributing aid as babysitters or offering assistance at crisis times in the families of their adult children.

In observing productivity of the elderly, one is cautioned to consider social policy constraints (for example, retirement) that inhibit productivity, as well as the lack of pertinent facilities (for example, transportation). Despite the physical and psychological decrements experienced by many elderly people and despite discouragement and financial penalty, it may be concluded that a significant number of older persons are engaged in contributive altruistic and volunteer services, while at least 15% are reportedly employed. The removal of arbitrary retirement restrictions augurs well for the increase of the elderly among those whom society regards as productive.

The Myth of the Golden Years

It is interesting that conflicting guiding fictions or mythical stereotypes and expectancies can be held simultaneously. Projecting a positive stereotype on the background of ageism may be required from time to time by a society that sometimes consciously but more often unconsciously seeks to deny its punitive aspects. Further, seeing the elderly as being in the golden years of their lives may protect many who are increasingly confronted with the painful aspects of their own mortality. More cynically, the "golden years" myth provides a youth-oriented society with the rationalization that the stated needs of the elderly have been addressed sufficiently with current and existing programs.

Despite technological advances, growth in the humane elements of responding to basic survival needs (such as food, shelter, and health care) lags behind. The "golden years" myth seeks to deny the physiological and emotional decompetence and deficits experienced by the older person. The need to believe in a serene senescence overlooks the loss of roles related to vocation and family. These personal losses are not only multiple but also quite often successive and hence cumulative, so as to impede the grieving process required for adjustment. Some older people never overcome the effects of reactive depression associated with consecutive losses.

Despite cost-of-living adjustments in Social Security, Supplemental Security Income (SSI), Medicare, Medicaid, and other income and health maintenance programs, almost 50% of older persons are living at or below the poverty levels. The "golden years of their lives" is a projection that applies only to those who have income sufficient to maintain a standard of living similar to that of their preretirement years and who, in addition, enjoy a state of physical, emotional, and social well-being.

The Myth That Their Needs Are Few

"Their needs are few," like the "golden age" myth, is a reflection of a life-satisfaction image projected by a youth-oriented, "ageistic" society experiencing intermittent guilt and pain as it grows older itself. Surveys have reported that financial security is a major factor for preretirees in experiencing a sense of personal autonomy and independence. Yet, social policy has focused on transferring control of individuals' lives from themselves to the public without adequate financial commitment or time to develop and implement programs responsive to basic survival needs. Society has ignored the pride of self-determination found in the older generation and has instead fostered a dependency of retired and older persons on community determination for their general well-being.

Upon retiring, income reductions for individuals and families range from 50 to 65%. Yet, despite their eligibility, only 10% of Social Security recipients come forward to claim Supplemental Security Income or other public assistance benefits—this despite government estimates that more than 65% of those receiving Social Security benefits are trying to live on incomes less than minimum as established by federal agencies (Atchley, 1977). It is at best cynical to suggest that because a group is mandatorily pauperized (that is, retired), it requires less for basic survival and life satisfaction.

Old age does not obviate the basic needs for survival—for example, shelter, food, health care, and clothing. In an urban couple's income, shelter accounts for an average of 35%, food for 33%, and clothing and personal care for an average of 8%. Health care as a percentage of income is difficult to determine; however, per capita health care expenditures indicate that older persons (who compose only 10% of the population) spend more than three times as much as those under 65. In 1975 almost 50% of all older noninstitutionalized elderly were either poor or marginally poor (Bureau of Labor Statistics). Although the total number of poor is decreasing, the aged poor account for one half of the poor of all ages and compose a slowly increasing proportion of the population. "One's needs are few when one's income is low" is perhaps the most appropriate image projected by the elderly, who, as a group, remain strong in their commitment to the ethic of individual responsibility and self-help. Pride in self-management may be the last bastion of declining self-esteem.

Self-defeating behaviors over time generally develop into self-destructive behaviors. Although intervention may inhibit, if not deter, the final outcome for those younger, the elderly are more vulnerable because they experience the most negative expectancies over a shorter time frame, thus making it difficult, if not impossible, to recoup losses.

I have explicated the myths of ageism to raise the level of awareness of counselors and other health care providers that stereotypes often influence and guide us without our awareness. They are also utilized consciously. They constrict attitudes and behaviors and, when projected as negative expectancies, tend to lead the client to the self-fulfilling prophecies of hopelessness and helplessness.

Implications for Counseling Older Adults

The elderly are a variegated population whose particular needs and concerns warrant the attention of counselors and other helping professionals. The decline of school enrollments, taken together with the rapid and continuing increase of the elderly in addition to the heightened social awareness of the needs of special groups, makes the potential service opportunities for counselors with older people seem logical and meaningful as well as humane. When facts about the life conditions of older people are added to the facts of the numbers of people and families involved, the needs for counseling seem obvious.

The age of retirement correlates with the emergence, almost simultaneously, of a number of biomedical, psychosocial, and socioeconomic losses, all of which combine to shrink the environment and curtail the interpersonal relationships of older persons. The elderly are affected more often than any other age group by accumulated grief and related depressions, occurring simultaneously or at best consecutively over a short time frame. Surviving into old age virtually ensures that a person will experience stress related to adaptation and change associated with certain developmental life transitions. Hence, in addition to understanding psychosocial aspects of aging and related helping skills, counselors for the 1980s and beyond will require knowledge about such developmental life events as retirement, dying and bereavement, remarriage, diminished sexuality and health, and institutionalization.

Retirement

The impact of retirement on life-style, attitude toward life, and sense of personhood is so significant that the necessity for thoughtful preparation is compelling. Yet, preretirement programs are few and at best cursory. To confuse the issue further, attitudes toward retirement support the concept that the elderly as a group reveal more heterogeneity than homogeneity. Atchley (1977) indicated that those among the elderly with higher job status, greater income, and more education are generally also in better health and are reluctant to consider retirement. Hence, they avoid information and programs related to this threatening or denigrating life event. Those on the lower end of the job status (mechanized labor), often with lower income and less education, view retirement as beyond their control and therefore see no need to engage in efforts that they perceive as beyond their ability to plan. It is regrettable that the vast majority of those in the labor force, many of whom would be most benefited, are the least likely to engage in appropriate planning and continue to resist it. Only those in the middle-income group are most willing participants in preretirement education and planning.

Addressing the variant needs of men and of women from upper, middle, and lower income brackets in programs pertinent to their interests is another obstacle to appropriate planning.

Counselors who are sensitive to the grieving process associated with separation from work roles and career roles, in addition to anxiety related to unknown future prospects, could do much to acquaint the older man or woman with new roles such as volunteerism or new careers (that is, rehirement). Much could be done to facilitate a worthy adaptation to the last stage of human development.

Physical and Emotional Decompetence

Planning for physical and emotional wellness should occur throughout life. It is probable that, with heightened social awareness about the effects of alcohol, tobacco, lack of exercise, and so on, increasing emphasis will be placed on prevention of impairment and disease rather than on *post facto* intervention. Despite the irreversibility of many chronic ailments that accompany a person into old age (for example, coronary heart disease, hypertension, diabetes, arthritis), health counseling, which would include nutrition, physical fitness, and stress-management strategies, could do much to prevent exacerbation as well as improve the related physical and emotional status of the older person.

Mental health has since its inception been the domain of the more clinical professional—for example, the psychiatrist and psychologist. Unfortunately, the mental-health needs of older clients have been largely ignored. Butler (1973) indicated that while a small number of older persons could benefit from psychiatric intervention, a more significant number could derive improvements with such strategies as life review, reminiscence, and supportive counseling during reactive depressions (to encourage release of feelings related to such losses as those associated with retirement, loss of income, role reversal, separation, illness, and death). Although intense analysis with emphasis on intrapsychic forces might not often be required, counselors for the 1980s and beyond cannot ignore requirements for additional training related to life review and supportive counseling.

Dying

The care of terminally ill persons is incomplete without counseling the dying persons as well as their survivors. Advances in medical technology have changed the nature and the causes of death. Hence dying and death have become more dramatically associated with aging and related diseases. The time span of dying has been extended, increasing concomitantly the duration of pain, fear, family trauma, and uncertainty. Society's negative attitude toward the elderly, accompanied by its inability to deal with persons who anticipate a limited future, has compounded the difficulty of dealing with death.

Counselors may witness the daily deterioration of a person beset by pain and emotional distress in addition to related family crises and upheaval. Many of the difficulties experienced by the dying person related to the continued conception of death as a biomedical rather than a psychosocial event. The avoidance of the terminally ill person by traditional health care providers and the conspiratorial conversations usually held by them with family members increase dying persons' heightened sense of aloneness and declining control over themselves.

The accelerated development of the hospice, as a distinct institution, as a unit within a hospital, or as a home-service concept, responds to the need of the terminal person to carry out the activities of daily life while he continues to die. Being in control of one's pain management, deciding where to die, constructing a funeral service to one's own liking, choosing cremation or burial are all choices that, if exercised, allow the dying person to maintain control and hence dignity. Hospitals, hospices, and the homes of the elderly who are dying will be the counseling settings for many in the 1980s. Sensitivity to facilitating choices for the dying older person is a requirement for those who would counsel them and their survivors.

Marriage and Remarriage

Historically, even as late as the early 1930s, marriages terminated by the death of the spouse, often by the time the first child left home. First marriages thus lasted no more than perhaps 18–20 years. The extension of life expectancy at birth brought with it at first a corresponding extension of marital years. However, the envisioned fantasy of the constant companionship of the retired partner did not always materialize. Work, for some spouses, legitimized their avoidance of intimacy and their failure to care and share. In addition, the communication skills absent during the working years rarely, if ever, appear full-blown upon retirement.

Being together in later life confronts many surviving couples with boredom, friction, anger, and frustration. Although an increasing number of marriages survive because of extended life expectancy, divorce after

25-30 years of marriage is on the rise. Counseling couples in midlife and old age must focus on such dimensions as the use of leisure time and possibilities of reemployment, in addition to the long-established areas of concern related to sexuality and communication.

Second marriages in later life are not uncommon. According to a recent census, more than 53% of the elderly are married. Most men (75%) 65+ are married (Gabe, 1981). Contrary to the May-December myth, men who remarry tend to marry someone of the same age or only somewhat younger (U.S. Bureau of Census, 1975a). Most women (62½%) are widowed, divorced, or otherwise single (Gabe, 1981). Problems related to remarriage may develop from unique concerns. Some emerge when idealized memories of former spouses are compared, often unfavorably, with the newest spouse. The sudden development of chronic or crippling illness of a new spouse may also contribute problems to a second marriage. In addition, adult offspring may provoke discord because the new spouse is seen as replacing a deceased mother or father. The new spouse may also be regarded jealously by adult offspring who now see their surviving parent "lavishing" attention on a stranger who may also share an inheritance that is seen as belonging in the family. Counseling for the 1980s and beyond will call for knowledge about relating to older couples who remain married or remarry and to their adult offspring and about the special concerns associated with this stage of marital development or status.

Sex and Sexuality

It is important to recognize that because of their socialization, many elderly people are not very comfortable in talking to anyone, let alone younger persons, about such private matters as sexuality. Yet the desire for sexual relations is a natural response at any age, and coitus remains a natural function for many into their eighth decade and beyond (Masters & Johnson, 1966; Burnside, 1975). Sexual relations are rather restricted when they are limited to coitus. In its broad sense sexuality includes holding, touching, caressing, stroking, kissing, embracing, making romantic, affectionate, and admiring remarks, and other aspects of intimacy. Very often the older person is unaware of his or her own physiology. In addition to knowledge about the psychology and physiology of sexual development, counselors need training and understanding in values clarification so that they can come to grips with their own sexuality and be comfortable in discussing sex with others. Further, the counselor needs to become an advocate on behalf of the older person, dispelling myths related to ageism, including the myth of sexual impotence.

Institutionalization

Older people apply to or are placed in extended-care facilities (that is, nursing homes) for at least three reasons: (1) physical or mental deterioration, (2) inability or unwillingness of family or friends to provide (or most often to continue to provide) necessary care, or (3) inability of the current system of services to assure independent living (Tobin and Lieberman, 1976). Although some alternatives to institutionalization, such as home health aides, adult day care, and friendly visitors, do exist in many communities, the most frequently utilized alternatives are daughters and daughters-in-law. It should be emphasized that the vast majority of the institutionalized elderly are not simply dumped into nursing homes. Very often institutionalization occurs because financial as well as emotional resources have been stretched to the breaking point and survival of the last caregivers (the adult offspring and their families) becomes critical.

Since nursing homes exist for persons who can no longer function independently (that is, perform the required activities of daily living), they are often viewed as the last alternative. These feelings are reinforced by the reports that 85% of those entering nursing homes die there—one-half within three years and one-half after three years (Butler, 1975).

Despite its negative view of the elderly, society yet holds the unrealistic expectation that all families should be able to care for their own. Where families find themselves unable to comply with society's expectation as well as their own, they feel shame, guilt, and anger. The older person also feels rejected, abandoned, and isolated. Frequently he or she strikes out in rage and anger at visitors, who experience guilt added to that generated by the decision to institutionalize.

Counselors for the elderly could assist nursing-home staff in developing orientation and other group meetings for adult family members where feelings of guilt and shame could be discharged and where a more appropriate understanding of a family's ability to care for the impaired older person could be developed. In addition, it should be noted that communication skills for the very impaired include touching, speaking slowly and clearly, placing oneself so that the person can view facial expressions, and a willingness to be directive in conversation so as to avoid unnecessary rambling. In counseling the institutionalized elderly, health care professionals should have resolved problems with their own elderly relatives and should have confronted their own potential frailty. To be effective for the older person, the counselor needs to be available to family members who will be dealing with the feelings of their older family member as well as their own feelings.

Adaptations to Retirement: Life Enhancement

Separation from the work force (retirement) often correlates with critical life events that include losses and declines in biopsychosocial well-being associated with lowered self-esteem. However, the corresponding freedom from work roles and related stresses provides time and opportunities for more than 80% of the elderly (that is, those functionally independent) to engage in life-enhancement strategies that can be used as buffers against negative feelings and attitudes of worthlessness associated with declines and losses. An examination of the related literature suggests at least three major life-enhancement areas that deserve attention: leisure, education, and rehirement.

Leisure

Among the alternatives facing the new retiree are continuing employment, doing nothing (which often leads to deterioration), and engaging in leisure activities. Leisure is not a new concept. The Greeks and Romans observed contemplation, rest, and recreation as significant aspects of leisure. The Chinese raised leisure to a status equivalent with the gift of immortality. While these ancient cultures relegated leisure to the aristocrats and philosophers of that day, the Hebrew scriptures attributed leisure even to the Divine, who rested on the seventh day and ordained one day weekly for rest and recreation for all who labored. Despite these early teachings, the Puritan work ethic, which still obtains, interprets leisure to mean nonproductiveness and idleness leading to sin.

Leisure counseling and advisement is complicated not only by heterogeneity of the elderly as a group but also by disagreement among authorities over what activities should be included. Kaplan (1979) includes physical, social, intellectual, mass media, spiritual, civic, esthetic, and touristic activities as related to leisure pursuits. Physical activities (for example, games and sports) and touristic activities (for example, vacations) have been defined as recreational and have been separated from leisure by Atchley (1976). In addition, leisure has been related to vocational enhancement activities (for example, reading scientific papers) or vocational compensatory activities (for example, yoga, jogging).

Unconditional leisure activities (Kelly, 1972) and autonomous leisure activities (Grobe, 1979) have been identified as those most pertinent to the retired elderly in that they are freely chosen and are totally unrelated to job or vocation. Unconditional, or autonomous, leisure can become the means by which older persons begin to regain and maintain self-esteem, self-control, social status, and confidence. Leisure thus can be not only life-enhancing but also preventive of maladaptive attitudes and behaviors such as alcoholism, abuse of medications, and suicide.

Engaging in leisure requires planning and preparation. Counselors will find it useful to learn about the Avocational Activities Inventory (Overs, Taylor, & Adkins, 1977), which organizes leisure into nine major categories: (1) games, (2) sports, (3) nature, (4) collections, (5) crafts, (6) art and music, (7) educational, entertainment, and cultural activities, (8) volunteerism, and (9) organization. The older person's finances, transportation, and past experiences are critical factors in interest and leisure-activity selection. Leisure has the potential to enrich the later years with meaningful and pleasurable activities and to provide the older person

SOMETHING OLD, SOMETHING NEW

Pastors have been counseling people in trouble during all of human history. We stand in a long tradition as caring persons in our society. In the last 20 years, some 2000-plus pastors have sought special designation by their denominations, by the American Association of Pastoral Counselors, by the Association for Clinical Pastoral Education, and by licensure to work full-time seeing individuals, couples, families, and groups in the counseling relationship.

The process of professional certification is long; the satisfactions are tremendous. After graduation from college, all pastoral counselors have secured a graduate degree in theology, some years of professional pastoral experience, a year of clincial internship in a hospital, and two years of supervision in a pastoral counseling center. Only after this training can they practice unsupervised. Usually this training period includes an extensive (two years) and intensive experience in personal psychotherapy. Pastoral counselors stand in the tradition of ministry—community caregivers. Accordingly, referrals come most often from other pastors. The pastoral counselor respects the religious dimension of the person seeking help, functions nonjudgmentally, and encourages self-definition, exploration, and decision making. As such, the counselor is a professional friend—a person of integrity and a caring partner in the pilgrimage of life.

Pastoral counselors generally see normal people with normal problems of living. Areas of expertise include grief, dying, guilt, self-confidence, depression, anxiety, marital conflicts, family communication, scrupulosity, and reason for being. As pastoral persons, we welcome the opportunity to look at religious dimensions of living in addition to other human concerns. The counseling session is not a time for religious persuasion in any direction but an opportunity to appreciate the whole person—physical, emotional, and spiritual. As such, we work closely with physicians for the body, with counselors and other psychologically oriented professionals for the mind, and with priests, rabbis, and ministers for the faith. We like our work and find real satisfaction in demonstrating love and empathy by being with individuals for tender moments as they travel through this very brief, once-lived life.

—A Pastoral Counselor

---

with a sense of reward for fulfilling the responsibilities of citizenship and family. The counselor for the 1980s will find it useful to review also Leisure: Lifestyle and Lifespan (Kaplan, 1979).

Education

Education for older adults has been regarded by some as only one among many categories of leisure. Yet many regard formal and nonformal learning as much more than leisure. Lifelong learning by adults may be essential to the well-being of society and the individual. It is for this reason that this chapter considers education as a life-enhancing strategy independent of leisure.

A national survey in 1974 showed that 5% of those between 55 and 64 and 2% of persons 65 and over were enrolled in educational institutions or were taking a course of some kind. Yet adults learn in varied settings—some solely educational (for example, schools, universities) or other settings (for example, churches, synagogues, hospitals, museums, libraries, industrial firms, labor unions) or at home with or without mass media. No systematic knowledge is currently available concerning participation of older adults in this varied range of settings.

A major question relates to the folkloristic mythology of the older person's ability to learn. The relation between laboratory studies and everyday learning has not been established. Even when declines in intellectual abilities are observed, learning by older persons may not be significantly affected because they can often reorganize their activities to compensate for or minimize declines.

Lack of education as well as obsolescence of much of their schooling may dispose the elderly to ignore educational opportunities. Level of formal education is significantly related to level of educational participation in adulthood. Because level of education has been increasing dramatically since the 1940s in the population at large, participation of the elderly in formal schooling is expected to increase in the 1980s and beyond. Studies show that those who have been educationally active suffer less decline in learning competence with age. Apparently learning skills can be established or renewed in old age.

The educational needs of the elderly have been categorized by McCluskey (1971). He lists four major areas:

1. *Coping needs:* Educational programs responding to social adjustment, psychological health, and physical well-being. Curricular subjects responding to coping needs include adult basic education, health education, income maintenance, legal arrangements, housing choices, family adjustment, and successful use of leisure.
2. *Expressive needs:* These include learning activities that are engaged in for intrinsic meaning and pleasure. Curricular programs responding to expressive needs include physical education, liberal education, and personal enrichment programs such as hobbies (for example, painting, photography).
3. *Contributive needs:* Programming in this area encourages the older person to repay society for the generosities he has experienced in the past. Curricula are offered through in-service training in leadership and community awareness education.
4. *Influence needs:* Education in this area responds to needs of the elderly to affect the direction and quality of their own lives (that is, to maintain control over their destiny as far as possible). Training in this area is approached through civic and political organizations. This is accompan-

ied by educational or in-service programs for leadership, community action, and problem solving (Peterson, 1971).

Counselors to the elderly not only should focus on the known competencies and needs of a long-neglected clientele but should assist in coordinating and consulting with adult educators and the elderly themselves in developing and implementing programs essential to the growth, development, and maintenance of the older person.

Knowles (1970) documented not only that the aged retain learning competencies but, moreover, that they learn best when they are involved in managing and implementing their own learning. To this date some modest efforts (for example, tuition reduction or omission) have been initiated. In addition, emphasis on opportunities for learning by the elderly is illustrated by such ongoing programs as the Institute for Retired Persons, New York; Institute for Post Retirement Studies, Cleveland; Institute for Continued Training, San Diego; and Institute for Lifelong Learning, Los Angeles.

One of the newest ideas in education for elderly retirees is the Elderhostel. The concept, in week-long units, includes study in noncredit courses, hostel-style accomodations in dormitories, meals in college dining halls, and participation in ongoing campus life. With the level of formal education increasing dramatically, the future participation of old people in educational pursuits is expected to increase steadily. Counselors for the 1980s and beyond may well be engaged in advising and guiding older students through such programs or curricula, addressing the various needs referred to by McCluskey. In addition, many older persons may use their free time to pursue a degree for its own worth or to engage in educational opportunities to explore and to enter new occupations.

Rehirement (Reemployment)

In recent decades retirement from work at age 65 or below had been a growing trend. Various studies indicate that labor-force participation by those 65 and over during the period 1950–1970 declined by 31% (Fisher, 1975). Retirement by age 65 was caused in part by the adoption of 65 by business, government, and unions as the "usual" (mandatory) age. Further, 65 was the age when full Social Security benefits became available. The incremental increase in benefits, as well as the extension of coverage to almost all of the working population, was influential in accelerating retirement trends in recent years. Even though Congress raised mandatory retirement to age 70 in 1978, the average retirement age continues to be about age 62.

Despite the increase in benefits, more than 30% of those over 65 recalled they had been forced out. When probed further about their regrets in retirement, many indicated the loss of friends and feelings of uselessness. But the overwhelming loss for many (35% of the men and 27% of the women) was money.

White-collar workers in middle management who traditionally retire to engage in recreational pursuits or hobbies are, according to *Business Week* (August 20, 1979), starting to have second thoughts about leaving the work force. Because the promise of people being able to retire in their early to mid-sixties is much less viable in the current and in the anticipated inflationary economy, an increasing number of older Americans are concluding that rehirement into a new career combines the best elements of retirement and continued full employment.

A second career may well involve a new field of interest and the use of skills different from those developed in previous employment. The options are almost as numerous as those seeking new careers. While real estate and motor, radio, or television repair are the new career choices of a majority, some are turning to painting, graphics, photography, teaching, professional singing. In many cases "rehirement" is in an interest area that had been cultivated before retirement.

Industry is responding to this growing need. IBM, through its Retirement Education Assistance Plan, provides potential retirees and their spouses $2500 each in tuition assitance for the three years prior to and the two years following retirement. Other large companies are responding in a similar way. A 1978 study by a social research institute found that 46% of middle- and upper-level management retirees work at some point after they retire.

The growing demand for second careers is currently turning senior-citizen job placement into a booming business. The rise in the number of elderly job applicants varies across the country, but it is estimated to range between 33 and 60% in recent years.

Rehirement into new careers often requires fewer hours of work and less interference with private life. Thus, second careers provide the supplemental income that is essential as inflation continues without infringing excessively on the extra leisure time traditionally the goal of retirement. Counselors for the 1980s and beyond may well find themselves interpreting personality checklists and interest tests to the senior as well as seasoned client.

The Psalmist (Psalm 90:12) reflects on the wise use of time in order to obtain wisdom. Life-enhancement strategies for the appropriate use of leisure activities, education, or reemployment could do much to improve feelings of self-worth, health, and financial status in addition to adding life to the gift of extended years.

Perspectives for the '80s

The increase in the number of aged citizens in our society will be matched by an increase in their problems unless a commitment is made to address them. Unfortunately for many of our aging citizens, the trend is not toward expanded social welfare services. The same economic factors, especially inflation, that restrict real-dollar public funds available to address the problems of our senior citizens present special problems for this large group who must continue to exist on low fixed incomes.

The costs of medical services continue to lead in inflation, and many elderly people have inadequate insurance coverage to close the Medicare gap. In fact, a large number who have problems related to aging do not qualify for Medicare. To catalogue the other rising costs, such as energy, that present special problems for the elderly would be only to restate the obvious.

The same economic factors that may cause many workers to continue past the typical traditional retirement age may force employers to press workers whose productivity slips to retire. Even workers who are financially prepared for retirement may find that they are not mentally prepared for their new life. Retirement planning will become a necessity as the choices faced by the senior worker become more complex.

Another serious issue of concern to many aging persons is quality of life. No one looks forward to completing her years in the typical nursing-care facility. Even those facilities that provide adequate physical care often fail to provide psychological maintenance other than a TV set to help their clients "kill time." However, the typical American family is not set up so that even a semidependent relative can be accepted into the household without major trauma. As the number of two-income families grows with inflation, the opportunity for older persons to be cared for in a home environment decreases.

The issue of helping the elderly cope with the ultimate reality of death will face the counselor who chooses to work with this group. The interest in the hospice movement demonstrates our rejection of the sterile, impersonal hospital passing for those who can avoid such an end of life.

On a more positive note, the increasing educational and recreational outlets available to senior citizens will require that someone provide information about the choices available and help choices be wisely made.

Professional counselors who work with the elderly in the '80s and beyond will need to assume a number of roles. Counselors will need to be *resource persons,* who can provide information and direction to clients in the areas of rehirement, second careers, and educational opportunities as well as methods of getting basic needs met. This will require counselor familiarity with the resources of the community and with current public policy. Counselors will need to be *planners of programs* and *educators* to work with the elderly themselves as well as the larger community. These counselor functions can facilitate understanding and awareness of developmental needs and reduce stereotyping and other negative forms of ageism, in addition to generating possible solutions to existing problems. Counselors will need to be *trainers,* who provide the skills to prepare the elderly for life changes while helping them maintain their own individual competence and productivity. Finally, counselors will need to be *counselors* for the elderly and their families. Counseling will provide the necessary support for the inevitable transitions that accompany aging.

Summary

Gerontological perspectives on counseling the elderly have been presented. The elderly, who compose 11% of the population at large, are also its most rapidly increasing segment. Associated chronic diseases and related psychosocial and economic declines and losses experienced by older persons make it inevitable that they will become a significant client group for counselors.

Aging can be defined from chronological, psychosocial, and biological perspectives and is an interactive as well as a multivariate process. Despite chronic ailments and gradual declines in system integrity (decompetence), the vast majority of elderly people remain relatively unrestricted in performing their daily activities.

The myths of aging or negative stereotyping include the phenomena of expectancy and learned helplessness, which exacerbate self-defeating and self-destructive behaviors. In this chapter these myths were refuted and were more appropriately interpreted in relation to research rather than folklore.

Critical life events coinciding with retirement include declines in health and sexuality, remarriage, institutionalization, and bereavement. The life-enhancement adaptations of leisure, education, and rehirement (reemployment) are vital areas for counselors to engage in with their older clients.

Knowledge of traditional counseling as illustrated by Rogers (1961) and Carkhuff (1979), enhanced by formal training in gerontology, and knowledge of and skills in accessing pertinent community resources are basic to maximizing the benefits of retirement and ameliorating despair, depression, and behaviors shown by clients in crisis.

In helping the older client, counselors will require flexibility in attitudes in addition to innovative use of existing knowledge and skills so as to more effectively respond to the heterogeneous needs of society's oldest but newest client group, the elderly.

Now It's Your Turn

1. *Dying*

A health-education-agency counselor who had been visiting a patient in a proprietary nursing home learned that his client, Herman, was expected to die shortly. In visiting that patient, the counselor, an older person himself, determined that Herman was not fully aware of his condition and his impending death. He had received little or no information about his health status and at best was confused. Although family and friends had not yet been informed, Herman's belongings had already been packed in anticipation of his death. How would you expect the counselor to proceed, building on the rapport he had already established with Herman?

1. Discuss the procedures you would follow in helping Herman to learn about his condition.
2. Whom else might you call on?
3. How would you as a counselor follow through once Herman was made aware of his condition?
   a. with Herman
   b. with family
   c. with staff

2. Retirement

Jack is 62 years old. He has been a high-powered executive at the Miniflex Company for more than 20 years. A new president was brought into the company and has indicated it would be a good idea, what with pension benefits and other fringes, for Jack to take early retirement. Jack becomes despondent, begins to drink, takes sleeping medication, and becomes depressed. His work suffers. Jack has been referred to you as the company's personnel counselor. You have known Jack for several years, and so to some extent basic foundations for rapport already exist. In what kinds of ways can you be helpful?

1. Encourage Jack to take his money and run?
2. Explore feelings of loss and separation from job role?
3. Explore what these feelings mean in relation to self-esteem, to family, to wife?
4. Discuss at a later date various leisure activities?
5. Determine interests or need in relation to continued employment, new employment, and so on?
6. What other activities would you use to explore Jack's needs?

3. Institutionalization

You have been involved with the Jones family as a family-service-agency counselor. Mrs. Jones, 78 years of age and widowed, has been living with her unmarried daughter, Sally, for the past eight years. Other adult children come and visit occasionally and offer some assistance, but by and large, the single daughter is the major caregiver to her mother, in addition to working as a full-time secretary. Since her last birthday, Mrs. Jones has manifested many symptoms of disorientation in time, place, and person. Her daughter has become concerned about leaving her alone for fear she will fall, turn on the gas forgetfully, or go wandering aimlessly in the neighborhood, as she has done several times in the past. The family cannot pay to have a full-time caretaker, and institutionalization is being considered. Although Sally's resources, emotional and financial, have been stretched to the breaking point, she feels a great deal of guilt in considering the idea of putting her mother away, especially since Mrs. Jones refuses to consider it and accuses Sally of wanting her to die. There are potentially two clients. How would you facilitate?

1. Which is the true client? Why?
2. What would you do to establish rapport?
3. Are there other alternatives to consider?
4. How would you go about finding them?
5. If institutionalization is agreed on, to what extent would Mrs. Jones be involved in the decision?
6. What kinds of things could be done to calm Mrs. Jones' fears and relieve Sally's guilt?

4. *Divorce*

I'm feeling distressed. My wife and I have been separated for six months—this after she found out I had a girlfriend at the office. Because of my age, 60, and the length of our marriage, she believes that this was not a single occurrence and that she'll never be able to trust me again. With the encouragement of our daughter, she moved to New York into her home. She refuses to talk to me. My daughter, with whom I never really got along too well, refuses to communicate also. I am sorry. I want my wife back. I want my old life back as it was. My wife expects me to support her but won't even talk to me. I feel sad, powerless, and angry and don't know what to do.

1. Define the problem(s) presented.
2. What are the issues involved?
3. What questions would you like to ask?
4. What are some possible topics for discussion?
5. What are the feelings you would explore?

References

Arenberg, D., & Robertson-Tachabo, E. A. Learning and aging. In J. E. Birren & K. W. Schaie (Eds.), *Handbook of psychology of aging.* New York: Van Nostrand Reinhold, 1977.

Atchley, R. *Sociology of retirement.* New York: Wiley, 1976.

Atchley, R. Retirement: Continuity or crisis. In R. Kaish (Ed.), *The later years.* Belmont, Calif.: Wadsworth, 1977.

Bengston, V. *The social psychology of aging.* New York: Bobbs-Merrill, 1973.

Birren, J., & Woodruff, D. (Eds.) *Aging: Scientific perspectives and social issues.* New York: D. Van Nostrand, 1975.

Botwinick, J. *Cognitive processes in maturity and old age.* New York: Springer, 1967.

Burnside, I. M. *Psychosocial nursing care of the aged* (2nd ed.). New York: McGraw-Hill, 1980.

Burnside, I. M. (Ed.). *Sexuality and aging.* Los Angeles: Andrus Gerontology Center, University of Southern California, 1975.

Busse, E. Theories of aging. In E. Busse & E. Pfeiffer (Eds.), *Behavior and adaptation in late life.* Boston: Little, Brown, 1977.

Butler, R. N. *Sex after 60.* In L. Brown & E. Ellis (Eds.), *The Later Years.* Acton, Mass.: Publishing Sciences, 1975a.

Butler, R. N. *Why survive: Being old in America.* New York: Harper & Row, 1975b.

Butler, R. N., & Lewis, M. I. *Aging and mental health: Positive psychological approaches* (2nd ed.). St. Louis: C. V. Mosby, 1977.

Carkhuff, R. *The skills of helping.* Amherst, Mass.: Human Resource Development Press, 1979.

Cattell, R. B., & Horn, J. Age differences in fluid and crystalized intelligence. *AcTa Psychologica,* 1967, 26(2), 107-129.

Eisdorfer, C. Intelligence and cognitive changes in the aged. In E. W. Busse & E. Pfeiffer (Eds.). *Behavior and adaptation in late life.* Boston: Little, Brown, 1977.

Finn, J. The educational environment: Expectations. Paper presented to American Educational Research Association, Minneapolis, March 1970.

Finn, J. Expectations and the educational environment. *Review of Educational Research,* 1974, 42, 3.

Fisher, P. Labor force participation of the aged and the social security system in nine countries. *Industrial Gerontology,* 1975, 2(1), 1-13.

Friedman, H. J. Patient expectancy and symptom reduction. *Archives of General Psychiatry,* 1963, 8(1), 61-67.

Gabe, T. *Social characteristics and economic status of U.S. age population* (Congressional Research Service Publication (L.O.C.), Report No. 81-32 ETW). Washington D. C.: U. S. Government Printing Office, 1981.

Goldstein, A. P. Patient's expectancies and non-specific therapy as a basis for symptom reduction. *Journal of Clinical Psychology,* 1960, 16(4), 399-403.

Goldstein, A. P., & Shipman, W. C. Patient expectancies, symptom reduction and aspects of the initial psychoterapeutic interview. *Journal of Clinical Psychology,* 1961, 17(2), 129-133.

Grobe, P. *Preretirement education.* Paper presented at the Norfolk Housing Authority Seminar, Norfolk, Va., Winter 1979.

Hendricks, J. & Hendricks, C. *Aging in mass society.* Cambridge, Mass.: Winthrop Publishers, 1977.

Kaplan, M. *Leisure: Lifestyle and lifespan.* Philadelphia: Saunders, 1979.

Kelly, J. R. Work and leisure: A simplified paradigm. *Journal of Leisure Research,* 1972, 4(1), 50-62.

Knowles, M. *The modern practice of adult education: Andragogy versus pedagogy.* New York: Association Press, 1970.

Krech, D., Crutchfield, R. S., & Egerton, L. B. *Individual in society.* New York: McGraw-Hill, 1962.

Masters, W., & Johnson, V. *Human sexual response.* Boston: Little, Brown, 1966.

McCluskey, H. *Education: Background and issues.* White House Conference on Aging. Washington, D. C.: U. S. Government Printing Office, 1971.

McKain, W. *Retirement marriage.* Storrs: University of Connecticut, 1969.

Neugarten, B., Moore, J. W., & Lowe, J. C. Age norms, age constraints and adult socialization. *American Journal of Sociology,* 1965, 70, 710-717.

Overs, R., Taylor, S., & Adkins, C. *Avocational counseling manual* (Rev.). Washington, D. C.: Hawkins and Associates, 1977.

Peterson, D. A. Education and the older American. *Adult Leadership,* 1971, *19,* 263.

Riegel, K. F., Riegel, R. M., & Meyer, G. A study of dropout rates in longitudinal research and aging and prediction of death. In B. L. Neugarten (Ed.). *Middle age and aging.* Chicago: University of Chicago Press, 1968.

Riley, M. R., & Foner, A. *Aging and society.* New York: Russell Sage Foundation, 1968.

Rogers, C. R. *On becoming a person.* Boston: Houghton Mifflin, 1961.

Rosenthal, R., & Jacobson, L. F. *Pygmalion in the classroom.* New York: Holt, Rinehart and Winston, 1968a.

Rosenthal, R., & Jacobson, L. F. Teacher expectations for the disadvantaged. *Scientific American,* 1968b, *218*(16), 19–23.

Seligman, M. E. P. *Helplessness: On depression, development, and death.* San Francisco: W. H. Freeman, 1975.

Tobin, S., & Lieberman, M. A. *Last home for the aged: Critical implications of institutionalization.* San Francisco: Jossey-Bass, 1976.

Weg, R. Changing physiology and aging. In R. H. Davis (Ed.), *Aging: Prospects and issues.* Los Angeles: Andrus Gerontology Center, University of Southern California, 1976.

CHAPTER **13**

Special Populations

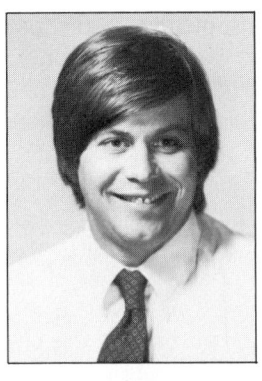

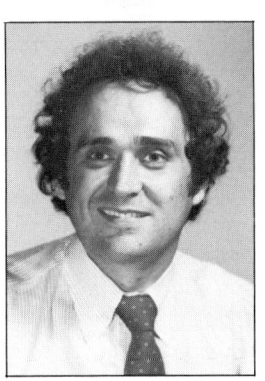

Charles F. Gressard
Keith R. Hume

Charles F. Gressard is an assistant professor in the Counselor Education Department at the University of Virginia. After graduating from the University of Iowa, he worked as a rehabilitation counselor in Ohio and then worked with drug addicts and alcoholics in the Boston area. He also taught in the Rehabilitation Counseling Program at the State University of New York at Buffalo before assuming his teaching responsibilities in rehabilitation counseling and substance abuse at the University of Virginia.

Keith R. Hume is a clinical psychologist currently specializing in drug and alcohol rehabilitation. He has lectured extensively in the fields of mental health and rehabilitation and has provided numerous workshops for both professionals and nonprofessionals. Currently he is director of clinical services at MountainWood Ltd., a residential drug and alcohol treatment program in Charlottesville, Virginia.

Although the process of counseling is usually associated with the "normal" person, counselors in all settings frequently encounter persons who deviate somehow from the norm. This is increasingly so as more students are mainstreamed and as institutions of higher education and buildings in other settings become more accessible to those with disabilities. In addition to these factors, more counselors are choosing to work in noneducational settings in which those who are labeled as deviant are more likely to be encountered. These are counselors who work in mental health, drug and alcohol abuse, rehabilitation, corrections, and other community agencies.

For these reasons, it is becoming more important for counselors to be aware of the particular problems and capabilities of these "special" populations. It is also important for counselors to be aware that those who differ from the norm can benefit from the services of the counselor. Although counselors have traditionally been defined as those who work with normal populations, they need to remember that many members of "deviant" populations aspire to normality and wish to have lives similar to the rest of the population and deal with the same developmental patterns. Those classified as different encounter the same developmental, social, and career problems as the rest of the population and consequently will require counseling services. Even psychiatric populations, which have traditionally been served by psychologists and psychiatrists, need assistance from the counselor near the end of therapy to adjust back to a normal routine of daily living.

We can understand, then, that all persons, regardless of disability, lifestyle, or difficulty, can benefit from the counselor's expertise if they aspire to reach their full potential and work, live, and play in our society. Therefore, counselors must have an understanding of the particular difficulties of special populations and of the ways they can be of assistance to persons in such classifications. It is the purpose of this chapter to give you an introduction to the issues of special populations that are relevant to the counselor and to explore how the counselor might work with special populations.

Deviance

All the individuals included under the term *special populations*—that is, those with physical disabilities, alcoholics, drug abusers, offenders, and so on—have in common the fact that they are somehow labeled by the rest of society as deviant. This labeling of deviance and the resulting implications are some of the main barriers to full participation by these individuals in society, and accordingly deviance is a concept that should be understood by those in the field of counseling.

Reactions of Society

To understand deviance and its implications, one must look at how society reacts to people who somehow deviate from the norm. Perhaps the best way to identify this reaction would be to say that those who deviate from the norm are *stigmatized* (Goffman, 1963). Goffman defined a stigma as an attribute that is deeply discrediting and taints the person's identity in a particular society.

Society's definition of stigma is a reflection of the values of the society at that point in time. If you look at what has been stigmatizing through history, the resulting list seems quite diverse and rather arbitrary. This can be seen in our own lives. Look at what has been stigmatizing to you. The facial blemish that may have caused a person anguish and embarrassment as an adolescent does not create much of a problem in later years, and the behavior or dress that may have been the norm in adolescence might be quite stigmatizing as an adult.

What is perhaps most important for the counselor to be aware of in working with persons who may be classified as deviant or stigmatized is the reaction of society to those persons. Throughout history all societies and cultures have had varied reactions to those who somehow deviate from the norm. Wolfensberger (1972) listed the following categories in which the disabled, retarded, and mentally ill have been placed:

- A subhuman organism
- A menace
- An unspeakable object of dread
- An object of pity
- A holy innocent
- A diseased organism
- An object of ridicule
- An eternal child

All these attitudes still exist in varied amounts today and help shape the reactions of society toward those in these deviant subgroups.

Although these responses are quite diverse, the common threat that ties them together is that society attempts to maintain the difference between normals and "deviants." All these responses tend to keep the ones who are different at a distance, either psychologically or physically, from the mainstream of society. We seem to feel more comfortable when deviants are furthest from us. An example of this response can be seen today whenever any kind of residence for a deviant group is proposed for a neighborhood. It makes little difference whether the proposed residents are alcoholics, offenders, the retarded, or the disabled. There is usually strong opposition among those in the area to the establishment of such a residence.

This reaction seems to be the common thread that connects those labeled as deviant. Reflect on your own feelings when you encounter someone who is visibly different. Most of us at some point, when encountering such a person, feel somewhat uneasy and try to avoid that person if possible. It is this feeling of discomfort when encountering someone who somehow deviates from social norms that seems to motivate society to isolate such persons.

Several theories have been proposed to explain this discomfort. Some have postulated a neuropsychological theory for our reaction to those with disabilities. Yamamoto (1971) hypothesized that those who are different disrupt our rituals of normal interaction. There are also socioeconomic and psychoanalytic theories for this reaction. Whatever the reasons, the effect is the same: those who are different are often isolated, institutionalized, and abandoned by the rest of society.

Reactions of the Stigmatized

The effects of the isolation of these special populations are spelled out in Goffman's book *Stigma* (1963). Goffman notes that those who find themselves, by virtue of their difference, stigmatized by society have few options, none of which are optimal. One choice is to withdraw and accept the limitations imposed on them by society. Another is to band together with those who have a similar stigma and reject the rest of society as society has rejected them. A third is for the stigmatized to take responsibility for interactions and assertively try to make others feel at ease through humor or downplaying their stigmatizing characteristic. A fourth option, if the stigma is not clearly visible, is to try to "pass," or hide the stigmatizing characteristic from others. Unfortunately, all these options have attendant pressures or disadvantages. Even the assertive approach, which Goffman believes is most often prescribed by professionals and helpers, leads only to, at best, a phantom acceptance. Phantom acceptance occurs when a person with a stigma can, through various strategies, become involved with normals but learns that there are limits to this interaction. For example, a crowd might tolerate a person with a disability attending a dance but might get quite upset should the person attempt to become involved in the activity of dancing. In other words, people are accepted as long as they stay within certain limits.

We can see that the social burden of those who are different in society is heavy. Because of this burden, it is important that counselors be trained to help people deal with the causes and effects of differentness. We need to remember that differentness and stigma are common to all of us. Who has not encountered the time when she stood out in a crowd or felt the pain of differentness during adolescence? The state of being special, different, or stigmatized is a universal human experience, and counselors generally encounter many differing categories of people who have been classified as "special." It would be impossible to discuss the characteristics of all these populations, and so only the largest and most common of the "special" populations will be examined. These are the physically disabled and retarded, alcoholics, other substance abusers, and offenders.

Physically Disabled and Retarded

Many of the difficulties of the physically disabled and retarded stem from the attitudes of society already discussed. However, both have unique problems beyond the stigmatizing effects of their condition. For the physically disabled, the functional limitations such as the inability to walk or the absence of motor coordination are certainly limitations that have to be dealt with. However, the person's own psychological reactions to the disability are perhaps even more limiting and are the ones of most concern to the counselor.

One of the most common reactions to disability is what Wright (1960) termed "as if" behavior. "As if" behavior occurs when someone with a disability idolizes the normal standards for appearance and function and therefore tries to appear normal at all costs. Examples of this type of behavior would be a person with a missing leg or some other type of gait problem attempting to walk without a cane, crutches, or other aids, or a person with a missing arm wearing a cosmetic artificial hand even though it is less functional than some other type of device. The difficulty of this type of attitude is that the person may be so concerned with appearing normal that he never becomes aware of what his actual capabilities are, thus eclipsing some of his behavioral potential.

Another common reaction to disability is overcompensation. You are probably aware of stories about people with a disability who have compensated in some way to become heroic or outstanding in some respect. Although these efforts are to be admired, whether the person involved really achieved a positive adjustment to the disability might be questioned. Overcompensating behaviors can serve as a constant reminder of the disability. While engaging in compensating activities, the person may be constantly aware of the disability and its negative meaning to her. This not only will create stress for her but may preclude the possibility of exploring other areas of competence and interest. The overcompensation becomes an obsession, which makes an acceptance of the disability very difficult. We certainly are not implying that people with disabilities should not aspire to great heights. There would be no more justification to imply this for the population of individuals with disabilities than there would be for an able-bodied population. However, when the aspiration relates only to the effects of the disability, there may often be a problem with full acceptance of the disability.

A third common reaction to disability is what Wright termed "spread." Spread is the process of extending the negative feelings about the particular disability to the rest of one's being. In other words, the person feels that because he has a disability, he is no longer a worthwhile person in any respect. Examples are males who lose a limb or the functioning of a limb and therefore feel that they are no longer "men" or some people with disabilities who feel that they no longer deserve to live or be loved. This failure to confine the effects of the disability to the actual loss of functioning can lead to a loss of motivation and depression.

A fourth common reaction to disability is responding to the disability in a succumbing mode. When people react in a succumbing mode, they tend to see only the things they cannot do rather than those they are able to do. This is a common reaction for all of us. When we run into a barrier to achieving a goal, we often see only that barrier for a period of time, rather than all the other options that we have left. The negative implications of this behavior are obvious. As long as we are in this mode of thinking, we cannot explore options that may lead to alternative routes to achieving our goals. Succumbing to the effects of disability is closely related to the reactions of compensation and spread.

The last negative reaction to disability is mourning. This reaction to loss is common to most of us when we lose something of value or someone who is close to us. Many (Kerr, 1961; Wright, 1960; McDaniel, 1976) believe that there are stages of mourning, such as shock, anger, guilt, denial, and depression, through which we must pass before we can fully adjust to the loss. Although there is disagreement on what exactly the stages are and whether everyone must pass through all the stages, it does seem clear that those who have disabilities often go through a stage of mourning, which must be resolved before they can begin to respond more positively to the disability.

This list of psychological difficulties in adjusting to disability is not exhaustive, nor do we imply that these occur in every case. The list should, however, give the reader some idea of the difficulties encountered by those with disabilities.

In many ways the psychological problems of persons classified as retarded are similar to those of the physically disabled. The problems revolve around an inferior status in society and the problem of self-image. Particularly important is the concept of spread. Because people encounter problems in one sector of their life, they feel that they are inferior in all areas of their life. As a result, a common reaction to retardation is passivity and a low self-concept.

Other problems center on the family. Overprotection or rejection of a retarded person often leads to problems in adapting to society. Overprotected persons will not have the opportunity to discover what they are capable of doing, and rejected persons will not have the support to fully develop their capabilities as human beings.

SPECIAL IS VERY SPECIAL

Counselors who work with handicapped persons have to help them learn a lot of things other people don't have to worry about or never even thought of. Did you ever wonder what it's like not to be able to do the things you always took for granted, like dressing yourself, feeding yourself, bathing yourself, riding a bus, or getting in and out of buildings? If you're going to be a counselor for the physically handicapped, then you've got to learn how to help them deal with these problems physically and emotionally.

But you have to learn how to do a lot more than counsel with them about self-acceptance. You've got to help them learn job-seeking and job-finding skills. You've got to provide consultation sessions with their families so that they can learn more about the family member with a problem. You've got to work with community agencies and organizations, not just for referral purposes but also for public-relations reasons. You have to plan, monitor, and coordinate your program of services, write progress reports, keep caseload records, do public speaking, and still find time to stay up to date on the latest legislative regulations for the handicapped.

As a counselor who works with handicapped individuals, your job won't be easy. You have to know what you want to do and why you want to do it. Sympathy is the wrong reason. Your counselees don't need it, and most of them don't want it. Also, you have to know whether you can accept what you are supposed to help them learn how to accept. A lot of counselors have had to admit they couldn't. So find out early just how "shockproof" you are. Later may be too late.

This "special" population of counselees is very special, mostly because they don't want to be treated as special. They would rather do it themselves, and most want nothing more than help in learning how. You've got to have patience with small steps and slow progress, and you've got to know when to "raise or lower the grapes"—within reach but just out of reach. Most of all, you've got to be able to deal with your own disappointments. The satisfactions you get if you do will outweigh everything else.

—*A Rehabilitation Counselor*

Counselor Settings

Although counselors encounter the disabled and retarded in all settings, there are certain organizations and agencies that are specifically oriented toward working with these populations. Perhaps the largest of these agencies is the state-federal vocational rehabilitation system. This is a system established by the federal government to provide rehabilitation services to people with disabilities. Its agency, the Rehabilitation Services Administration, provides states with matching funds and guidelines for the administration of services. Services provided include training, prosthetics, medical services, counseling, psychotherapy, tools and materials needed for training, and any other services needed for rehabilitation. To be eligible for these services, a client must meet the following criteria: (1) the existence of a medically certifiable disability, (2) the existence of a substantial handicap, and (3) the reasonable expectation that rehabilitation services will benefit the person.

The overall goal of rehabilitation agencies has changed in the last decade. Before 1973, these services were directed toward the *vocational* rehabilitation of the person with a disability. However, since the Rehabilitation Act of 1973, the services need not be vocationally oriented but can be directed toward improvement of functioning in other areas of life as well. This change is a response to an increased emphasis on the rehabilitation of the severely disabled person who may not be appropriate for vocational rehabilitation. Although the emphasis is now on the severely disabled person, all persons with disabilities, including retardation, are eligible for services.

There are rehabilitation agencies in all 50 states, and there are offices in most major cities.

Another setting in which counselors work with people with disabilities is sheltered workshops. Sheltered workshops usually provide such services as evaluation of vocational potential (work evaluation), vocational adjustment training, job-skill training, and, in some cases, employment for those capable of functioning in the sheltered shop but unable to work in a competitive environment. In addition to trainers and vocational evaluators, workshops have a staff of counselors to assist clients with vocational planning and personal problems. These workshops usually provide services for the state rehabilitation agency. The result is a close association between these two types of service providers.

Other types of organizations provide services to people with disabilities. Comprehensive rehabilitation centers provide medical services, physical therapy, occupational therapy, vocational evaluation, vocational adjustment, prosthetic training, vocational training, counseling, and placement, all under one roof. Local associations such as those for the blind or the deaf provide advocacy, counseling, and sometimes funds for the needs of the particular population.

Counselor Role

The role of the counselor in these agencies varies, depending on the type of the agency. In the state rehabilitation agency, the rehabilitation counselors not only engage in face-to-face counseling with the client but also coordinate other client services. Because they must coordinate a variety of services and professionals such as physicians and psychologists, rehabilitation counselors must be "jacks of all trades." To help provide for the varied needs of people with disabilities, they must not only be skilled counselors but also be knowledgeable in areas including the medical aspects of disability, psychopathology, vocational information, prosthetics, and the full range of services in the community. Counselors in other rehabilitation settings have somewhat different roles. Usually rehabilitation counselors in settings such as sheltered workshops and comprehensive rehabilitation centers have more client contact than counselors in the state agencies, but they must also coordinate the efforts of the staff and must also have a wide range of knowledge concerning the person with a disability. What should be clear by now is that the counselor in the rehabilitation setting is the person who is usually closest to the client and is the one who must see the whole picture of the rehabilitation effort.

Another role of the rehabilitation counselor is that of advocate. The first part of this chapter outlined some of the difficulties a person has in our society if he or she is classified as different. The person with a disability will never have equal opportunity until these attitudes are changed. Consequently, part of the role of rehabilitation counselors is to do everything in their power to change these negative attitudes toward those with disabilities.

In addition to changing attitudes of society, the rehabilitation counselor must help the person with a disability change his attitude toward himself. The reactions of the person that were discussed previously must be changed if the person is to take advantage of the rehabilitation effort. As Wright (1960) has outlined, the counselor must help the person develop a coping rather than a succumbing attitude toward the disability. The counselor must help the person contain the effects of disability by combating the spread effect. In addition, the counselor must help the person overcome the effects of mourning by helping him see that there is more to his life than just the disability and, finally, help him discover that there are values beyond just appearing and acting normal in every way. This applies not only to the person with a physical disability but to the retarded as well. These people must discover their capabilities and discover personal values beyond their limitations.

Counselor Competencies

Rehabilitation counselors must have a wide range of capabilities and knowledge. The training of rehabilitation counselors, therefore, must encompass many areas. In addition to counseling courses, there must be training in medical aspects of disabilities, psychological aspects of disabilities, and the practice of counseling people with disabilities. Most rehabilitation counselors have training at the master's level, although there are some programs at the bachelor's level. To ensure that rehabilitation counselors have the wide range of competencies needed for the job, national certification of rehabilitation counselors by the Commission on Rehabilitation Counselor Certification now requires a master's degree from an accredited program and passing performance on a national certification examination.

In addition to the academic requirements needed to counsel those with disabilities, rehabilitation counselors should have other characteristics. First of all, they must understand their own prejudices and attitudes toward disability. This requires intensive self-examination. Rehabilitation counselors must have an optimistic attitude about the rehabilitation effort and should be constantly focusing on their clients' abilities rather than disabilities. They must also have a commitment to the rehabilitation effort in order to be a successful advocate for their clients. Finally, they must be able to tolerate the paperwork that is a part of most rehabilitation counselors' jobs. The rehabilitation effort requires money, and with money comes accountability. The accountability, in turn, creates the need for numerous forms. The forms can seem overwhelming at times, and at these times counselors must remember that the financial aid for which the paperwork is required allows them to be a potent force in the lives of those with disabilities.

Overall, the rehabilitation counselor must be a knowledgable, highly competent person who is able to tolerate the many frustrations that accompany the rehabilitation effort. Despite the frustrations involved, however, it is a highly rewarding career that offers many satisfactions.

Alcoholics

Alcoholism and alcohol abuse is one of the nation's most severe health problems. Perhaps as much as 10% of our population has problems with alcohol (U.S. Department of Health, Education and Welfare, 1974), costing the country about $25 billion each year (Berry, Bolland, Laxson, Hayler, Sillman, Fein, & Feldstein, 1971). Unfortunately, the problem is getting worse. There seems to be a rise in drinking among youth, in particular, and most other segments of the population. With a problem of this magnitude, it is likely that counselors in all settings will encounter an alcoholic or someone close to an alcoholic.

Alcoholism is not easily defined. No one seems to have been able to define it successfully on the basis of quantity consumed, what happens to alcoholics once they do drink, or the specific effects of alcohol on their lives. There also seems to be no definable alcoholic personality. The most acceptable definition seems to be that alcoholics are people whose consumption of alcohol causes problems in their lives. Although this definition is quite simple and general, there is no better one at this time.

The problems faced by the alcoholic are in some ways similar to those faced by people with disabilities. During the rehabilitation process the alcoholic faces much of the stigma that all deviant members of society face. Those who have problems with alcohol, however, have many problems that are unique to them.

One of the problems the alcoholic faces is the progressive nature of the disease. Until an alcoholic stops drinking or dies, the condition seems to get continuously worse, causing not only a deterioration of health but a deterioration of relationships, career, financial status, and psychological health as well. By the time alcoholics accept that they have a problem, they are often in such bad shape that they are in need of rehabilitation in all these areas.

It is impossible to classify all the problems alcoholics face, because the psychological dynamics of alcoholism are not fully understood. There are, however, some general statements about these problems that seem to fit most alcoholics. Many alcoholics are bothered by excessive guilt, low self-esteem, and impaired interpersonal relationships.

One factor that makes these problems even worse is the lack of recognition by the alcoholic that a problem with alcohol even exists. Part of the progressive nature of alcoholism is an elaborate system of denial that the alcoholic and sometimes the family of the alcoholic use to protect themselves. This system of denial is the reason that alcoholics often have to "hit bottom" or encounter some personal disaster before they recognize that they are caught in a destructive drinking pattern.

In sum, alcoholics are people who usually have financial, family, and health problems. They often deny their drinking problem, but those who do admit their alcoholism suffer from guilt and low self-esteem. The problem is a challenge to any counselor who encounters alcoholics.

Counselor Settings

The settings in which counselors most often work with alcoholics and the treatment process of alcoholics will be covered in the order in which they would be encountered by a person going through the treatment process. Before describing this process, though, it should again be emphasized that counselors working in any setting will probably encounter an alcoholic or a member of an alcoholic's family. All counselors should therefore be familiar with the treatment process for alcoholism.

The first step in the rehabilitation process is usually detoxification. This occurs in a medical setting because of the possibility of seizures and other dangerous effects of withdrawal from alcohol. Medication can also be dispensed to make the process more tolerable. The purpose of detoxification is withdrawal from the physical effects of sustained alcohol consumption. This process usually takes about 3–5 days, during which the person rests and allows the effects of the alcohol to wear off. During detoxification there is usually a series of meetings with counselors to set up a postdetoxification rehabilitation program. In addition to counseling, the person receives education about alcoholism and exposure to Alcoholics Anonymous.

Upon release there are several treatment options. One of these is inpatient treatment. Under this option clients go directly from detoxification to the inpatient setting, where they stay for a specified period of time (usually 3–6 weeks). In this setting, they receive intensive individual and group counseling, education, family counseling, and sometimes regular exposure to Alcoholics Anonymous meetings. They may also be referred for vocational rehabilitation counseling if they are having work-related problems. After completing the inpatient program they return home and are often referred for outpatient counseling.

Outpatient counseling is also an option directly after detoxification and may be used without any inpatient treatment at all. This type of referral would depend on the needs and situation of the particular client. In outpatient counseling the person is usually seen once or twice weekly for group, family, or individual counseling or a combination of the three. Usually clients are also encouraged to attend AA meetings on their own. Outpatient clinics are usually attached to a detoxification unit or a mental-health clinic.

A third option after release from detoxification is placement at a halfway house. A halfway house is a residential treatment modality in which residents are encouraged to become more involved in the community over time. Time spent in a halfway house usually lasts from about three months to a year, depending on the needs of the resident. A person is usually referred to a halfway house if the alcoholism has had a severe effect on his social and vocational functioning. The halfway house allows individuals to slowly integrate themselves into the community at their own rate. During the stay at a halfway house, group and individual counseling is usually required, and attendance at AA meetings is encouraged.

These are the main types of treatment for alcoholism. Treatment usually consists of a combination of these types, the sequence and particular combination depending on the needs of the alcoholic.

Counselor Role

Counselors in the field of alcoholism can be broken down into two basic types. One is the person with a bachelor's or master's degree who has had training in both counseling and the treatment of alcoholism. The other type is a recovering alcoholic who may or may not have the academic degrees but who has shown good interpersonal skills and who may have received appropriate training. This distinction may not always be clear, since duties and roles are often interchangeable; however, the discussion here will be oriented as much as possible to the professionally trained counselor.

Professional counselors are usually found in outpatient settings and in inpatient treatment programs, while recovering alcoholic counselors are usually found in detoxification centers and the halfway houses. There are, of course, many exceptions to this generalization. In an outpatient setting the counselor is usually involved in regular visits by the client to participate in individual, group, or family counseling. Because groups are commonly used with alcoholics and because of frequent involvement of the family, the alcoholism counselor should have group and family counseling skills. The outpatient counselor will also be involved with Alcoholics Anonymous. Because AA is one of the oldest and most successful forms of treatment for alcoholism, counselors should be very familiar with the organization and how it functions. They should be open to referring clients to AA and should not feel threatened by it as a competing type of treatment. Counselors who do not refer to AA lose a valuable ally for their treatment effort. Outpatient counselors also act as consultants to other agencies and educational institutions. They conduct training programs for teachers, ministers, physicians, and personnel from related fields. They may also spend time in the classroom with high school or elementary students.

In inpatient settings, the counselor performs many of the same functions, including individual, group, and family counseling. The inpatient counselor, however, has a more intense involvement because of daily contact with the client. The inpatient counselor must also be concerned with the milieu at the treatment settings. The inpatient counselor will also be involved with efforts to educate the alcoholic on the nature of alcoholism and the importance of treatment.

Counselor Competencies

It should be obvious that the counselor who works with alcoholics must have good counseling skills and be trained in the dynamics of alcoholism and alcoholism treatment. Just as important, though, the counselor must also be extremely persistent and tolerant. Alcoholism, like other addictions, is a problem that does not usually disappear after a single treatment effort. The treatment process usually involves a number of attempts at sobriety, with a similar number of relapses. Through this series of attempts, alcoholics, it is hoped, learn about themselves and maintain progressively longer periods of sobriety. Success, however, is never guaranteed. Clients may die before they succeed with the problem. The tenacity of the problem can be extremely frustrating to the counselor. All counselors need to feel some degree of success on their jobs, and the frequent relapses do not help this need to be met. Alcoholism counselors must have faith that their efforts are helping clients attain their goals in the absence of any tangible results.

In addition to persistence, the counselor who works with alcoholics must feel comfortable with confrontation. The alcoholic's denial system can be resistant to all but the strongest confrontation. The counselor must be able to make or arrange such a confrontation with family and friends in a way that not only confronts but also provides the support necessary for the client to make the difficult step of admitting that he or she has a problem and needs help (Johnson, 1980).

In sum, counselors should be aware that counseling alcoholics takes a great deal of skill, persistence, and knowledge of alcoholism. They should also be aware, though, that helping alcoholics and their families piece their lives back together can be a gratifying experience.

Other Substance Abusers

Like alcoholism, abuse of other drugs has been on the rise in the United States in recent years. Drug users are getting younger and more numerous (Blum, 1979). Unfortunately, there seem to be few effective ideas on how to control or treat drug abuse (Brecher, 1972).

Identifying the particular problems of drug abusers is difficult because of the many patterns of drug abuse. On one hand, there are narcotic addicts who use illegal drugs and who are often involved in criminal activities to pay for the costly drugs. On the other hand are those who have come addicted to drugs such as sedatives and tranquilizers that have been prescribed by physicians. These drug abusers are not necessarily involved in a criminal life-style. Obviously the patterns of problems in these cases will be quite different.

With people who are addicted to illegal drugs, such as heroin, the lifestyle can be as much a problem as the addiction. Such persons are usually involved in a subculture that condones not only the use of the drug but the illegal activities that are needed to support the expensive habit. In some groups a very expensive habit is seen as a status symbol. The illegal activities usually lead to involvement with the criminal justice system, which, in turn, can lead to incarceration. By the time addicts see counselors, many are entrenched in a criminal subculture. They have little incentive to eliminate the drug habit because drug use does not run counter to the addict's value system. They may lose more prestige and acceptance among peers by eliminating the habit than by keeping it. Quite frequently the only motivations to come to treatment are legal pressures or the unavailability of drugs. These types of motivation do not usually make for an enthusiastic client.

Although these barriers are, perhaps, fewer when counseling people who are addicted to prescribed drugs, a major problem area seems to be the identification of such persons. Because the practice of using barbituates and sedatives is condoned by society, these persons rarely stand out until the use of the drug has severely impaired their functioning. Once they are identified, however, treatment can usually be successful unless there are some severe underlying problems. This group is also less affected by the stigma of deviance.

Other drug users present problems particular to the specifc substance used. Users of marijuana, LSD, PCP, and other hallucinogens do not become physically addicted but may use the drug to the extent that it interferes with their social, vocational, or family functioning. It may be difficult to persuade these users to seek treatment because of the seeming harmlessness of the drug and the fact that they are not physically addicted.

People using amphetamines, cocaine, and other "uppers" constitute another group of drug abusers. These drugs are usually not considered physically addictive either, but prolonged use can create physical and psychological problems. Physical problems center on prolonged stimulation of the central nervous system. Extreme exhaustion and physical deterioration may result. Psychological problems include an increased tendency to violence and, with long-term use, symptoms of paranoia. Drug users in this category may seek treatment during withdrawal, when they often experience depression and suicidal thoughts.

Counselor Settings

Treatment of drug abusers begins with detoxification. The purpose is much the same as it is with alcoholics—to help the person physically withdraw from the effects of the drug. This must be done in a medical setting because of the potentially dangerous effects of withdrawal. In addition to the actual detoxification, the clients receive counseling regarding their postdischarge plans. There is not much time for more than this, since detoxification usually takes only 7–10 days. The options after detoxification are similar to the options for alcoholism treatment. Inpatient treatment, outpatient counseling, and halfway houses are all routes that one can follow.

One option that is somewhat different from those usually used with alcoholics is the therapeutic community. The therapeutic community is a residential program that is normally staffed by ex-addicts. The program usually utilizes a process whereby the residents can attain increased privileges and responsibilities by demonstrating behavior that conforms to the norms established for the community. When a resident first enters the community, he has the lowest status in the community and usually performs the most menial tasks, such as cleaning floors and bathrooms. If he demonstrates a cooperative attutide, he can move up by progressing through specified stages and eventually "graduate" or become one of the staff. The primary mode of counseling in therapeutic communities is groups that usually involve a direct verbal attack on the defenses and denial of the resident. The theory guiding the therapeutic community is that the addict's personality and defenses must be broken down and then slowly rebuilt in a more positive manner through the system of privileges an increased responsibility.

One alternative to the entire system outlined so far is treatment with methadone. Methadone is a synthetic narcotic that is administered to narcotic addicts on a regular basis. The assumption behind this administration is that the addict is not capable of functioning totally drug-free. It is therefore better to prescribe a substitute that will eliminate the need for narcotics and the resulting criminal behavior. Some addicts are put on methadone for an indefinite period of time; others are put on methadone and are then slowly withdrawn. Along with the administration of methadone is mandatory counseling on an outpatient basis. Methadone treatment is highly controversial, and its effectiveness is still not clear (Brecher, 1972).

Many substance-abuse counselors spend part of their time as consultants and educators. In this role, they help schools, law enforcement agencies, and other human service agencies to work effectively with the drug abusers they encounter. They may also educate the public about drug abuse and prevention. Workshops and lectures are oriented toward elementary and high school students, parent groups, church groups, and public service groups.

The roles and duties of the drug-abuse counselor are obviously quite diverse, ranging from the actual counseling to the coordination, consultation, and prevention roles. Add to these the administrative functions such as supervision and the ubiquitous paperwork connected with public funding, and you have a counselor who is very busy, active, and involved in the community.

Counselor Competencies

Counselors who work with drug abusers must have good counseling skills and must be knowledgeable about the problems of the population with which they are working. There are, however, some additional characteristics that are particularly important for the drug-abuse counselor.

The first of these characteristics is tolerance. This is particularly true for counselors working with clients involved with illegal drugs. Counselors may find that such clients have values quite different from, even diametrically opposed to, their own. If they are not able to accept these values or refrain from condemning, they will immediately alienate their clients. This does not mean that they should accept these values for themselves, but they must recognize the rights of others to have their own.

Another characteristic needed by drug-abuse counselors is a high frustration level. The course of drug-abuse treatment is similar to the course of treatment for alcoholics. Immediate success is rare and relapses are frequent. Counselors must be patient enough to realize that their efforts may have no immediate effect but may have some effect ten years later. A counselor with a need for immediate reinforcement may not last long in drug-abuse counseling.

One last characteristic needed by those counseling with this population is a certain toughness. Often drug abusers are forced by external pressures to enter counseling. In these cases the counselor must be able to handle the negative attitudes that the client may have about counseling and turn the relationship into a positive experience. Given the life-styles and values of many of these clients, this is no job for the meek. The counselor must have a strong commitment and a positive outlook to work with drug abusers.

Offenders

It is not easy to delineate the characteristics and problems of the offender because the category includes such a wide range of people. As yet there has been little success in classifying the "criminal" personality (Hatcher, 1978). Specifics are therefore difficult, but some general problems of the offender can be identified.

The first of these is the offender's behavior. By definition, offenders have behaved in a fashion deviant enough to bring them into contact with the criminal justice system. The offender is normally a person who has developed an extended pattern of antisocial behavior that has become an integral part of his or her life-style. The problem, then, is not just the correction of a few isolated problems but the change of an entire life-style.

The magnitude of this problem for the offender, counselors, and the criminal justice system can be understood if you look at the difficulty of changing some of your own habits, such as eating, studying, sleeping, or smoking. These are usually only small segments of one's life, but they can still be quite resistant to change. You can imagine that the resistance to changing an entire life-style is many times stronger.

As we have discovered about drug abusers, offenders may be involved in a subculture that actually values criminal behavior. Changing their own long-established behavior patterns is extremely difficult with a network of peers and friends actually reinforcing such deviant patterns.

Another difficulty encountered by offenders is a lack of vocational and educational skills. In many cases, there is a strong relationship between crime and poverty, lack of education, and lack of employment. Criminal behavior is often the result of not having the skills to receive adequate reinforcement from society. Those without such skills often look to antisocial means of meeting their needs for acceptance, companionship, and economic survival. The problem, therefore, is not merely one of changing existing behavior but one of teaching or exploring new skills that will enable offenders to survive in society through socially acceptable means.

For offenders who have been imprisoned, readjusting to society after a period of forced isolation may create additional problems. The initial difficulty of readjustment is learning to cope with their own freedom and autonomy. During such a period they may feel overwhelmed by the lack of constraints and freedom of choice. Self-control of behavior may be particularly difficult at this time. The loss of time, freedom, relationships, status, vocational potential, and individuality that occurs during imprisonment leads many to a period of resentment. Although this is quite understandable, these feelings may lead to further antisocial behavior, difficulties with relationships, and lack of motivation to find employment. This is particularly difficult to alleviate because the anger may be seen as appropriate action in response to the loss that has occurred. Many offenders returning to society need assistance in directing the anger in acceptable ways and in minimizing the negative effect it may have on their lives.

Resuming old relationships is another concern. Because offenders and those close to them have all adjusted to living without each other, it may be difficult or impossible to resume the relationships where they left off. In a sense, they have all become different people. Once offenders are released, they are faced with the task of restructuring old relationships or forming new ones. The difficulty of this task is similar to one we all experience at times when we encounter someone whom we have not seen for a while. After catching up on news, we often find that we have little to say. You can imagine how isolated the offenders feel when this happens with everyone around them. It can be an alienating, lonely experience.

Finally, the offender experiences the previously mentioned stigma. In addition to feeling isolated from friends and family, the offender tends to be isolated from the rest of society. This only adds to the loneliness, anger, and fear that follow release from imprisonment.

Counselor Settings

There are several settings in which counselors work primarily with offenders. These will be listed in the order that they might be encountered by the offender.

Presentence services are usually conducted after conviction and before sentencing. It is at this point that counselors (and other professionals) try to get to know the clients, their families, and the circumstances surrounding the crime in order to advise the court on an appropriate sentence. For first or second offenders, counselors often recommend referral for counseling rather than confinement if they believe that the offenders or their families can be helped. In some locations such counseling services are offered by the court, particularly for juvenile offenders.

If the offender is given probation, he or she is placed under the supervision of a probation officer. Although probation officers are seen by many courts as extensions of the enforcement system, many others view the probation officer as a worker who provides counseling and rehabilitation. In the latter case, it is common to find trained counselors hired as probation officers. When the probation officer does not have training in counseling, then offenders may be referred to counselors who can help them with their particular problems.

Offenders who are institutionalized may encounter counselors in prison. Whether counselors are present depends on the size and location of the prison and the philosophy of correctional administrators. In the absence of trained counselors there may be peer counselors, guards, or other personnel who may function in that capacity, or surrounding human service agencies may be utilized.

After release, parole officers may function as counselors, or they may perform mostly supervisory duties. Offenders may also encounter counselors in vocational rehabilitation agencies, halfway houses, or agencies that specialize in services to offenders, such as Offender Aid and Restoration (OAR).

Counselor Role

As with other populations, counselors who work with offenders have various roles, depending on the setting in which they work. Probation and parole officers are primarily responsible for enforcing rules and imposing sanctions for violations, as well as for counseling. Counselors in halfway houses must help enforce house rules as well as be concerned about the atmosphere and general functioning of the house. Counselors in institutions are often responsible for many functions besides counseling.

Since there are so many possible roles, we will focus on a few that seem to be most strongly related to working with an offender population. Others, such as individual and group counseling, are possible functions of professional counselors in all the previously mentioned settings.

One of the roles for counselors hired by the court, by insitutions, and by probation and parole officers is diagnosis and classification. When offenders are sentenced or put up for probation, information must be gathered to determine the appropriate sentencing and/or the appropriate type of treatment. This requires a thorough investigation of the offender's background, family situation, work situation, motivation, personality, and general level of functioning. Usually the counselor or officer must spend time interviewing friends, family, and the offender himself. Although the focus here is on obtaining information, some brief counseling is often required, and it is particularly important that the worker be sensitive to the stress that those being interviewed are under.

Two other important functions are treatment planning and postdischarge planning. After the diagnosis and classification process, the recommendations must be translated into a workable treatment plan. If institutional placement is recommended, the particular institution and the type of program within the institution must be specified. Offenders who are not institutionalized are often referred to a community agency for treatment of problems such as drug and alcohol abuse. All these arrangements require an extensive knowledge of the correctional system and the human service delivery system. In postdischarge planning, counselors must work out a plan involving living arrangement, follow-up, and vocational rehabilitation. Again, this requires a thorough knowledge of the community and available resources.

Another role is that of a juvenile-court counselor. In many juvenile

LOVE IS NOT A ONE-WAY STREET

This job involves working with people with low IQs, low educational backgrounds, poor work records, and low incomes. The people I deal with are very manipulative. I have to be very direct, quick to assess what I think they should do and not hesitate to tell them to do it. If you are planning to do correctional work, you should be aware that this job involves many failures and that you can't help everyone. Sometimes when you can't help them adjust to the community, then the best help you can give them is to keep them out of the community—by holding them in jail.

Most of the people that I work with have no great desire to see me. They feel that probation is not an opportunity. It is just an obligation they must complete for the court or the parole board. Many of them do not trust me and never will. And I must say that many of them I cannot trust either. A lot of my job involves verifying, through other sources, what my probationers and parolees have told me. I have found that the best way to develop rapport in dealing with these people is to be stern, not let them manipulate you, and above all be fair.

Did my counselor education program prepare me for working in the field of corrections? Sure, it did. It helped me to communicate with the people I deal with by being concrete and truthful in what I say to them and by making me a more active listener. It helped me know how to show my feelings and concerns in dealing with people. It also helped me to know how to write concise, meaningful reports and understand the results of tests I must verify. It did not prepare me for the people I work with. Being warm, accepting, and trusting won't work with people who haven't learned self-acceptance and a sense of social responsibility. You've got to start them at another level and try to work them up to the other ones. Love is a two-way street, and if you don't believe it, you'll break your neck and maybe your heart too.

I don't get much sleep, but I sleep sound. Counselors, no matter where they work, are responsible to lots of people, not just their counselees. We're responsible to our profession, to ourselves, and to our society. So I'd stack my kind of counseling against all the rest when it comes to measuring up to responsibility. Sure, my kind of counseling may lose a few counselees along the way, but just count up how many others we saved.

—*A Probation and Parole Counselor*

courts there is an emphasis on resolving the particular individual and family problems rather than institutionalizing the offender. As a result, some courts have units that work closely with juvenile offenders and their families to alleviate sources of stress. Obviously counselors in this position engage in frequent individual and family counseling as well as report writing and completion of the necessary paperwork.

These are a few of the roles for counselors who work with offenders. There are others, the nature of which depends on the locality and the philosophy of the administrators in the particular state or region. Most, however, have elements similar to those outlined.

Counselor Competencies

The competencies needed to counsel offenders are similar to those needed for counseling drug abusers. Openness, tolerance, and a certain "toughness" are requisite attributes. In addition, counselors who work with offenders must have a thorough knowledge of criminal law and the legal and correctional system. Because they will be working closely with courts, lawyers, and judges, they must know the workings of the system and be able to discuss the law intelligently.

One last attribute is perseverance. Counseling offenders does not often provide tangible rewards. The clients are usually reluctant and often resent the role that counselors are playing in their lives. To counter these factors, offender counselors must have a well-defined philosophy of what they are doing and a strong belief that their actions will ultimately benefit society. Without these qualities, counselors will not last long in this field.

Perspectives for the '80s

As in all areas of counseling, there are no safe predictions of the direction in which the counseling of special populations will go in the next decade. The field of counseling in human services is closely tied to the directions of federal and state funding. An example of this tie is the state-federal rehabilitation system. Although the purpose of the program has always been the rehabilitation of the disabled, exactly who the disabled are and what rehabilitation means have been determined by federal acts and policies. During the 1950s and 1960s, the definition of disability expanded rapidly under relatively liberal administrations. The retarded, offenders, substance abusers, and even the socially disadvantaged were considered disabled and therefore became recipients of rehabilitation services. Since the early '70s, however, the target population has narrowed. The Rehabilitation Act of 1973 mandated that the severely physically disabled should be the main focus of rehabilitation services. This was a reversal of the trend toward rehabilitation of the nonphysically disabled. All these trends have been the result of decisions made at the federal level by those in power in Washington. Since this is likely to be the situation in the future, it must be understood that any trends in the '80s will depend largely on who is in power and the general political climate of the country.

Rehabilitation

There are, however, some trends that seem likely to continue for a while. For rehabilitation, it seems that the emphasis on the severely disabled will continue. The extent of the services to this population will be determined by the extent of budget cuts for the field of rehabilitation in the early 1980s. The impact of these cuts will not be determined for several years, but there will probably be some curtailment of services in rehabilitation.

Barring any drastic changes in the system, the role of the rehabilitation counselor will probably remain the same. The position of being the coordinator of medical, psychological, and supportive services is one for which rehabilitation counselors are still being trained. It is also likely that the rehabilitation counselor will still need strong counseling skills to be able to communicate with and support those encountering the difficulties of disability. In addition, rehabilitation counselors will continue to perform other functions such as work evaluation and work-adjustment training.

One factor that will probably affect rehabilitation counseling is licensing and certification. National certification for rehabilitation counselors is becoming more significant as increasing numbers of counselors become certified. The day may be coming when counselors must be certified to obtain employment in many agencies. State licensing of rehabilitation counselors has also occurred in several states and will also probably be a force affecting the practice of rehabilitation counseling.

One last influence that will affect counseling of persons with disabilities is the current emphasis on independent living for those with severe disabilities. Professionals in the field have become increasingly aware that people with disabilities have the right to function on their own. As more people select this type of life-style, the issues in counseling will shift from purely vocational ones to those related to an entire life-style. This will require a change in counselors' skills and attitudes and the type of training that rehabilitation counselors receive.

Alcoholism

The field of alcoholism counseling is unlikely to change much in the next decade. Despite preventive efforts, the problem of alcoholism in our society is not fading. Detoxification units, public and private treatment centers, and halfway houses all seem likely to be integral parts of the alcoholism treatment network, as does the alcoholism counselor.

One trend which received its initial push during the '70s and which will probably continue to be a factor in alcoholism treatment in the '80s is early detection of alcoholism. An important component of this effort is the Employee Assistance Program. Employee assistance programs have been established in business and industry to detect and treat problems with alcohol and other employee difficulties that affect job performance. Early signs of such difficulties, such as absenteeism, lack of production, and interpersonal or supervisory difficulties, are all followed up by the personnel of these programs to detect the existence of alcholism or problem drinking. If problems with alcohol are found to exist, the employee is referred for treatment. These programs not only provide early detection of alcohol problems but save industry thousands of dollars each year. We expect that the cost-effectiveness of such programs will guarantee their growth through the '80s.

Drug Abuse

A review of drug-abuse treatment (Sells, 1979) reveals that the 1960s and 1970s were decades in which treatment of drug abusers, as opposed to legal actions against drug abusers, reached a peak. However, as questions about the effectiveness of such treatment begin to grow, counselors' roles in dealing with drug abuse become increasingly uncertain. As federal funding gets tighter, the need for accountability of drug-abuse programs increases. Since the evaluatory data coming from drug-abuse treatment have called into question the effectiveness of the treatment, the future becomes more cloudy. It is quite possible that legal action against drug abusers will be seen as a more viable alternative to solving this problem.

Even if federal funds become scarce, there will still be a need for counseling programs funded at a local level. Although treatment may not receive high priority in the '80s, it is likely that educational efforts aimed at prevention will still be needed. In addition, counselors in all other settings may have to be knowledgeable about drug abuse, since the problem is not likely to vanish. Whether counselors are located in schools, mental-health centers, colleges, or rehabilitation agencies, they are likely to encounter problems related to drug abuse.

Offenders

The role of counseling with offenders in the 1980s is difficult to predict. During the past 20 years several trends have come and gone in a search for a solution to recidivism; despite these efforts, there seems to be no solution. It does seem clear that there will be a continued need for counselors regardless of the current trends for rehabilitation. The need will come from the inherent nature of incarceration and the rest of the justice system. The person who is put in jail or is labeled an offender must attempt to integrate himself into society if he is to attain a productive life-style and not come into contact with the criminal justice system again. Because the process of reintegration can be frustrating and full of roadblocks, there is a need for counselors, whether they are parole or probation officers or counselors in related agencies. The counselor's purpose is to guide the offender through the process and assist him in resolving his own conflicts in adapting to a new life-style. It is unlikely that this basic role will change in the future.

In summary, there will be a continued need for counselors to work with special populations in the '80s. The form of this counseling and the setting in which the counseling will take place will depend on further developments in the field and the trends and policies of government bodies.

Summary

Although there are several differences among the populations covered, what makes them similar is that they are all classified as deviant. As a result, they all have to deal with the implications and difficulties of such a classification. All these individuals present counselors with the challenge of either helping them find ways of reintegrating themselves into the rest of society or helping them cope with remaining outside the mainstream of society. Since most counselors will work with people in all these categories at one time or another, it is important that counselors be flexible enough in their outlook toward deviance to enable them to work with these clients in a positive and accepting manner. If counselors attempt to work with these populations without broadening their view of what is acceptable, their moralizing or condemning behavior may do the client considerable harm.

In addition to the difficulties shared by all these groups, each group has its own particular difficulties. People with disabilities must deal with their functional limitations and isolation, alcoholics must deal with the damage that has occurred to their family and other relationships, other drug abusers must work on deviant life-styles, and offenders have to cope with a readjustment to society after incarceration. Counselors must take the time and effort to understand these problems and explore the impact on the client. These varied problems present a challenge to all those in the field of counseling.

Finally, the counselor must understand that people who are classified as deviant have more in common with the rest of society than they have differences. First, we are all human beings. This common denominator transcends all our differences. Second, being different is an experience we all have in common. We all have some characteristic of our personalities or bodies that we or others see as being significantly different on some dimension. Since being different is a common experience, it is one that counselors should understand and be able to work with regardless of the work setting.

Now It's Your Turn

1. There are many other "special populations" that have not been covered in this chapter. Discuss in small groups which of these populations

might be served by counselors. Answer the following questions for each group.
   a. What are the particular problems for this population?
   b. What are their options for solving these problems?
   c. What agencies or institutions serve this population in your area?
   d. What role can counselors play in providing services to this population?

2. The counselor's role in working with special populations cannot be completely understood without talking with someone who works in the field. Pick one of the populations we discussed and visit an agency in your community that serves this population. Arrange for an interview with one of the counselors to discuss:
   a. The counselor's perception of the problems encountered by the population.
   b. The counselor's philosophy of counseling this population.
   c. The duties of his or her job and what he or she enjoys the most.
   d. The difficulties he or she encounters.
   e. The type of training and experiences the counselor would recommend for someone who wants to work with this population.

3. One of the best ways to understand what it means to be different is to experience it yourself. With another person, assume a disability or deviance. This can be done with a wheelchair, with dark glasses to appear blind, or by some other means. Be creative. Go someplace where you will interact with others, such as a mall, a shopping center, or a restaurant, and engage in an activity that will bring you into contact with others. While you are assuming the disability, the other person observes the reactions of those around you. Once you have finished, switch roles. Be aware of your feelings before, during, and after the experience. Note the reactions of others to you and to your partner when he or she assumes the disability. Take notes and discuss these experiences in class.

4. One of the sources of assistance for many of the special populations we have discussed is the self-help group. Arrange to visit one of these groups (Alcoholics Anonymous is the most prevalent) and observe what makes these groups helpful to their members.

References

Berry, R., Bolland, J., Laxson, J., Hayler, D., Sillman, M., Fein, R., & Feldstein, P. *The economic costs of alcohol abuse and alcoholism—1971*. Prepared for the National Institute on Alcohol Abuse and Alcoholism (Contract no. HSM-42-73-114), 1974.

Brecher, E. M. *Licit & illicit drugs*. Mt. Vernon, N.Y.: Consumers Union, 1972

Blum, R., & Richards, L. Youthful drug use. In R. L. DuPont, A. Goldstein, & J.

O'Donnell (Eds.), *Handbook on drug abuse*. Washington, D.C.: National Institute on Drug Abuse, 1979.

Goffman, E. *Stigma: Notes on the management of a spoiled identity*. Englewood Cliffs, N.J.: Prentice-Hall, 1963.

Hatcher, H. A. *Correctional casework and counseling*. Englewood Cliffs, N.J.: Prentice-Hall, 1978.

Johnson, V. E. *I'll quit tomorrow*. New York: Harper & Row, 1980.

Kerr, N. Understanding the process of adjustment to disability. *Journal of Rehabilitation,* 1961, *27,* 16–18.

McDaniel, J. W. *Physical disability and human behavior*. New York: Pergamon Press, 1976.

Sells, S. B. Treatment effectiveness. In R. L. DuPont, A. Goldstein, & J. O'Donnell (Eds.), *Handbook on drug abuse*. Washington, D.C.: National Institute on Drug Abuse, 1979.

U.S. Department of Health, Education and Welfare. *Second special report to the U.S. Congress on alcohol and health from the Secretary of Health, Education, and Welfare, 1974*. DHEW Publ. No. (ADM) 74-124. Washington, D.C.: U.S. Government Printing Office, 1974.

Wolfensberger, W. *Normalization: The principle of normalization in the human services*. Toronto: National Institute on Mental Retardation, 1972.

Wright, B. A. *Physical disability—a psychological approach*. New York: Harper & Row, 1960.

Yamamoto, K. To be different. *Rehabilitation Counseling Bulletin,* 1971, *14,* 180–189.

PART *4*

The Decisions of the Counselor

Your training as a counselor is just beginning, but our effort to introduce you to your new career is about to end. What we have shared with you is only an overview of your future professional responsibilities and heritage. Your in-depth study of the topics we have explored will come from other courses, but we hope that the material in this text will be helpful to you in those other encounters. Now, somewhat like anxious parents, perhaps we can be forgiven our need to know how well we have done our job.

This section of your text includes a series of exercises that try to run the gamut of human experience. They are our attempt to provide you with "fail-safe" conditions for discovering not only how much you have learned but how much you have yet to learn. The experiences allow you to test yourself against yourself at this point in your training. You are asked to think and behave like a full-fledged counselor although you are now only a fledgling.

We accept this paradox. And we hope you will accept the exercises as an opportunity *to learn how* to fly. The skills and depth of understanding needed to earn your wings must come from other courses and other training experiences. But now you should be asked to use the information you have to speculate about alternative responses to future problem situations. Our exercises were designed for that purpose only. So be forewarned. They may tax your decision-making skills but only as they seek to challenge you into more reasoned judgments about the work of the professional counselor you are about to become.

Here, in this section, are exercises that allow you to test the worth and meaning to you of the notions we have presented. Here, also, is your chance to discover how well you *might* perform in all those other professional-preparation experiences you are scheduled for. Involve yourself in our little games. Discover whether you have merely memorized the material presented or whether you have internalized it so completely that you can generalize it and apply it to the many aspects of a professional counselor's work.

All societies impose certain trials on their members before allowing them to assume a new status. If it is helpful, then consider the exercises that follow as only the first in a series of rites of passage that must be gracefully tolerated. But we strongly suspect that you will enjoy your vicarious excursion into the work world of professional counselors.

CHAPTER *14*

Practical Exercises

Jeannette A. Brown

Throughout your text we have tried to help you understand what a professional counselor does and what skills and knowledge a professional counselor needs in order to be competent. Now we want to help you try to *experience* some of the things we have been talking about.

Simulated and/or contrived experiences are never as good as the real thing, but they certainly will make your first encounter with the real thing a lot easier to handle. So if it was important to learn all this material we presented, then it is important that we give you a chance to learn what you will be able to do with it.

We have represented the exercises in this chapter as games, and we have described them as fun. We do not mean, however, that they are "fun and games." We do not mean to caricature the work of professional counselors. Our only motive in providing gaming opportunities for learning the serious business of professional counseling is to provide you with an action-oriented foretaste of the exciting, satisfying, challenging, and tentative world of professional counselors.

And herein is our first effort to create in you one of the most important of your professional attributes. It's a state of mind. It's *tentative insecurity*. It's the opposite of knowing. It's being able to know that you *don't* know but still being able to act. It is the stuff out of which wisdom is made. And contrary to popular opinion, you don't have to be old to be wise—but you do have to be courageous.

Courage is an interesting concept. It implies a tolerance for ambiguity, an excitement for problem solving, and a creativity for defining the ill-defined. Put another way, it implies *risk taking,* the most critical single factor contributing to success in life (Cronbach, 1963; White, 1965). As our contribution to your future success, we suggest that your risk-taking experiences begin right now.

What follow are ambiguous, highly speculative, sometimes frustrating, but always challenging situational propositions concerning the most success-defying puzzle in the world—human behavior. But here is your chance to exercise your reasoning power by creating alternative responses to questions for which you may never find satisfying or conclusive answers.

Because things are never as they seem, you must be on guard. Like some of your future clients, we will deceive you if we can. This is our continuing effort to develop in you what we perceive to be a prime attribute of competent counselors—tentative insecurity. Absolute certainty and right answers are rarely a part of the professional world you are about to enter. And they have never been the better part of wisdom. There simply are no right answers.

Sarah

Sarah, a 16-year-old tenth-grade student, is waiting to see you. Inside your office you are examining the information prepared for you by your receptionist. Sarah's father is a building contractor and her mother is a homemaker. Neither has a high school diploma. Her 39-year-old father ended his formal education with the eighth grade, and her mother, aged 37, completed ten years of schooling. Sarah has two older brothers; one is 17 years old and is in the 11th grade, the other is a freshman in college and is 19 years old.

At this point, what do you *also* know about Sarah? A professional counselor's answer to this question should be "Very little!" Why? Because you will recall from Chapter 4 that counselors never prejudge their counselees. If they do, they risk intruding their own biases and values, which can result in their projecting onto others the attributes and characteristics they secretly resent in themselves.

But aren't counselors supposed to understand human behavior and to be able to know why people behave the way they do? Not exactly! You see, it's because counselors *are* experts in human behavior that they appreciate its diversity of expression. They know that even though several people may share the same talents, traits, and experiences, they may be quite different. Each of them almost certainly has some unique talent, trait, or experience that the others do not have. Our work would be much easier if we could lump everybody into definitive, predictable categories, but we can't. That luxury is reserved for those who sort data.

You create categories for the purpose of organizing data, but such efforts are useless when it comes to people. If you try to put people in boxes, you will usually run into trouble. People have a way of not staying in the neat little boxes you designed for them. They have a way of moving from one box to another as their circumstances change. So don't be caught in the trap of believing you have your counselee all figured out. You haven't, even if your counselee is willing to reinforce you in your mistakes.

Exercise 1

What, then, *do* you know, not about Sarah but about your options? First you know that you can and should formulate a series of tentative hypotheses about Sarah, her family, and the problem she wants to discuss with you. What are they? With the information you have thus far, what kinds of tentative hypotheses could be formulated? Perhaps we should do a little "dry run" with you to let you get the feel of what we're talking about. For example:

Tentative hypotheses about Sarah:

1. Sarah is a 16-year-old young woman struggling with the perfectly normal "abnormalities" of adolescence.
2. Sarah is striving for independence and autonomy as they conflict with her status as a dependent.
3. Sarah is aware of the discrepancies between her family's values and those of her peer group.
4. Sarah is intolerant of ambiguity.
5. Sarah is self-conscious and often self-centered in her interactions with young men.

Now back to Sarah's reason for coming to see you. Some tentative hypotheses might include:

1. She's been caught with pot. (There has been a growing problem among the tenth-grade students at None Greater High. Several have been suspended for possessing, smoking, and/or distributing marijuana.)
2. She wants you to intercede for her with her parents. (They are upwardly mobile and have a high regard for education, and she may be failing some of her courses.)
3. She wants you to intercede for her with one of her teachers. (Adolescents are anxious to demonstrate their independence, and sometimes their coping skills are not as selective as those needed for effective interactions with adults. Perhaps she has "blown up" in one of her classes, regrets it, and wants the teacher to forgive and forget the incident.)
4. She wants you to get her a job. (The summer vacation is coming up, and a lot of the 16-year-old students want to earn some money during the school holidays.)
5. She wants you to solve her "love affair" problem. (Adolescents often have some difficulty in accepting the emotions they are beginning to

experience. They don't always relate to the opposite sex in productive ways.)

This time we have shared with you the reasoning we used to formulate our tentative hypotheses. Perhaps you recognized some of the information. It came from Chapter 10. How about reviewing that discussion of adolescence and designing some additional tentative hypotheses about Sarah's problem? The chapter is full of information for speculating about why she came to visit you. Try your hand. It's rather interesting—and it can be fun. Betting against yourself usually is, since there is no way you can lose. Now, for a moment, in your mind's eye imagine 16-year-old Sarah sitting outside your door, and rehearse with yourself the developmental tasks discussed in Chapter 10 about adolescence. What mental images can you conjure up? What *developmentally based* tentative hypotheses can you postulate about the adolescent who is waiting to talk with you?

Were your tentative hypotheses more informed than ours? Your classmates'? How well did yours withstand your classmates' critical review? More to the point, how much have you really learned about adolescent behavior and the problems adolescents might face?

One last consideration: Did you notice that each of our tentative hypotheses began with the notion that Sarah wanted *you* to solve her problem? What's wrong with Sarah's expecting you to intercede for her? Some of the material in Chapter 6 might give you a little help here.

Enough! Sarah is waiting. Your tentative insecurity is well organized, and you are now ready for almost any adolescent concern Sarah could want to share. And because you remember something from Chapter 4 about how to establish good working relationships, you know how to begin. So you go out to greet her.

But what do you do now that you are both there in your office? And how do you do it? You will, of course, begin with some of the notions discussed in Chapter 4 about the difference between *counseling* and *conversation*.

Exercise 2

Sarah is an attractive, blond, blue-eyed, well-developed teenager. She is well-mannered and tastefully dressed. During your interview she tells you that:

1. Her mother and father were never married.
2. Her father has a violent temper and hasn't been able to land any building contracts for as far back as she can remember, and the family is on welfare.
3. Their house is a shambles because her mother is always drunk.
4. Nobody cares whether she comes home or not because nobody is there except her mother, and she's usually passed out, sometimes on the floor.

5. She wishes she could "space out" too, but she can't stand pot, and that's what most of her friends use.
6. She's been a straight-A student since the third grade. She thought it would help because that's how her older brother got to college and because her teachers are so good about helping her learn. They are very nice to her.
7. She has a job for the summer because the money will help out at home, but she may have to use it for herself because she is pregnant.

OK, counselor, what do you do now? Do you throw out all those tentative hypotheses and show your unconditional positive regard for your counselee by accepting, unconditionally, Sarah's account of her life? Of course you don't. You know that what you must do now is go after more information that will either confirm or deny each of the various propositions in the two sets of conflicting data.

A counselor's tentative hypotheses are merely speculative data requiring verification. This is also true for the data presented by your clients. For example, does the information shared by Sarah represent (1) reality, (2) Sarah's perception of reality, or (3) Sarah's deliberate attempt to distort reality? You cannot proceed effectively and competently without examining these three questions and trying to resolve them. Sometimes we have been so concerned to be supportive that we have failed to be objective about the information shared with us. Do not be caught in this trap. Instead, you must always examine each possible alternative and derive its implications for your interactions with your counselees.

For example:

1. If the information shared by Sarah does, in fact, represent reality, then what are your legal, ethical, and professional responsibilities?
2. If the information is only Sarah's perceptions of reality, then why would this young woman deceive herself?
3. If Sarah is deliberately distorting the facts, then why would she deceive her counselor?

Put another way, what are the risks involved *for both of you* if you check out the information? What are the risks if you don't?

Now let's focus on the two exercises themselves. Specifically, we would like you to speculate about our purposes and our intended outcomes.

For example:

1. What did we mean to share with you? Can you explain the mind set we were trying to encourage you to adopt? Can you generate arguments for adopting it, and what would they include? What arguments would you like to propose for rejecting our motions?
2. What parts of the two exercises were worth remembering, and why? What parts were a waste of your time, and why?
3. Would you agree or disagree that a necessary first step for counselors-

in-training is a healthy respect for the diversity of human behavior and the fallibility of human beings? Why? Why not?

The next exercise is an exciting one because it puts you right in the middle of the action. To this point, your role has been relatively passive, but now you will be actively involved in a few risk-taking encounters.

Exercise 3

The members of your class should be sorted into pairs, so choose a partner. Now:

1. Decide who is Sarah and who is the counselor. (Sex doesn't matter.)
2. Practice the first phase of the counseling process, "establishing the relationship."
3. Allow Sarah to give the counselor feedback about how well the counselor performed as a counselor.
4. Switch roles. (Sarah becomes the counselor, and the counselor becomes Sarah.)
5. Repeat steps 2 and 3.

Remember, only the establishment of the counselor/counselee relationship is to be role-played. No more. Take it through that process and cut it off. After everyone has had a chance to rehearse implementing the first phase of the counseling process, you are ready to perform in front of the entire class. So, two by two, take turns getting feedback from your classmates about:

1. What you did well, and why they thought so?
2. What you could improve, and how?
3. What you should try *not ever* to do again, and why?

Isn't that dreadful? We bet you were scared to death—before you tried it. We also bet you are exhilarated and pleased with yourself now that you've experienced what it's like.

Our Gang

Even if you don't hate statistics, we think you are going to hate these. We are imposing them on you to set you up for your group counseling session with a bunch of kids. Zero-population-growth campaign efforts notwithstanding, there are 66 million children in the United States, and almost 18 million of them live in dire poverty. More than half a million are born to teenage mothers every year, and 1 million run away from home each year. The number of *reported* cases of child abuse totals 1 million, and more than 5 million children are living with a single divorced parent (National

Commission on the International Year of the Child Preliminary Report, 1979.)

The problems of these kids are the problems of society, which are, in turn, the problems of professional counselors. Our intervention attempts are organized on many levels in order to reach the many differing individuals involved in the problem. As you learned from Chapter 7, you must create *programs* of services for all the problem participants— mothers, fathers, community members and agencies, and so on—not merely those who *seem to be* the problem recipients. Therefore, this exercise must be understood as only one of the many programmatic efforts you would implement to help children lead more satisfying lives and achieve their goals as productive and contributing members of society as children and as adults.

Your final preparation for this exercise is a review of the material in Chapters 9, 5, and 11. Chapter 9, a discussion of children, may help you in your approach to the children you are about to meet, and the material in Chapter 11 may stimulate some notions about their parents' behavior. But Chapter 5 is your "without which, nothing." You see, you are going to work with a *group* of children, so sharpen your group counseling skills and approaches and sit down with:

1. A fourth-grade girl who was raped by a 42-year-old man who rented a room in her home.
2. A second-grade boy who has run away from home twice within the last month.
3. A 9-year-old extortionist who beats or threatens other children on their way to school and takes money and other possessions from them. She has been suspended several times for this behavior.
4. A 10-year-old first-grade girl who lives with her grandmother because her father was accused of incestuous activity with her.
5. Two other behind-grade-level girls, both 12 years old, who are disruptive in the classroom and have been reported for a series of fights in the school environment.
6. Two sixth-grade girls who assaulted their teacher.

Your first step might be to *not* step into such a ridiculous plot. Characters like those exist in soap operas, not in real life. You might also protest that the proposed group composition is similarly unrealistic. Some group-counseling authorities argue that your groups must be homogeneously composed. You could probably pose many other arguments, and one of them would certainly be your right as a fledgling counselor to refuse to take on all those problems in one and the same group.

Do we have rebuttal privileges? All the children described are real live children, and when we first met them, they were all in the same group. We admit we were not novices in the group counseling process, but we must also admit our panic and our attempt to disguise it as indignation.

Unfortunately, there was no opportunity for indignant protests. There we were, right in the middle of problems that others—teachers, principals, school psychologists, social workers, community agents, and parents—thought we were capable of solving. We know what *we* did, but we don't know what you would do.

Exercise 4

So what will you do?

1. Absolutely nothing! This is a ridiculous exercise, and I refuse to dignify it by becoming involved with it.
2. Sit there and seethe.
3. Make a speech about my unconditional positive regard for children and my empathy with their abused and misused conditions.
4. Tell them that I am going to reorganize them into different groups because their group, as it exists, has too many different ages and kinds of problems. And it might even help if the girls were separated from the boys.
5. Tell them who I am and why I'm there and invite them to do the same.

We want to express our empathy with those of you who chose the first option by assuring you it will not cause us to withhold our unconditional positive regard for you. Rather, we would like to reaffirm your right to make your own decisions. At the same time, you are reminded of a discussion about decision making in Chapter 6.

Why would you have selected option 2? Why not? How many counterproductive consequences might follow from this response to the problem? Name some and discuss your reasoning. And before deciding on the legitimacy of #3, since empathy and unconditional positive regard are highly respected attributes for professional counselors, try to decide whether these attributes are more highly respected as words or as *deeds*.

What's your opinion about #4? What's wrong with reconstituting the group? What would be right about *not* reconstituting it? Some of your reasoning ought to be guided by the material in Chapter 5. And the material in Chapter 9 that discusses how children learn from, and teach, one another should also give you some help. Chapter 5 reinforces these observations about the value of group interactions. Still another consideration is your definition of homogeneity. Aren't all groups homogeneous on at least one dimension? Each person in the group has something in common with everyone else in the group. All of them are experiencing a problem that they need to solve. Your problem is to decide which environmental characteristics have the greatest potential for problem solving. What do you think and why?

Option #5 could have been an obvious giveaway. Was it? Do you think this is an effective way to begin? Why? Do you think you could have sat down with the described group of children and implemented the process implied in #5? Of course you could have, and here's your chance to prove it.

Exercise 5

Divide your class into groups of nine. Index cards indicating the identity of each of the eight children—sex, age, grade, problem—together with a ninth card that identifies the counselor must be prepared for each of your groups. Once you are settled in your groups, draw a card from the face-down stack. Keep your identity to yourself unless you are one of those pairs of girls or pairs of boys who knew each other before the group meeting. (These two pairs of cards will have been paper-clipped together, so that if you draw one of these, find a classmate who is willing to take your extra card.)

Your next step is to study the brief description of the child you are to role-play and project yourself into an artistic performance of the behaviors believed to be characteristic. You must discover what you would do and how if the problem described were your problem. And then you must behave that way during this stage of the group process. If you have drawn the counselor's card, then you must withdraw from the group until it is seated so that you can make your grand entrance and begin your performance. Places, everyone! Let the play begin!

Rave reviews, you did not get! The only howling successes were those "rotten kids." But, counselor, before you slash both wrists and slit your throat, remember what is going on here. This is role playing. These exercises were designed only to *introduce* you to the specific training experiences you are yet to have. This is your chance to take chances without any fear of failure. Nobody expects you to be a pro in a skill you've never had any training for. So take a few risks now, and your yet-to-come skill training will be much more satisfying.

Now, let's get back to your exercise. At this point you must get rid of your self-conscious false fears and listen carefully to everything the people in your group can tell you. You want to learn from them:

1. Why they behaved as they did and what approaches they would have used on themselves if they had been you, and *why. (Note:* The material in many chapters is relevant and useful here. Try pulling it all together and putting it to work.)
2. What happened that could have been prevented, and how. *(Note:* Don't confuse this question with #1. The first question focused on the behavior of the group members. This one focuses on the behavior of the group leader.)
3. What the counselor did well, should capitalize on, and should continue to do. *(Note:* Don't be deceived into thinking nothing went right. Try to learn that there is something good in everything. Competent counselors are known for their skill in this arena. Also, as you identify certain

effective behaviors, try to design a variety of different interpretations of them, because each of us has a different *style* of doing what all of us must do.)

When you have performed enough dress rehearsals to have assured yourself of your familiarity with the initial stage of group counseling, you may want to—

1. Take your show on the road. You and the other groups in your class can perform for, and get feedback from, one another.
2. Extend your group-process experiences to include other (a) stages of the process, (b) age groups, (c) problem areas, (d) group sizes—that is, group consulting and/or guidance.

If not, then take off your makeup, strike the set, and move out.

Final Report

In this exercise you are asked to put together all the material presented, directly or indirectly, in Parts 1, 2, and 3. This is your chance to organize it for its practical applications to your future work as a professional counselor. This is your chance to hypothetically test your competence as a staff member of an organization.

You are in the conference room of your mental-health clinic. Around the table are seated the other staff members and your director. The purpose of the meeting is to allocate the various tasks involved in preparing the annual report for the board of directors, federal, state, and local governing agencies. The tasks have been sorted into (1) program of services, (2) budget, (3) grants sought and received, (4) research and evaluation activities and data, and (5) recommendations.

One way to proceed, at this point, would require that your class be divided into four groups. (Not five: recommendations can't be written until after the report has been prepared and shared.) Now, each group must assume responsibility for one of the four tasks listed above. So accept your differing assignments, and as you begin your work together, remind yourself of the characteristics of groups, responsibilities of group membership, and the necessary conditions described for productive working groups. Now you are ready to go to work.

Exercise 6

Suppose you were assigned *program of services*. What would you need to consider?

1. What counseling services do you provide? Individual and/or group? Young, middle, and/or senior adults? (*Note:* The topics of counseling,

except as they relate to special group-counseling offerings, are not pertinent to your assignment. Your agency may be very proud that it provided individual counseling for so many different problem needs, but your funding source doesn't see it that way. It sees it as only one task. Don't make the mistake of representing it to others, or yourself, as more than that.)
2. What consulting services do you provide? Individual and/or group? In-house and/or out? Do you offer community outreach programs? If so, what is included? For whom? How? (*Note:* Remember, counselors have a lot to offer, and a lot of people need what we have to offer. We need to learn better ways of giving our skills away to everybody. Otherwise, our contribution to society will be more limited than our potential. We need to use more efficient approaches to our work, approaches that will reach and help an ever-increasing number of people—not merely for their benefit but for our own.)
3. Why are you offering the services you are offering? How are they integrated with each other? Who is managing and coordinating things, or is each of you merely minding your own little store without concern for, or knowledge of, what anyone else on the staff is doing? Or do the tasks each of you perform result from a comprehensive examination of your agency's mission and a coordinated response to it? (*Note:* You know, of course, that the question posed in #3 should have been resolved before you dealt with the questions in #1 and #2. Why something should be undertaken, your rationale, always precedes an explication of what and how. At least it does theoretically. Unfortunately, this sequencing of development is rare in the real live world of work. Almost all professional groups have an upside-down evolutionary pattern. First they tried to learn *what* they should do, then they trained others to do it and asked themselves how well they did what they were doing, and finally they got around to formulating their philosophies about *why* they should do what they had been doing. If that explanation of our ordering of your responses does not seem sufficient, then how about this one? We put these questions in their presented sequence because you might come up with better answers to them *after* we had provided you with a frame of reference—questions #1 and #2. However you resolve *our* dilemma, please put your answers to question #3 *at the beginning of your report.*)

But what if you were assigned to *budget?* That would require you to consider—

1. How great, or small, is your total budget?
2. What are the sources of your financial support?
3. Are they categorical funds, or can they be developed without restriction? Some of each? How much for what?
4. What categories were established by your agency this year, and what percentage of the available funds was used for each?

5. What surpluses and/or deficits have accrued in the past year? Why? (*Note:* Called for here is a whole series of *projections* about your imaginary agency. Set it up however you like: number of staff members, phones, offices, clerks, secretaries, receptionists, hotlines, office supplies, instructional materials, office equipment, travel allowances, office furniture, maintenance, utility bills, and so on. Are all your people *paid* employees? What is the cost of your fringe-benefit program, and is this shared by members of the plan? Do you get the point? It may be fun to project a high-cost budget, but in the real world, bills must be paid. The higher the budget, the harder it is to meet.)

Now, on to more about money. For example, if you were assigned the task of describing *the grants* your agency sought and/or received, then what would you have to consider? You might want to describe—

1. The federal agencies you submitted proposals to, the titles under which they could have been or were funded, the arm of the federal government that supported them, the amount of support requested, the objectives to be achieved by the funding, and the current status of the proposal.
2. The state agencies you submitted proposals to, and so forth (same as above).
3. The private foundations (Ford, Rockefeller, and so on).
4. Local community organizations, philanthropic and service institutions. (It's your turn. Name some money sources and describe *how you told them* why you asked them for money and why they should give it to you.) (*Note:* Counselors help people deal with various crippling consequences of their interactions with their environments. Counselors themselves are not supposed to accept a helpless condition. Start your professional career with a deep appreciation of the maxim that God helps those who help themselves. Every budget of every setting in which you will work will have its limits and its priorities. Your priorities may not be among them—not because they are unimportant but because no one but you may realize their importance. Sitting around and complaining about it will never change any but weak minds. Taking the initiative and providing for your own special needs might change a lot of minds. The message here is don't whine about what *others* won't let you do. You control you. So reach out and inform yourself of the sources of your supply, and don't be surprised when you discover that the greatest of these is *you*. Your financial resources may always be limited, but your own unique resources are unlimited.)

All right, all you *researchers and evaluators,* what are you going to do, and how are you going to do it? As you begin your search for research and evaluation data, you might want to consider—

1. What populations does your agency provide services for?
2. What service needs exist for the individuals represented in these populations?

3. What do previous research and evaluation attempts indicate as productive areas of inquiry?
4. Were the approaches of your agency conducive to the methods and procedures previously undertaken? If not, drop your consideration of them.
5. What are the goals and objectives of your agency? What research and/or evaluation designs could be formulated to measure each of them?
6. Which of these have the potential for yielding objective rather than subjective data? Given a choice, choose the former. Our profession already has more of the latter than it is proud to claim.
7. How do you demonstrate your worth? If your individual counseling sessions produced insignificant behavior changes in your counselees, then don't beat that poor horse to death; look instead to your other services. What changes occurred in one or another of your group-counseling programmatic offerings? *Behavior* changes, not *attitude* changes. Grandiose statements of love and affection for the counselors involved won't hack it with those who hold the pursestrings. It's not hearts and flowers that you are after here. It's hard, cold, concrete evidence that the majority of individuals you were employed to help received more than empathy, unconditional positive regard, refuge from the enemy, Kleenex, and a shoulder to cry on. The taxpaying public is not at all eager to support public servants who cannot prove their worth. (Have you failed to identify yourself as a public employee? Have you forgotten some of the material in Chapter 1? Did you read too quickly the material in Chapter 2 about private practice? And how about Chapter 3? All the standards in the world will not an honest counselor make.) So what *do* you do? What can you measure?
8. What differences might have been observed for your consultees? How did you measure the changes? Were your data objective or only "love letters"? How many of which populations did what? When? Which among your outreach programs were most heavily attended? At the last season as opposed to the first? What other measures were, or should have been, useful if employed here?
9. Do you have evaluation measures of the management and organizational skill of your director? How about the cooperative working relationships among the staff members? Do the other working-force members have any conflicting and/or supporting *objective,* though *second-hand,* evidence to contribute?
10. What expectations about, and motives for, counseling are held by (a) counselees, (b) society, and (c) counselors? (*Note:* Expand your view of society's expectations for you and you will come closer to the mark described for professional counselor behavior. Do not limit your expectations for yourself. You can and must provide more than "snuzzle sessions" for counselees who may want to withdraw and

luxuriate in a freedom from social obligations and responsibility. Prolonged dependency relationships may feed your ego, but they will also destroy your credibility. Counselors must hold *themselves* accountable and learn new ways of meeting this challenge. Our professional reputation rests in your skillful research and evaluation hands.)

Now that all the work groups have completed their separate assignments, let's return to the conference room and present your report. This is the time for sharing your views, offering your interpretations of your agency's work and worth. You will realize that all your individual vested interests are important but only the director has the *big* picture. The final decisions belong to that person because it is to the director that the final blame also belongs. The director is the only one ultimately responsible for your program of services, and so the decisions must be *agency-*, not *staff-* oriented. So share your recommendations knowing these things. Whether or not your recommendations were incorporated in the report would have nothing to do with you as a person. If we must help others learn not to personalize incidents in their lives, then we should begin by learning it for ourselves.

Exercise 7

For Exercise 7, a self-exploration of your management skills to set the stage for Exercise 8, consider the following:

1. What do you know about yourself? Do you have a need to order the lives of others or to help them learn how to order their own?
2. What do you know about how you perceive others? Do you believe others are self-centered, dependent, and devious, or do you view others as self-directed, resourceful, and committed?
3. What do you know about your own resourcefulness? Are you able to identify the special talents and skills that are unique to all those you live, work, or study with? And are you able and/or willing to provide opportunities for each of them to express these attributes and increased understandings of them?
4. Do you believe that getting to "the top of the ladder" requires you to keep everyone else at the bottom? Or have you learned that success should not be characterized as a ladder but as an escalator? In order to go up, others don't have to go down. If you want to move up, you must take everyone else with you.
5. Will you surround yourself with minimally competent people so that you will look highly competent? Or will you want to be associated with the most competent so that the work you're responsible for will be competently performed?

6. Will you make equitable allocations and assign them with respect to individual skills and talents? Will you explain the task and not its solution? And will you hold each person responsible for promptly and effectively completing all assigned tasks? Will you ask for opinions, give them due consideration, and assume responsibility for the decisions ultimately made?
7. Will you provide opportunities for others to learn of your respect for them and your appreciation of their efforts? And will these positive reinforcements include more than "lip service"? What *concrete* rewards—advancement, salary increase, advanced training—would you consider?
8. Would you realize that leadership, even in democratically organized systems, requires strength and courage? You alone are the one ultimately responsible for the record achieved by your unit, and unless you assume responsibility for ultimately making the final decisions, you risk the loss of your leadership status. If your staff decide you are not "running the show," then *they* will "run the show" and you.
9. What if I don't want to lead, manage, control and/or be responsible for anyone or anything?

Some of the notions in Chapters 5, 6, 7, and 11 might be useful here, but the only meaningful resources are your own. Who are you? Who are all those others with whom you will be working? What do you respect in the *leaders and managers* you have known? What did you find counterproductive in their behavior? Think back to those interactions. They may become the best material for formulating your own list of leadership and management objectives. What would your list include? Which do you already possess? Which would fall into the "must acquire" column?

Exercise 8

Leadership and management skills

I admire	*I possess*	*I must acquire*
1.		
2.		
3.		
Etc.		

Do any of your projections reflect a need to respond to what you have learned about adulthood, its characteristics and concerns? Good! Now you're prepared for a closer look at, and a more personal involvement with, a group of adults. However, your involvement does not begin with them. It begins with a child.

Timothy

A 10-year-old boy who is an only child has been referred to you because he is falling behind in his school work. Timothy had been at the top of his class in previous years, but now he doesn't participate in class recitations, fails to present his homework, doesn't respond to his classmates' urgings to play with them during recess, is often absent, and seems withdrawn and unhappy. His teacher has suggested that something may have gone wrong at home but has no certain knowledge of this.

Exercise 9

After you have introduced yourself, you try to get the young man to share his problem with you by—

1. observing that he is unhappy?

Not unless you want to reinforce him in his unhappiness and *not* if he is proud and independent. *Not* unless you want to force him into lying about it, and particularly *not,* unless you want to get egg all over your face for what might turn out to be a faulty projection.

2. asking whether his mother and father get along very well with each other and him? Whether they have fights? Sleep in the same bed? Tuck him in bed and kiss him goodnight? Hurt him or leave him alone in the house?

Wrong again! What do you remember from Chapter 2 about the laws assuring rights of privacy? And whose privacy is being invaded when we question minors about their home lives? Under these circumstances, you would also have difficulty taking refuge in child-protection laws. They stipulate that you *report* your suspicions, not *verify* them. Your immunity from civil and criminal liability has not been described to include other than "reporting in good faith." You have a mandate to report, but you should be cautious about attempting to extend this mandate to include information-seeking activities with minors. What if your suspicions were groundless, and what if the child told his parents the questions you asked? What would you, as a responsible parent, do if you learned your child's counselor was asking such questions?

3. telling him that counselors never tell secrets and if he has a secret he wants to tell you, then it will be all right because you won't tell anyone else?

Absolutely right! You would *not* tell him this, because professional counselors do not "bait" kids into relationships. The literature is full of what's right about confidentiality, but its bad spinoffs are rarely discussed. This is one. Another is the protection it provides incompetence. If you have a need to hide what you are doing or a need to feel important and omniscient, then confidentiality is something you will not be able to do without. If you keep a kid's or anyone else's secret, how are you going to help him? The meaningful help he needs must come not merely from you but from all those others who are a part of the secret. How can all those others provide the needed help if you don't provide the needed information? But here's the biggie. You must have accurate information if you are going to be helpful. How will you know you are operating with accurate information if you can't check it out? And don't think the concept of confidentiality is a *sometime* thing. It is an *at all times* thing. You can't have your cake and eat it too. You can't become the judge of what should be confidential or under which circumstances it should be set aside. Confidentiality is confidentiality. Will it help or hinder your work as a professional counselor?

4. telling him that counselors are child advocates, that they help children and protect them when they need help and want it?

"Baiting" again? You sure are, but there's something else here. Attorneys are advocates. They are *directed by their courts* to be advocates. Do you know what an advocate is? An advocate must defend another person's actions regardless of whether they are right or wrong, good for society or bad, good for the person or self-defeating. Do *you* believe an advocate's role is an appropriate one for professional counselors?

5. telling him that his teacher has noticed that he doesn't seem to be enjoying school as much as he used to and that his teacher wants to help him, that his teacher thought he might want to talk it over with you?

Why not? It's the way things really are, isn't it? The teacher *noticed,* and the teacher *wants to help* him, so level with the kid and give the teacher credit for his affectionate concern. Counselors don't have a corner on the love market, and they shouldn't spend their lives trying to persuade their counselees that "only my counselor loves and understands me."

From the material in Chapter 4 you learned that some of us stereotype kids as nonverbal. If you've listened to them at play with their friends, you might want to quarrel with this view. If kids don't talk, it is usually because they don't want to talk. The reasons vary. Sometimes it is because the counselor has turned them off by not leveling with them, baiting them, asking embarrassing questions, or otherwise invading their privacy. They can be turned off by the same things that turn off adults. Their response to inconsiderate behavior may differ. Whereas adults may tell you in *words* what they think of you and your approach to them, a child may tell you in *silence.*

There are other reasons for a child's silence. Often children are still trying to figure it out for themselves, and they are not ready to talk about it. But let's assume that our young man was both willing and able to share with you what was bothering him and he told you that his mother and father had got a divorce. After you have let him tell you what he thinks *divorce* means, offered some factual information to correct his misconceptions about divorce—not his perceptions of its consequences—then you might ask whether he thinks his mother and father would like to talk with him and you about it. If so, then all four of you could talk about some of the things that he would like to know more about.

1. Why would you do that? Why wouldn't you do that? Which of your two sets of answers seemed better?
2. If you decided it was worth a try, what *else* would you do?
3. Do you suppose he's the only kid in his school whose parents are divorced or the only kid who is struggling with his new status and trying to sort it out? What about helping all of them? Or will you simply wait for each of them or someone else to ask for your help? Will you help them individually, or have you discovered a more efficient *and* effective way of delivering your services? Do kids learn from kids, or do they learn only from interacting with counselors? And could children of divorce learn anything helpful by talking with adults who were once children of divorce? Could such people be enlisted? How?
4. If you believe that a kid's happiness is intimately related to the happiness of loved ones, then what are you going to do for, and with, the parents and/or loved ones? How? Perhaps you've decided a group of divorced parents would want to meet with one another to share their thoughts about their new marital state, their children, and the ways they have managed their new lives and responsibilities.
5. You may also have realized that divorced parents aren't the only single parents. There are widows and abandoned or separated spouses, as well as a growing number of never-married parents, who are bringing up their children alone. What about them? Does this require that a separate group be organized because they are different? Or because your projected group would be too large if you added these people? If they all share the same problem, single parenting, then they all should be able to share something profitable with one another. Rather than considering a different group, why not consider a different group approach? What's wrong with implementing large-group sessions? What's right about it? Remember, your consulting skills are the same as your counseling skills. The level of your *obvious* interaction is significantly decreased, but the degree of your influence is significantly increased. If you want to be really successful in "giving your skills away," then find yourself some large groups. Children, adolescents, adults, or seniors—it doesn't matter. It's the medium, not the message.
6. Listening to concerns such as day care, babysitting, male and female role models, after-school supervision, and self-preservation and self-renewal, you might have wondered about possible sources of help. You might also have wondered about some of the material you read in Chapter 12. Why wouldn't it work? Why might it? Why not try it? But because you remember your lessons in Chapter 6, why not let someone in the group suggest inviting seniors to help out? Remember, if it was *the*

group's idea, then the group will make it work. What kind of "wonder whether . . ." pump-priming statements could you make in the group that could help them discover the idea themselves and propose it? Try some out on your classmates. What kind of characteristics of seniors led you to believe they could or would help? Trade a few of these with your classmates.

Surely, by now you have realized that our bombardment of questions was designed to help you understand how programs of services are created. All you need is an appreciation of the multifaceted nature of problems, the multifaceted nature of your counseling skills, and your unlimited capacity for discovering new ways of helping people learn how to solve their own problems.

How do you get all these things done? You don't, if you try to do them all yourself. Remember always that your unique leadership skills require you to be a manager of *programs,* not people. Your skills make it possible for you to become a resource person to, and a facilitator of, people in search of solutions to problems. Your leadership and management skills make it possible for you to help people learn how to identify the tasks that need performing, allocate those tasks, monitor them, and hold themselves accountable for the performance of them. You make all those things possible by creating *the system* within which all these things must operate. This is your responsibility, and it results from your talent for interacting with others at a level of imperceptibility. They learned how to do what they were capable of doing because you created a fail-safe system within which they could learn.

So how do you implement your program of services? You involve all those people who are the recipients of your services. They must become responsible for themselves, and there is only one way. You must let go and let them run their own show. In this case, "them" would be your single-parent group members.

They must determine when they meet, where, for how long, and for what purpose, and they must be responsible for getting themselves to *their* sessions. They must create their own senior support system, and they must be responsible for its trouble-free functioning. They must organize their own babysitting cooperative and discover the joy that comes from realizing their own inner resources.

And what do *you* do? You secretly savor the gratification you feel—from knowing that yours were the resources that helped so many people resolve some of their daily living problems. You also secretly experience a sense of satisfaction in knowing that you were not limited in your understanding of a child's problem or in your response to his problem. You are rewarded by your realization that so many lives were enriched because you didn't stop with the child. More to the point, you enriched your own because you were willing to let a little child lead you to an enlarged expression of *your own* potential.

Are you beginning to understand what it would be like to be a counselor? And are you still interested in joining this group of professionals? Then you are ready for your final "rite of passage."

The Convention

You are about to attend your first national convention. The APGA has sent you, as one of its members, preregistration and housing materials. Also included are *Call for Programs* materials.

Exercise 10

Here you are at your desk, and spread out on top of your desk are all those materials (see Appendixes F & G). As you examine the—

1. housing form and note the descriptions of the facilities you can request space from, you ask: "Why should counselors spread themselves out in so many different hotels? Why do ACPA, ASCA, ACES, NVGA, AMHCA, and so on have different headquarters hotels? Am I supposed to stay in the one where my division headquarters is? Will there be anybody else at the convention who feels as uninformed as I?" (*Note:* Try a review of Chapter 1. It may help you with these questions. Chapter 1 is a must for the big picture and should assuage your doubts about your ability to hold your own and establish new relationships with colleagues. If appropriate behavior is your problem doubt, then get yourself up on Chapter 2).
2. forms on which you could propose a program you would like to present, you find they require your program title; the names, addresses, telephone numbers, and titles of others who may assist you in your program presentations; the titles of your and their presentations; the amount of time you think you need for your presentations; the room size, arrangements, and audiovisual support systems you will require; and the APGA division that you think would be interested in sponsoring your proposed program. You say: "Good grief! If conventions are organized for the purpose of sharing professional information, then why should the opportunity to share be made so difficult? Why should I do all this work—organize the program, get all the participants' letters of acceptance and summaries together and perhaps have to hound them to get them, duplicate all the materials and get them in before the deadline, which is only about a week after the end of summer vacation? Only to ask 'Please, may I share something I think is useful to counselors?' Who needs this hassle? I can go off to the convention and be the audience for somebody else's program." (*Note:* Sure you can, and so can everybody else, but if everybody else *did*, where would *all of us* be? We are professionals, and the material in Chapter 1 should help you to accept the responsibilities associated with your membership in a

profession that your colleague group worked hard to develop. All programs need an audience. Your fullest appreciation of this will come when you find yourself with none. But you don't die when this happens to you. You resolve to make your future programs more responsive to the needs of your colleagues. So don't resent those colleagues who not only didn't show for your program but didn't show for *any* programs because another inclusion in your convention registration materials invited you to register for—

3. special luncheons sponsored by the division in which you hold membership, the convention banquet, special tours organized by your colleagues who work in the host city of the convention. "I'm strapped for money. I extended my budget to be able to go to the national convention. And don't tell me all about how tax-deductible it will be. Tell me instead where I'm going to get the money to get there, stay there, and get home again. Tell me why "my leaders" negotiated for divisional luncheons, banquets, and room rates that compromise my budget and family responsibilities. Tell me why a professional organization with 40,000 members doesn't have sufficient clout to negotiate economical and reasonable convention contracts. I want to participate in my national conventions. It's my responsibility. Why must the cost be so high?" (*Note:* These are tough questions. We don't know all the answers. We are a *big* association providing a great number of services, and it takes a lot of money to keep it running. Perhaps, as we move along in this exercise, you will discover what some of these expenditures are. Nevertheless, in most budgets there is some fat that might be trimmed. All of us older and not as wise colleagues take hope that you may find ways to do it.)

Once your ventilating is complete, you complete your registration and housing-request forms, enclose your check, and put everything in the mail. You resolve your travel arrangements and submit your program proposal, and soon there you are at your first APGA national convention.

The hotel lobby is jammed, the room clerks are harassed, and you are exhilarated. When you finally get to your room, you leave it immediately for the registration center, which also is jammed with people wearing buttons and badges and ribbons. You and your unadorned chest feel almost naked until you claim your registration packet. Inside are tons of things. Among them is your badge. It has your name, whom you work for, and the city you come from, typed in big bold letters. If your program proposal was accepted, there will also be a ribbon inside marked *Speaker* or *Presenter,* which is attached to your badge. Now, you are *dressed* for the occasion, but are you all dressed up with no place to go? Not on your life!

1. Just standing there, you have run into people you never expected to see, but you're curious whether anyone else you know is there, too. So you—
   a. ask the people behind the registration desks to look them up for you.

(We do *not* recommend this solution. They are counselors from the host city who volunteered to work with registration, not lost and found. And even counselors are not always warm and accepting.)
  b. run up to everyone you see and ask whether he or she knows your friends and has seen them. (This might work. But it seems a rather unsystematic way of going about it. And this kind of behavior could raise a few eyebrows.)
  c. go to the information center and check the computer printouts of preregistrants. (Very good! The printout includes the names of all preregistered members. It also indicates the hotels in which they are staying. If your friends did not preregister, all is not lost. There's a big bulletin board for messages. Check it. It could have one for you, or you could leave one for each of them. What have you got to lose?)
2. Now take a look at some of the other things in your handsome, plastic convention portfolio embossed with the APGA logo. One of them is the program, which lists all the programs and events of the convention by dates, times, and locations. It also includes an alphabetical listing of all the presenters and a categorical listing by interest areas of all the programs; group, women, non-white concerns, children, adolescents, death and dying, drugs, gays, marriage and family, and so on. Excluding preconvention activities, the convention usually runs for three days. There is a lot to do and very little time to do it in, and so you decide to—
  a. forget the whole thing and just enjoy yourself. After all, this is costing a bundle, and so you might as well give yourself a holiday. (Why not? There's a Special Tours booth right over there, and you could book yourself on *all* of them. But how about booking yourself on just one? It's true that you ought to have a little fun while you're here, but shouldn't your major purpose be *professional?*)
  b. introduce yourself to someone who looks friendly and ask him which programs he is going to attend and whether you can go with him? (It might work out even better than you hoped—but only if the programs he planned to attend were programs of interest and concern to you. Otherwise, you are about to have a wasted convention.)
  c. sit down somewhere and study your program. (What a dreadful thing to suggest! *Study* is a *work* word. That's right, and that's what you must spend some time doing. Discover what is happening when. If several programs that sound interesting to you are scheduled at the same time or in settings too remote to accommodate your scheduling, then you've got to decide among them. Use your pen. Mark up your program and then go back and review your first impressions. Finally, compile, by dates, times, and locations, your personal conference schedule. When you have all this written, go back and fill in all the special events—opening session, president's receptions, divisional luncheons, banquet, and so on.)

You are now dressed for the occasion, and you are prepared for the occasion. What do you do now? You check your schedule, of course.

If you feel the need to get a *better* feel for what we have been talking about, we suggest you get an old convention program and try a dry run. Flip through the one you were able to find. Orient yourself to it and then run through the steps we discussed for planning your personal convention agenda. Talk it over with your classmates and get your prof to fill you in on all those things we left unclarified.

Find out what all those Delegate Assembly, Board of Governors, and special committee meetings are all about. Find out which ones you are able to attend. Is attendance by nonmembers prohibited? If not, then why not schedule yourself into them? You may think politics has no place in your life. If you do, you could be making a very big mistake. The politics of your profession *is* you. It needs your input and your concerned involvement. So get involved at the very beginning of your career.

As a "hail and farewell" gesture, may we commend you for your—

1. *Courage* to do battle with the forces of society that create in its members a variety of developmental struggles.
2. *Commitment* to developmental counseling approaches that provide alternative ways of helping not only your counselees but others.
3. *Good judgment* for selecting this as one of the most rewarding of all careers.

And may we assure you of our confidence in your long and successful, satisfying and edifying career.

Welcome to the distinguished and proud community of professional counselors!

References

Cronbach, L. J. *Educational psychology* (2nd ed.). New York: Harcourt Brace Jovanovich, 1963.

National Commission on the International Year of the Child, Preliminary Report, 1979.

White, R. W. Competence as a basic concept in the growth of psychology. Paper presented to the Social Science Research Council at the Conference on Socialization and Evocation of Competence, San Juan, Puerto Rico, April-May 1965.

Appendix A
Professional Organizations of Interest to Counselors

Note: The information presented in this compilation reflects primarily the brochures, pamphlets, and other publications received from the organizations listed. Most notably, this consideration applies to the "Focus" section. Some data may have changed since this information was assembled during the Fall of 1981.

Membership categories often number more than those presented. Listed are the major categories and any student arrangements. Students must have graduate status and not be employed full-time.

Name & Address	Focus	Membership Requirements	Benefits	Structure
AMERICAN ASSOCIATION FOR MARRIAGE AND FAMILY THERAPY (AAMFT) 924 W. Ninth Upland, CA 91786	Serving as the professional membership organization for the field of marriage and family therapy	Clinical members: Masters or doctorate degree in marital/family therapy or related field, specified clinical experience, $90-110 dues Associate members: Degree complete, in process of becoming a clinical member, $50.00 annual dues, 5 year limit Student members: Currently enrolled in specified program, $25.00 annual dues, 5 year limit	Publications: *Journal of Marital and Family Therapy*, *Family Therapy News* professional meetings, credentialing information	National organization; 40 regional, state and provincial divisions throughout North America
AMERICAN ASSOCIATION OF COLLEGIATE REGISTRARS AND ADMISSIONS OFFICERS (AACRAO) One Dupont Circle Suite 330 Washington, D.C. 22036	Enhancing the professional growth of college admissions officers	Institutional (no individual memberships)	Access to publications, conferences, and special projects	National organization; President, vice presidents (5), regional associations (29), admissions and financial aid, records and registration, data management and research, international education, ad hoc committees

APPENDIX A

Name & Address	Focus	Membership Requirements	Benefits	Structure
AMERICAN ASSOCIATION OF SCHOOL ADMINISTRATORS (AASA) 1801 North Moore St. Arlington, VA 22209	Serving the public interest through assuring the availability of high quality education for all through effective school administrators	Active (voting) members: School administrators, $125.00 dues Nonvoting members: Students, $20.00 dues	Publications: *The School Administrators*, Newsletters, retirement plans, insurance plans, reduced hotel/motel rates, travel service, auto rental discount, reduced rates to AASA-NASE seminars and workshops	National organization, AASA National Academy for School Executives offers workshops, seminars, contact programs to advance the knowledge and skills of school administrators. National Center for the Improvement of Learning (NCIL) promotes educational excellence.
AMERICAN CORRECTIONAL ASSOCIATION (ACA) 4321 Hartwick Road Suite L-208 College Park, MD 20740	To fulfill the needs of those who have an interest in acquiring knowledge in the field	Eleven different categories of membership, several for organizations but most for professional membership. Dues depend on services Associate membership: Students, retirees, inmates and interested persons, $12.50 dues.	Publications: *Corrections Today* Professional members vote; associates do not.	National organization
AMERICAN EDUCATIONAL RESEARCH ASSOCIATION (AERA) 1230 Seventeenth Street, N.W. Washington, DC 22036	Improvement of the educational process by encouragement of scholarly inquiry and application of the results	Active (voting) members: Master's degree, evidence of active interest in research, $35.00 dues. Nonvoting members: Students, three year limit, full time students only, $15.00 dues	Publications: *Educational Researcher* Placement service, group insurance, travel service, one divisional membership, (Placement service at annual meeting only)	National organization; Divisons: Administration, curriculum and objectives, learning and instruction, measurement and research methodology, counseling and human development, history and historiography, social context of education, school evaluation and program development, education in the professions

APPENDIX A   333

Name & Address	Focus	Membership Requirements	Benefits	Structure
AMERICAN PERSONNEL AND GUIDANCE ASSOCIATION (APGA) Two Skyline Place Suite 400 5203 Leesburg Pike Falls Church, VA 22041	Coordination and growth of the human development professions	Voting members: Professional counselors, $47.00 dues Nonvoting members: Students, $29.00 dues	Publications: *Personnel and Guidance Journal* Reference service, films, books, monographs and pamphlets, Career Information Center, workshops, group insurance, convention, Counselors Legal Defense Service	National organization; Divisions: American College Personnel Association, American Mental Health Counselor Association, American School Counselor Association, American Rehabilitation Counseling Association, Association for Counselor Education and Supervision, National Vocational Guidance Association, Association for Humanistic Education and Development, Association for Measurement and Evaluation Guidance, Association for Non-White Concerns in Personnel and Guidance, Association for Religious and Value Issues in Counseling, Association for Specialists in Group Work, National Employment Counselors Association, Public Offender Counselor Association, Regional Branch Assemblies (4), State Branches (56)

Name & Address	Focus	Membership Requirements	Benefits	Structure
AMERICAN PSYCHOLOGICAL ASSOCIATION 1200 Seventeenth Street, N.W. Washington, D.C. 200-36	To advance psychology as a science, as a profession, and as a means of promoting human welfare	Membership by election. Associates: Completion of two years of graduate study, or masters degree in psychology, and involvement in work or additional study that is primarily psychological in nature, $68.00 annual dues Members: Minimum of doctoral degree, $89.00 annual dues. Student Affiliates: Undergraduate/graduate, must be endorsed by a member, preferably from the school in which they're enrolled, $5.00 annual dues	Publications, research	National organization; State associations, forty specialized subject-matter divisions
AMERICAN VOCATIONAL ASSOCIATION (AVA) 2020 North 14th Street Arlington, VA 22201	Provide leadership in Washington in government affairs, and increase public understanding of vocational education	Affiliated: $20.00 dues (with membership in state association and payment of state dues) Student: $5.00 dues	Publications: *Vocational Education Update* Group insurance, membership in one division, conferences and workshops	National organization; Divisions: Administration, agriculture, business and office, distributive, guidance, health occupations, home economics, industrial arts, manpower training, technical, trade and industrials, State associations
ASSOCIATION FOR SUPERVISION AND CURRICULUM DEVELOPMENT (ASCD) 225 N. Washington Street Alexandria, VA 22314	Reshaping the future of education by studying and using innovative concepts and ideas	Open to all disciplines in the profession. Comprehensive: $35.00 dues Regular: $25.00 dues	Publications: *Educational Leadership* Group insurance, conference, choice of ASCD books (Regular membership does not include books)	National organization

APPENDIX A   335

Name & Address	Focus	Membership Requirements	Benefits	Structure
(THE) COLLEGE PLACEMENT COUNCIL, INC. (CPC) P.O. Box 2263 Bethlehem, PA 18001	Provide coordination of and information for career planning and placement personnel	Institutional/individual membership: Applicant must hold personal membership in one of the seven regional placement associations or in one of the CPC affiliates. Membership plan for individuals and institutions range from $100 to $300, depending on the number of College Placement Annuals needed	Publicatons: College placement annuals, salary surveys and recruiting, activity reports *Spotlight* (newspaper) *Directory of College Planning and Placement Officers, Directory of College Recruiting Personnel* Resource information center	National organization; Regional Associations (7) Affiliates (3) National Association for Law Placement, Association for School, College, and University Staffing, Employment Management Association
INTERNATIONAL ASSOCIATION OF PUPIL PERSONNEL WORKERS (IAPPW) c/o William E. Myer Executive Director Mt. View, P.O. Box 36 Barnesville, MD 20838	Provide leadership in the development of the field by research and professional growth in its members	Regular: $35.00 dues Student: $10.00 dues	Publications: *IAPPW Journal* Reduced journal advertising rates, travel service	Organization includes members from USA and Canada
NATIONAL ASSOCIATION OF COLLEGE ADMISSIONS COUNSELORS (NACAA) 9933 Lawler Avenue Suite 500 Skokie, IL 60077	Serve the needs of all professional counselors in college admissions areas	Voting membership for institutions and employees of member institutions only. Nonvoting membership for not-for-profit organizations, retired persons (past members), and individuals at non-member institutions, $15-$150	Inservice workshops, Publications: *Journal, Newsletter* Computerized college search data bank, college fairs	National organization; 1700 institutions, 850 individuals, state and regional, 18 associations

APPENDIX A

Name & Address	Focus	Membership Requirements	Benefits	Structure
NATIONAL ASSOCIATION OF SCHOOL FINANCIAL AID ADMINISTRATORS (NASFAA) 1766 Massachusetts Ave, NW Suite 100 Washington, D.C. 20036	Promoting effective financial aid administration throughout the nation	Voting members: Institution (designate voting representative) $100-$300 (based on enrollment) Nonvoting members: Nonmember administrator $100-$200 Student: $50.00	Publications: *Journal of Student Financial Aid* Staff training manuals	National organization; Regional associations (6)
NATIONAL REHABILITATION ASSOCIATION (NRA) 1522 K Street, NW Washington, DC 20005	Advance the rehabilitation of all handicapped persons	Professional members: Active in some aspects of vocational evaluation or adjustment training of handicapped persons, $42.00 dues Students: Full time enrollment in programs related to vocational evaluation or adjustment training of handicapped persons, $21.00 dues	Publications, group insurance, division membership	National organization; State chapters, divisions

Appendix B
Ethical Standards
American Personnel and Guidance Association

(Approved by Executive Committee upon referral of the Board of Directors, **January 17, 1981**).

PREAMBLE

The American Personnel and Guidance Association is an educational, scientific, and professional organization whose members are dedicated to the enhancement of the worth, dignity, potential, and uniqueness of each individual and thus to the service of society.

The Association recognizes that the role definitions and work settings of its members include a wide variety of academic disciplines, levels of academic preparation and agency services. This diversity reflects the breadth of the Association's interest and influence. It also poses challenging complexities in efforts to set standards for the performance of members, desired requisite preparation or practice, and supporting social, legal, and ethical controls.

The specification of ethical standards enables the Association to clarify to present and future members and to those served by members, the nature of ethical responsibilities held in common by its members.

The existence of such standards serves to stimulate greater concern by members for their own professional functioning and for the conduct of fellow professionals such as counselors, guidance and student personnel workers, and others in the helping professions. As the ethical code of the Association, this document establishes principles that define the ethical behavior of Association members.

Section A:
General

1. The member influences the development of the profession by continuous efforts to improve professional practices, teaching, services, and research. Professional growth is continuous throughout the member's career and is exemplified by the development of a philosophy that explains why and how a member functions in the helping relationship. Members must gather data on their effectiveness and be guided by the findings.

2. The member has a responsibility

both to the individual who is served and to the institution within which the service is performed to maintain high standards of professional conduct. The member strives to maintain the highest levels of professional services offered to the individuals to be served. The member also strives to assist the agency, organization, or institution in providing the highest caliber of professional services. The acceptance of employment in an institution implies that the member is in agreement with the general policies and principles of the institution. Therefore the professional activities of the member are also in accord with the objectives of the institution. If, despite concerted efforts, the member cannot reach agreement with the employer as to acceptable standards of conduct that allow for changes in institutional policy conducive to the positive growth and development of clients, then terminating the affiliation should be seriously considered.

3. Ethical behavior among professional associates, both members and nonmembers, must be expected at all times. When information is possessed that raises doubt as to the ethical behavior of professional colleagues, whether Association members or not, the member must take action to attempt to rectify such a condition. Such action shall use the institution's channels first and then use procedures established by the state Branch, Division, or Association.

4. The member neither claims nor implies professional qualifications exceeding those possessed and is responsible for correcting any misrepresentations of these qualifications by others.

5. In establishing fees for professional counseling services, members must consider the financial status of clients and locality. In the event that the established fee structure is inappropriate for a client, assistance must be provided in finding comparable services of acceptable cost.

6. When members provide information to the public or to subordinates, peers or supervisors, they have a responsibility to ensure that the content is general, unidentified client information that is accurate, unbiased, and consists of objective, factual data.

7. With regard to the delivery of professional services, members should accept only those positions for which they are professionally qualified.

8. In the counseling relationship the counselor is aware of the intimacy of the relationship and maintains respect for the client and avoids engaging in activities that seek to meet the counselor's personal needs at the expense of that client. Through awareness of the negative impact of both racial and sexual stereotyping and discrimination, the counselor guards the individual rights and personal dignity of the client in the counseling relationship.

Section B: Counseling Relationship

This section refers to practices and procedures of individual and/or group counseling relationships.

The member must recognize the need for client freedom of choice. Under those circumstances where this is not possible, the member must apprise clients of restrictions that may limit their freedom of choice.

1. The member's *primary* obligation is to respect the integrity and promote the welfare of the client(s), whether the client(s) is (are) assisted individually or in a group relationship. In a group setting, the member is also responsible for taking reasonable precautions to protect individuals from physical and/or psychological trauma resulting from interaction within the group.

2. The counseling relationship and information resulting therefrom be kept confidential, consistent with the obligations of the member as a professional person. In a group counseling setting, the counselor must set a norm of confidentiality regarding all group participants' disclosures.

3. If an individual is already in a counseling relationship with another professional person, the member does not enter into a counseling relationship without first contacting and receiving the approval of that other professional. If the member discovers that the client is in another counseling relationship after the counseling relationship begins, the member must gain the consent of the other professional or terminate the relationship, unless the client elects to terminate the other relationship.

4. When the client's condition indicates that there is clear and imminent danger to the client or others, the member must take reasonable personal action or inform responsible authorities. Consulation with other professionals must be used where possible. The assumption of responsibility for the client(s) behavior must be taken only after careful deliberation. The client must be involved in the resumption of responsibility as quickly as possible.

5 Records of the counseling relationship, including interview notes, test data, correspondence, tape recordings, and other documents, are to be considered professional information for use in counseling and they should not be considered a part of the records of the institution or agency in which the counselor is employed unless specified by state statute or regulation. Revelation to others of counseling material must occur only upon the expressed consent of the client.

6. Use of data derived from a counseling relationship for purposes of counselor training or research shall be confined to content that can be disguised to ensure full protection of the identity of the subject client.

7. The member must inform the client of the purposes, goals, techniques, rules of procedure and limitations that may affect the relationship at or before the time that the counseling relationship is entered.

8. The member must screen prospective group participants, especially when the emphasis is on self-understanding and growth through self-disclosure. The member must maintain an awareness of the group participants' compatibility throughout the life of the group.

9. The member may choose to consult with any other professionally competent person about a client. In choosing a consultant, the member must avoid placing the consultant in a conflict of interest situation that would preclude the consultant's being a proper party to the member's efforts to help the client.

10. If the member determines an inability to be of professional assistance to the client, the member must either avoid initiating the counseling relationship or immediately terminate that relationship. In either event, the member must suggest appropriate alternatives. (The member must be knowledgeable about referral resources so that a satisfactory referral can be initiated). In the event the client declines the suggested referral, the member is not obligated to continue the relationship.

11. When the member has other relationships, particularly of an administrative, supervisory and/or evaluative nature with an individual seeking counseling services, the member must not serve as the counselor but should refer the individual to another professional. Only in instances where such an alternative is unavailable and where the individual's situation warrants counseling intervention should the member enter into and/or maintain a counseling relationship. Dual relationships with clients that might impair the member's objectivity and professional judgment (e.g., as with close friends or relatives, sexual intimacies with any client) must be avoided and/or the counseling relationship terminated through referral to another competent professional.

12. All experimental methods of treatment must be clearly indicated to prospective recipients and safety precautions are to be adhered to by the member.

13. When the member is engaged in short-term group treatment/training programs (e.g., marathons and other encounter-type or growth groups), the member ensures that there is professional assistance available during and following the group experience.

14. Should the member be engaged in a work setting that calls for any variation from the above statements, the member is obligated to consult with other professionals whenever possible to consider justifiable alternatives.

Section C:

Measurement and Evaluation

The primary purpose of educational and psychological testing is to provide descriptive measures that are objective and interpretable in either comparative or absolute terms. The member must recognize the need to interpret the statements that follow as applying to the whole range of appraisal techniques including test and nontest data. Test results constitute only one of a variety of pertinent sources of information for personnel, guidance, and counseling decisions. .

1. The member must provide specific orientation or information to the examinee(s) prior to and following the test administration so that the results of testing may be placed in proper perspective with other relevant factors. In so doing, the member must recognize the effects of socioeconomic, ethnic and cultural factors on test scores. It is the member's professional responsibility to use additional unvalidated information carefully in modifying interpretation of the test results.

2. In selecting tests for use in a given situation or with a particular client, the member must consider carefully the specific validity, reliability, and appropriateness of the test(s). *General* validity, reliability and the like may be questioned legally as well as ethically when tests are used for vocational and educational selection, placement, or counseling.

3. When making any statements to the public about tests and testing, the member must give accurate information and avoid false claims or misconceptions. Special efforts are often required to avoid unwarranted connotations of such terms as *IQ* and *grade equivalent scores.*

4. Different tests demand different levels of competence for administration, scoring, and interpretation. Members must recognize the limits of their competence and perform only those functions for which they are prepared.

5. Tests must be administered under the same conditions that were established in their standardization. When tests are not administered under standard conditions or when unusual behavior or irregularities occur during the testing session, those conditions must be noted and the results designated as invalid or of questionable validity. Unsupervised or inadequately supervised test-taking, such as the use of tests through the mails, is considered unethical. On the other hand, the use of instruments that are so designed or standardized to be self-administered and self-scored, such as interest inventories, is to be encouraged.

6. The meaningfulness of test results used in personnel, guidance, and counseling functions generally depends on the examinee's unfamiliarity with the specific items on the test. Any prior coaching or dissemination of the test materials can invalidate test results. Therefore, test security is one of the professional obligations of the member. Conditions that produce most favorable test results must be made known to the examinee.

7. The purpose of testing and the explicit use of the results must be made known to the examinee prior to testing. The counselor must ensure that instrument limitations are not exceeded and that periodic review and/or retesting are made to prevent client stereotyping.

8. The examinee's welfare and explicit prior understanding must be the criteria for determining the recipients of the test results. The member must see that specific interpretation accompanies any release of individual or group test data. The interpretation of test data must be related to the examinee's particular concerns.

9. The member must be cautious when interpreting the results of research instruments possessing insufficient technical data. The specific purposes for the use of such instruments must be stated explicitly to examinees.

10. The member must proceed with caution when attempting to evaluate and interpret the performance of minority group members or other persons who are not represented in the norm group on which the instrument was standardized.

11. The member must guard against the appropriation, reproduction, or modifications of published tests or parts thereof without acknowledgment and permission from the previous publisher.

12. Regarding the preparation, publication and distribution of tests, reference should be made to:
a. *Standards for Educational and Psychological Tests and Manuals,* revised edition, 1974, published by the American Psychological Association on behalf of itself, the American Educational Research Association and the National Council on Measurement in Education.
b. The responsible use of tests: A

position paper of AMEG, APGA, and NCME. *Measurement and Evaluation in Guidance,* 1972, 5, 385-388.

    c. "Responsibilities of Users of Standardized Tests," APGA, *Guidepost,* October 5, 1978, pp. 5-8.

Section D:
Research and Publication

1. Guidelines on research with human subjects shall be adhered to, such as:

    a. *Ethical Principles in the Conduct of Research with Human Participants,* Washington, D.C.: American Psychological Association, Inc., 1973.

    b. Code of Federal Regulations, Title 45, Subtitle A, Part 46, as currently issued.

2. In planning any research activity dealing with human subjects, the member must be aware of and responsive to all pertinent ethical principles and ensure that the research problem, design, and execution are in full compliance with them.

3. Responsibility for ethical research practice lies with the principal researcher, while others involved in the research activities share ethical obligation and full responsibility for their own actions.

4. In research with human subjects, researchers are responsible for the subjects' welfare throughout the experiment and they must take all reasonable precautions to avoid causing injurious psychological, physical, or social effects on their subjects.

5. All research subjects must be informed of the purpose of the study except when withholding information or providing misinformation to them is essential to the investigation. In such research the member must be responsible for corrective action as soon as possible following completion of the research.

6. Participation in research must be voluntary. Involuntary participation is appropriate only when it can be demonstrated that participation will have no harmful effects on subjects and is essential to the investigation.

7. When reporting research results, explicit mention must be made of all variables and conditions known to the investigator that might affect the outcome of the investigation or the interpretation of the data.

8. The member must be responsible for conducting and reporting investigations in a manner that minimizes the possibility that results will be misleading.

9. The member has an obligation to make available sufficient original research data to qualified others who may wish to replicate the study.

10. When supplying data, aiding in the research of another person, reporting research results, or in making original data available, due care must be taken to disguise the identity of the subjects in the absence of specific authorization from such subjects to do otherwise.

11. When conducting and reporting research, the member must be familiar with, and give recognition to, previous work on the topic, as well as to observe all copyright laws and follow the principles of giving full credit to all to whom credit is due.

12. The member must give due credit through joint authorship, acknowledgment, footnote statements, or other appropriate means to those who have contributed significantly to the research and/or publication, in accordance with such contributions.

13. The member must communicate to other members the results of any research judged to be of professional or scientific value. Results reflecting unfavorably on institutions, programs, services, or vested interests must not be withheld for such reasons.

14. If members agree to cooperate with another individual in research and/or publication, they incur an obligation to cooperate as promised in terms of punctuality of performance and with full regard to the completeness and accuracy of the information required.

15 Ethical practice requires that authors not submit the same manuscript or one essentially similar in content, for simultaneous publication consideration

by two or more journals. In addition, manuscripts published in whole or in substantial part, in another journal or published work should not be submitted for publication without acknowledgment and permission from the previous publication.

Section E:
Consulting

Consultation refers to a voluntary relationship between a professional helper and help-needing individual, group or social unit in which the consultant is providing help to the client(s) in defining and solving a work-related problem or potential problem with a client or client system. (This definition is adapted from Kurpius, DeWayne. Consultation theory and process: An integrated model. *Personnel and Guidance Journal*, 1978, 56.)

1. The member acting as consultant must have a high degree of self-awareness of his-her own values, knowledge, skills, limitations, and needs in entering a helping relationship that involves human and-or organizational change and that the focus of the relationship be on the issues to be resolved and not on the person(s) presenting the problem.

2. There must be understanding and agreement between member and client for the problem definition, change goals, and predicated consequences of interventions selected.

3. The member must be reasonably certain that she/he or the organization represented has the necessary competencies and resources for giving the kind of help that is needed now or may develop later and that appropriate referral resources are available to the consultant.

4. The consulting relationship must be one in which client adaptability and growth toward self-direction are encouraged and cultivated. The member must maintain this role consistently and not become a decision maker for the client or create a future dependency on the consultant.

5. When announcing consultant availability for services, the member conscientiously adheres to the Association's *Ethical Standards*.

6. The member must refuse a private fee or other remuneration for consultation with persons who are entitled to these services through the member's employing institution or agency. The policies of a particular agency may make explicit provisions for private practice with agency clients by members of its staff. In such instances, the clients must be apprised of other options open to them should they seek private counseling services.

Section F:
Private Practice

1. The member should assist the profession by facilitating the availability of counseling services in private as well as public settings.

2. In advertising services as a private practitioner, the member must advertise the services in such a manner so as to accurately inform the public as to services, expertise, profession, and techniques of counseling in a professional manner. A member who assumes an executive leadership role in the organization shall not permit his/her name to be used in professional notices during periods when not actively engaged in the private practice of counseling.

The member may list the following: highest relevant degree, type and level of certification or license, type and/or description of services, and other relevant information, Such information must not contain false, inaccurate, misleading, partial, out-of-context, or deceptive material or statements.

3. Members may join in partnership/ corporation with other members and-or other professionals provided that each member of the partnership or corporation makes clear the separate specialties by name in compliance with the regulations of the locality.

4. A member has an obligation to withdraw from a counseling relationship if it is believed that employment will

result in violation of the *Ethical Standards*. If the mental or physical condition of the member renders it difficult to carry out an effective professional relationship or if the member is discharged by the client because the counseling relationship is no longer productive for the client, then the member is obligated to terminate the counseling relationship.

5. A member must adhere to the regulations for private practice of the locality where the services are offered.

6. It is unethical to use one's institutional affiliation to recruit clients for one's private practice.

Section G:
Personnel Administration

It is recognized that most members are employed in public or quasi-public institutions. The functioning of a member within an institution must contribute to the goals of the institution and vice versa if either is to accomplish their respective goals or objectives. It is therefore essential that the member and the institution function in ways to (a) make the institution's goals explicit and public; (b) make the member's contribution to institutional goals specific; and (c) foster mutual accountability for goal achievement.

To accomplish these objectives, it is recognized that the member and the employer must share responsibilities in the formulation and implementation of personnel policies.

1. Members must define and describe the parameters and levels of their professional competency.

2. Members must establish interpersonal relations and working agreements with supervisors and subordinates regarding counseling or clinical relationships, confidentiality, distinction between public and private material, maintenance, and dissemination of recorded information, work load and accountability. Working agreements in each instance must be specified and made known to those concerned.

3. Members must alert their employers to conditions that may be potentially disruptive or damaging.

4. Members must inform employers of conditions that may limit their effectiveness.

5. Members must submit regularly to professional review and evaluation.

6. Members must be responsible for inservice development of self and-or staff.

7. Members must inform their staff of goals and programs.

8. Members must provide personnel practices that guarantee and enhance the rights and welfare of each recipient of their service.

9. Members must select competent persons and assign responsibilities compatible with their skills and experiences.

Section H:
Preparation Standards

Members who are responsible for training others must be guided by the preparation standards of the Association and relevant Division(s). The member who functions in the capacity of trainer assumes unique ethical responsibilities that frequently go beyond that of the member who does not function in a training capacity. These ethical responsibilities are outlined as follows:

1. Members must orient students to program expectations, basic skills development, and employment prospects prior to admission to the program.

2. Members in charge of learning experiences must establish programs that integrate academic study and supervised practice.

3. Members must establish a program directed toward developing students' skills, knowledge, and self-understanding, stated whenever possible in competency or performance terms.

4. Members must identify the levels of competencies of their students in compliance with relevant Division standards. These competencies must accommodate the para-professional as well as the professional.

5. Members, through continual student evaluation and appraisal, must be aware of the personal limitations of the learner that might impede future performance. The instructor must not only assist the learner in securing remedial assistance but also screen from the program those individuals who are unable to provide competent services.

6. Members must provide a program that includes training in research commensurate with levels of role functioning. Para-professional and technician-level personnel must be trained as consumers of research. In addition, these personnel must learn how to evaluate their own and their program's effectiveness. Graduate training, especially at the doctoral level, would include preparation for original research by the member.

7. Members must make students aware of the ethical responsibilities and standards of the profession.

8. Preparatory programs must encourage students to value the ideals of service to individuals and to society. In this regard, direct financial remuneration or lack thereof must not influence the quality of service rendered. Monetary considerations must not be allowed to overshadow professional and humanitarian needs.

9. Members responsible for educational programs must be skilled as teachers and practitioners.

10. Members must present thoroughly varied theoretical positions so that students may make comparisons and have the opportunity to select a position.

11. Members must develop clear policies within their educational institutions regarding field placement and the roles of the student and the instructor in such placements.

12. Members must ensure that forms of learning focusing on self-understanding or growth are voluntary, or if required as part of the education program, are made known to prospective students prior to entering the program. When the education program offers a growth experience with an emphasis on self-disclosure or other relatively intimate or personal involvement, the member must have no administrative, supervisory, or evaluating authority regarding the participant.

13. Members must conduct an educational program in keeping with the current relevant guidelines of the American Personnel and Guidance Association and its Divisions.

Note: Reproduced with permission of the American Personnel and Guidance Association. Individual copies may be obtained by writing APGA, Professional Information Service, Suite 400, 5203 Leesburg Pike, Falls Church, VA 22041

Appendix C
Ethics Committee
Virginia Counselors Association
Responsibilities and Procedures

Section One   Introduction

The Virginia Counselors Association (VCA) is an educational, scientific, and professional organization whose members are dedicated to the enhancement of the worth, dignity, potential, and uniqueness of each individual, and thus to the service of society. The Association believes that those persons engaged in counseling, guidance, and student development services in the Commonwealth of Virginia should adhere to and be judged according to the ethical standards of the American Personnel and Guidance Association.

Counseling, guidance, and student development refers to those individual and group efforts designed to assist individuals in achieving more effective personal, social, educational and career development, and adjustment. It further refers to rendering or offering to render to individuals, groups, organizations, or the general public any service involving the application of principles, methods, or procedures of the counseling profession. These services include: (1) "counseling," which means assisting individuals through the counseling relationship, to develop understanding of personal problems, to define goals, and to plan action reflecting their interests, abilities, aptitudes, and needs as these are related to educational progress, occupations and careers, and personal-social concerns; (2) "appraisal activities," which means selecting, administering, scoring and interpreting instruments designed to assess individuals' aptitudes, and shall not include the use of projective techniques in the assessment of personality; (3) "counseling, guidance and student development consulting," which means interpreting or reporting upon scientific fact or theory in counseling, guidance and student development services to provide assistance in solving some current or potential problems of individuals, groups, or organizations; and (4) "referral activities," which means the evaluating of data to identify problems and to determine advisabilty of referral to other specialists.

Section Two   Responsibilities of the VCA Ethics Committee

The Ethics Committee of the Virginia Counselors Association has the responsibility to receive and investigate complaints of the unethical professional conduct of persons engaged in the practice of counseling, guidance, and student development services in Virginia; to attempt to resolve such complaints confidentially, and to take appropriate action when unethical practices are found to exist. Further, this committee shall:

1. Endeavor to provide information and advice on appropriate ethical practices of counselors.
2. Work to protect the public and the profession against unethical practices by counselors.
3. Monitor the professional conduct of counselors.
4. Investigate ethical complaints in an objective, factual, and confidential manner in order to avoid injury to the reputation or means of livelihood of the counselor in question.
5. Make periodic reports to the VCA Board of Directors focusing on general committee functioning, while maintaining investigative confidentiality.

The VCA Ethics Committee will concern itself with the ethical conduct of all persons engaged in the practice of counseling, guidance, and student development services in Virginia, with the following exceptions: (1) those persons who are Virginia licensed professional counselors, whose alleged misconduct will be referred to the Virginia Board of Professional Counselors; (2) those persons who are not licensed as Virginia professional counselors but who are engaged in private practice, whose alleged misconduct will also be referred to the Virginia Board of Professional Counselors; (3) those persons who are engaged in counseling, guidance, and student development services, who *are not* members of the Virginia Counselors Association but who *are* members of another Virginia professional association (e.g., Virginia Psychological Association, Virginia State Chapter of the National Association of Social Workers) whose alleged misconduct shall be referred to the ethics committee of that professional association; and (4) those persons who are engaged in counseling, guidance, and student development services, who *are not* members of the Virginia Counselors Association and who *are not* members of any other related professional group with an ethics committee. When a complaint is filed against such individuals, the person filing the complaint will be given suggested procedures to follow to redress the grievance individually.

In such cases as those listed above, the Virginia Counselors Association will prepare a follow-up report within ninety (90) days after the complaint referral is made.

If the person engaged in alleged misconduct is both a member of the Virginia Counselors Association and of another professional association, the VCA Ethics Committee will follow the procedures for dealing with complaints listed in Section Five.

Section Three   Committee Membership

The Ethics Committee shall consist of five members including a Chair appointed by the VCA president. The VCA president shall serve as an ex-officio member of the Committee. It is highly desirable to have this Committee as representative of the membership of VCA as possible. A majority of those members serving shall constitute a quorum, and when differences of opinion arise, the majority opinion shall prevail. To assist in an investigation the Chair may appoint an *ad hoc* fact-finding committee, composed of members from the VCA. This *ad hoc* committee shall be bound by the same standards of confidentiality as the VCA Ethics Committee.

Section Four   Guidelines for Ethical Conduct

The 1981 revision of *Ethical Standards of the American Personnel and Guidance Association* shall serve as the source for decision making about unethical behavior.

Section Five   Procedures for Receiving and Processing Complaints

5.1   Receiving Complaints

a. The Ethics Committee Chair will receive and act promptly upon all complaints from any responsible person or group.
b. All complaints must be in writing and signed by the complainant(s), but the name(s) will be kept confidential and written permission will be required for its use if any investigation is conducted.
c. Complaints of a counselor's unethical conduct should not only be signed but include the complainant's address and telephone number and include as much detail as possible about the incident being reported. Unsigned complaints will usually be destroyed upon receipt.
d. Exceptions to this rule may be receipt of evidence of questionable advertising or written evidence of unethical behavior, i.e., in a public document or newspaper article. In such cases, the Committee may act without a specific complaint.

5.2 Processing the Complaint

a. The Chair will determine whether the issue being reported falls within the jurisdiction of the Committee and shall notify complainant(s) of receipt of the complaint and of the next step, if any, to be taken by the Ethics Committee.
b. When the Committee determines the complaint does not constitute an ethical breach, the complainant(s) shall be so informed and the complaint will be dismissed.
c. When the Committee has reason to believe that an ethical violation may have occurred, it shall proceed with an investigation and secure written persmission from the complainant(s) to reveal the name(s) of the complainant(s) to the person against whom a complaint has been made, hereinafter referred to as the respondent.
d. If complainant(s) refuse to permit their name(s) to be used, this refusal may be used as a base for forfeiting the right to complain.
e. The Committee need not make its investigational files available to the respondent.

5.3 Investigating the Complaint

a. If the Committee decides that a breach of ethical standards may have occurred, the following steps shall be taken:
   1. The person against whom a complaint has been made, the respondent, shall be notified in writing. The respondent shall be furnished a copy of the *1981 APGA Ethical Standards* and relevant information pertaining to possible ethical violation. At the same time, the respondent will ordinarily be advised of who has made the complaint, or, in the case of other evidence, furnished documentation of the ethical questions raised.
   2. The respondent has thirty (30) calendar days to reply to the Committee. He/she may provide any information deemed pertinent to the issue. Further, respondent has the right to request, of the Chair, a hearing on the charges.
   3. If a response is not received from the respondent within thirty (30) calendar days, the Chair will send a second notification by Registered Mail. If at the end of fifteen (15) additional days the respondent has not yet replied, an investigation shall proceed, keeping in mind respondent's refusal to cooperate.

5.4 The Hearing

a. The purpose of the hearing is to determine whether an ethical violation has occurred. The total Committee, or a quorum as defined above, shall hold a formal meeting for the purpose of conducting the hearing.

b. Both the respondent and complainant(s) have a right to be present and to speak before the Committee.
c. Care will be taken to adhere to accepted rules of confidentiality.

5.5 Actions Taken On Complaints

a. If the VCA Ethics Committee determines that *no ethical violation has occurred,* the complaint will be destroyed. In cases so determined, the respondent shall be notified, and an apology will be offered.
b. If the VCA Ethics Committee finds that *an ethical violation has occurred,* it will be expected to take appropriate action. Possible actions will be restricted to one or more of the following:
   1. Advise respondent to stop the unethical practice and to take positive, corrective action. Require respondent's written agreement to stop the unethical practice. (If written agreement is not received within fifteen (15) calendar days, one or more of the following actions will be taken by the Committee.)
   2. Place respondent on probation as a member of VCA for a period of time to be determined by the Committee.
   3. Suspend membership from VCA for a period of time to be determined by the Committee.
   4. Expel respondent from VCA membership.
   5. Recommend to complainant that the complainant take legal action.
   6. Public disclosure of respondent's unethical practices and action taken by the Ethics Committee in the VCA newsletter.
c. The Chair of the Ethics Committee shall notify respondent, within thirty (30) calendar days, of the Committee's findings and actions.
d. After action has been taken, a case summary will be prepared by the Ethics Committee Chair, and the summary will be maintained in a safety desposit box. The remaining file will be destroyed.

Reprinted by permission of Virginia Counselors Association. The Plan for Implementing Ethical Standards was developed under a professional development grant from the Southern Regional Branch Assembly of APGA, Joseph A. Kloba, Grant Director.
Note: The Virginia Branch of the American Personnel and Guidance Association became the Virginia Counselors Association in 1981.

Appendix D
Regulations of Virginia Board of Professional Counselors

Section V: Ethical Standards.

POR 5.1: Code of Ethics.

Preamble

Professional Counselors believe in the dignity and worth of the individual. They are committed to increasing knowledge of human behavior and understanding of themselves and others. While pursuing these endeavors, they make every reasonable effort to protect the welfare of those who seek their services or of any subject that may be the object of study. They use their skills only for purposes consistent with these values and do not knowingly permit their misuse by others. While demanding for themselves freedom of inquiry and communication, Professional Counselors accept the responsibility this freedom confers; competence, objectivity in the application of skills and concern for the best interests of clients, colleagues, and society in general. In the pursuit of these ideals, Professional Counselors subscribe to the following principles:

PRINCIPLE I. RESPONSIBILITY

In their commitment to the understanding of human behavior, professional counselors value objectivity and integrity, and in providing services they maintain the highest standards. They accept responsibility for the consequences of their work and make every effort to insure that their services are used appropriately.
a. Professional Counselors accept the ultimate responsibility for selecting appropriate areas for investigation and the methods relevant to minimize the possibility that their findings will be misleading. They provide thorough discussion of the limitations of their data and alternative hypotheses, especially where their work touches on social policy or might be misconstrued to the detriment of specific age, sex,

ethnic, socio-economic, or other social categories. In publishing reports of their work, they never discard observations that may modify the interpretation of results. Professional Counselors take credit only for the work they have actually done. In pursuing research, Professional Counselors ascertain that their efforts will not lead to changes in individuals or organizations unless such changes are part of the agreement at the time of obtaining informed consent. Professional Counselors clarify in advance the expectations for sharing and utilizing research data. They avoid dual relationships which may limit objectivity, whether theoretical, political, or monetary, so that interference with data, subjects, and milieu is kept to a minimum.

b. As employees of an institution or agency, professional counselors have the responsibility of remaining alert to institutional pressures which may distort reports of counseling findings or use them in ways counter to the promotion of human welfare.

c. When serving as members of governmental or other organizational bodies, professional counselors remain accountable as individuals to the code of Ethics of the Virginia Board of Professional Counselors.

d. As teachers, Professional Counselors recognize their primary obligation to help others acquire knowledge and skill. They maintain high standards of scholarship and objectivity by presenting counseling information fully and accurately, and by giving appropriate recognition to alternative viewpoints.

e. As practitioners, Professional Counselors know that they bear a heavy social responsibility because their recommendations and professional actions may alter the lives of others. They, therefore, remain fully cognizant of their impact and alert to personal, social, organizational, financial or political situations or pressures which might lead to misuse of their influence.

f. Professional Counselors provide reasonable and timely feedback to employees, trainees, supervisees, students and others whose work they may evaluate.

PRINCIPLE 2. COMPETENCE

The maintenance of high standards of professional competence is a responsibility shared by all Professional Counselors in the interest of the public and the profession as a whole. Professional Counselors recognize the boundaries of their competence and the limitations of their techniques and only provide services, use techniques, or offer opinions as professionals that meet recognized standards. Throughout their careers, Professional Counselors maintain knowledge of professional information related to the services they render.

a. Professional Counselors accurately represent their competence, education, training and experience.

b. As teachers, Professional Counselors perform their duties based on careful preparation so that their instruction is accurate, up-to-date, and scholarly.

c. Professional Counselors recognize the need for continuing training to prepare themselves to serve persons of all ages and cultural backgrounds. They are open to new procedures and sensitive to differences between groups of people and changes in expectations and values over time.

d. Professional Counselors, with the responsibility for decisions involving individuals or policies based on test results, should have an understanding of counseling or educational measurement, validation problems and other test research. Test users should know and understand the literature relevant to the tests used and testing problems with which they deal.

e. Professional Counselors/practitioners recognize that their effectiveness depends in part upon their ability to maintain sound interpersonal relations, that temporary or more enduring aberrations on their part may interfere with their abilities or distort their appraisals or others. Therefore, they refrain from undertaking any activity in which their personal problems are likely to lead to inadequate professional services or harm to a client; or, if they are already engaged in such activity when they become aware of their personal problems, they would seek competent professional assistance to determine whether they should suspend or terminate services to one or all of their clients.

PRINCIPLE 3. MORAL AND LEGAL STANDARDS

Professional Counselors' moral, ethical and legal standards of behavior are a personal matter to the same degree as they are for any other citizen, except as these may compromise the fulfillment of their professional responsibilities, or reduce the trust in counseling or counselors held by the general public. Regarding their own behavior, Professional Counselors should always be aware of the prevailing community standards and of the possible impact upon the quality of professional services provided by their conformance to or deviation from these standards.

Professional Counselors should also be aware of the possible impact of their public behavior upon the ability of colleagues to perform their professional duties.

a. To protect public confidence in the profession of counseling, Professional Counselors will avoid the public behavior that is clearly in violation of accepted moral and legal standards.

b. To protect students, counselors/teachers will be aware of the diverse backgrounds of students and, when dealing with topics that may give offense, will see that the material is treated objectively, that it is clearly relevant to the course, and that it is treated in a manner for which the student is prepared.

c. Providers of counseling services conform to the statutes relating to such services as established by the Commonwealth of Virginia and the Virginia Board of Professional Counselors.

d. As employees, Professional Counselors refuse to participate in employer's practices which are inconsistent with the moral and legal standards established by federal or state legislation regarding the treatment of employees or of the public. In particular and for example, Professional Counselors will not condone practices which result in illegal or otherwise unjustifiable discrimination on the basis of race, sex, religion or national origin in hiring, promotion or training.

e. In providing counseling services to clients, Professional Counselors avoid any action that will violate or diminish the legal and civil rights of clients or of others who may be affected by the action.

PRINCIPLE 4. PUBLIC STATEMENTS

Professional Counselors in their professional roles may be expected or required to make public statements providing counseling information, professional opinions, or supply information about the availability of counseling products and services. In making such statements, Professional Counselors take full account of the limits and uncertainties of present counseling knowledge and techniques. They represent, as objectively as possible, their professional qualifications, affiliations, and functions, as well as those of the institutions or organizations with which the statements may be associated. All public statements, announcements of services, and promotional activities whould serve the purpose of providing sufficient information to aid the consumer public in making informed judgments and choices on matters that concern it.

a. When announcing professional services, Professional Counselors limit the information to: name, highest relevant degree conferred, certification or licensure, address, telephone number, office hours, cost of services, and a brief explanation of the types of services rendered. Such statements will be descriptive of services offered but not evaluative as to their quality of uniqueness. They will not claim uniqueness of skills or methods beyond those available to others in the profession unless determined by acceptable and public scientific evidence.

b. In announcing the availability of counseling services or products Professional Counselors will not display their affiliations with organizations or agencies in a manner that implies the sponsorship or certification of the organization or agency. They will not name their employer or professional associations unless the services are in fact to be provided by or under the responsible, direct supervision and continuing control of such organization or agencies.

c. Professional Counselors associated with the development or promotion of counseling devices, books, or other products offered for commercial sale will make every effort to insure that announcements and advertisement are presented in a professional and factually informative manner without unsupported claims of superiority over devices, books and products of similar purpose. Claims of superiority must be supported by scientifically acceptable evidence or by willingness to aid and encourage independent professional scrutiny or scientific test.

d. Professional Counselors engaged in radio, television or other public media activities will not participate in commercial announcements recommending to the general public the purchase or use of any proprietary or single-source product or service.

e. Professional Counselors who describe counseling or the services of Professional Counselors to the general public accept the obligation to present the material fairly and accurately, avoiding misrepresentation through sensationalism, exaggeration or superficiality. Professional Counselors will be guided by the primary obligation to aid the public in forming their own informed judgments, opinions and choices.

f. As teachers, Professional Counselors ensure that statements in catalogs and course outlines are accurate, particularly in terms of subject matter to be covered, bases for grading, and nature of classroom experiences, As practitioners providing private services, Professional Counselors avoid improper, direct solicitation of clients and the conflict of interest inherent therein.

g. Professional Counselors accept the obligation to correct others who may represent their professional qualifications or associations with products or services in a manner incompatible with these guidelines.

PRINCIPLE 5. CONFIDENTIALITY

Professional Counselors have a primary obligation to safeguard information about individuals obtained in the course of teaching, practice, or research. Personal information is communicated to others only with the person's written consent or in those circumstances where there is clear and imminent danger to the client, to others or to society. Disclosures of counseling information are restricted to what is necessary, relevant, and verifiable.

a. All materials in the official record shall be shared with the client who shall have the right to decide what information may be shared with anyone beyond the immediate provider of service and to be informed of the implications of the materials to be shared.
b. The anonymity of clients served in public and other agencies is preserved, if at all possible, by withholding names and personal identifying data. If external conditions require reporting such information, the client shall be so informed.
c. Information received in confidence by one agency or person shall not be forwarded to another person or agency without the client's written permission.
d. Service providers have a responsibility to insure the accuracy and to indicate the validity of data shared with their parties.
e. Case reports presented in classes, professional meetings, or in publications shall be so disguised that no information is possible unless the client or responsible authority has read the report and agreed in writing to its presentation or publication.
f. Counseling reports and records are maintained under conditions of security and provisions are made for their destruction when they have outlived their usefulness. Professional Counselors insure that privacy and confidentiality are maintained by all persons in the employ or volunteer services of the agency or office, including clerical staff, students, volunteers, and community aides.
g. Professional Counselors who ask that an individual reveal personal information in the course of interviewing, testing or evaluation, or who allow such information to be divulged, do so only after making certain that the person or authorized representative is fully aware of the purposes of the interview, testing or evaluation and of the ways in which the information will be used.
h. Sessions with clients are taped or otherwise recorded only with their written permission or the written permission of a responsible guardian. Even with guardian written consent one should not record a session against the expressed wishes of a client.
i. Where a child or adolescent is the primary client, the interests of the minor shall be paramount.
j. In work with families, the rights of each family member should be safeguarded. The provider of service also has the responsibility to discuss the contents of the record with the parent and/or child, as appropriate, and to keep separate those parts which should remain the property of each family member.

PRINICIPLE 6. WELFARE OF THE CONSUMER

Professional Counselors respect the integrity and protect the welfare of the people and groups with whom they work. When there is a conflict of interest between the client and the Professional Counselors' employing institution, the Professional Counselors clarify the nature and direction of their loyalties and responsibilities and keep all parties informed of their commitments. Professional Counselors fully inform consumers as to the purpose and nature of any evaluative, treatment, educational or training procedure, and they freely acknowledge that clients, students, or subjects have freedom of choice with regard to participation.

a. Professional Counselors are continually cognizant both of their own needs and of their inherently powerful position "vis-a-vis" clients, in order to avoid exploiting the client's trust and dependency. Professional Counselors make every effort to avoid dual relationships with clients and/or relationships which might impair their professional judgment or increase the risk of client exploitation. Examples of such dual relationships include treating an employee or supervisee, treating a close friend or family relative, and sexual relationships with clients.

b. Where Professional Counselors work with members of an organization goes beyond reasonable conditions of employment, Professional Counselors recognize possible conflicts of interests that may arise. When such conflicts occur, Professional Counselors clarify the nature of the conflict and inform all parties of the nature and directions of the loyalties and responsibilities involved.

c. When acting as supervisors, trainers, or employers, Professional Counselors accord recipients informed choice, confidentiality, and protection from physical and mental harm.

d. Financial arrangements in professional practice are in accord with professional standards that safeguard the best interests of the client and that are clearly understood by the client in advance of billing. This may best be done by the use of a contract. Professional Counselors are responsible for assisting clients in finding needed services in those instances where payment of the usual fee would be a hardship. No commission or rebate or other form of remuneration may be given or received for referral of clients for professional services, whether by an individual or by an agency.

e. Professional Counselors are responsible for making their services readily accessible to clients in a manner that facilitates the client's ability to make an informed choice when selecting a service provider. This responsibility includes a clear written description of what the client may expect in the way of tests, reports, billing, therapeutic regime and schedules.

f. Professional Counselors who find that their services are not beneficial to the client have the responsibility to make this known to the responsible persons.

g. Professional Counselors are accountable to the parties who refer and support counseling services and to the general public and are cognizant of the indirect or long-range effects of their intervention.

h. The Professional Counselor attempts to terminate a private service or consulting relationship when it is reasonably clear to the Professional Counselor that the consumer is not benefitting from it. If a consumer is receiving services from another mental health professional, Professional Counselors do not offer their services directly to the consumer without informing the professional persons already involved in order to avoid confusion and conflict for the consumer.

PRINCIPLE 7. PROFESSIONAL RELATIONSHIPS

Professional Counselors act with due regard to the needs and feelings of their colleagues in counseling and other professions. Professional Counselors respect the prerogatives and obligations of the institutions or organizations with which they are associated.

a. Professional Counselors understand the areas of competence of related professions and make full use of other professional, technical, and administrative resources which best serve the interests of consumers. The absence of formal relationship with other professional workers does not relieve Professional Counselors from the responsibility of securing for their clients the best possible professional service; indeed, this circumstance presents a challenge to the professional competence of Professional Counselors, requiring special sensitivity to problems outside their areas of training, and foresight, diligence, and tact in obtaining the professional assistance needed by clients.

b. Professional Counselors know and take into account the traditions and practices of other professional groups with which they work and cooperate fully with members of such groups when research, services, and other functions are shared or in working for the benefit of public welfare.

c. Professional Counselors strive to provide positive conditions for those they employ, and they spell out clearly the conditions of such employment. They encourage their employees to engage in activities that facilitate their further professional development.

d. Professional Counselors respect the viability, reputation, and the proprietary right of organizations which they serve. Professional Counselors show due regard for the interests of their present or prospective employers. In those instances where they are critical of programs or policies, they attempt to effect change by constructive action within the organization.

e. In the pursuit of research, Professional Counselors give sponsoring agencies, host institutions, and publication channels the same respect and opportunity for giving informed consent that they accord individual research participants. They are aware of their obligation to future research workers and insure that host institutions are given feedback information and proper acknowledgment.

f. Credit is assigned to those who have contributed to a publication, in proportion to their contribution.

g. When a Professional Counselor violates ethical standards, Professional Counselors who know first-hand of such activities should, if possible, attempt to rectify the situation. Failing an informal solution, Professional Counselors should bring such unethical activities to the attention of the Virginia Board of Profesional Counselors.

PRINCIPLE 8. UTILIZATION OF ASSESSMENT TECHNIQUES

In the development, publication, and utilization of counseling assessment techniques, Professional Counselors follow relevant standards. Individuals examined, or their legal guardians, have the right to know the

results, the interpretations made, and where appropriate, the particulars on which final judgment was based. Test users should take precautions to protect test security but not at the expense of an individual's right to understand the basis for decisions that adversely affect that individual or that individual's dependents.
 a. The client has the right to have and the provider has the responsibility to give explanations of test results in language the client can understand.
 b. When a test is published or otherwise made available for operational use, it should be accompanied by a manual (or other published or readily available information) that makes every reasonable effort to describe fully the development of the test, the rationale, specifications followed in writing items or selecting observations, and procedures and results of item analysis or other research. The test, the manual, the record forms and other accompanying material should help users make correct interpretations of the test results and should warn against common misuses. The test manual should state explicitly the purposes and applications for which the test is recommended and identify any special qualifications required to administer the test and to interpret it properly. Evidence of validity and reliability, along with other relevant research data, should be presented in support of any claims made.
 c. Norms presented in test manuals should refer to defined and clearly described populations. These populations should be the groups with whom users of the test will ordinarily wish to compare the persons tested. Test users should consider the possibility of bias in tests or in test items. When indicated, there should be an investigation of possible differences in validity for ethnic, sex, or other subsamples that can be identified when the test is given.
 d. Professional Counselors who have the responsibility for decisions about individuals or policies that are based on test results should have a thorough understanding of counseling or educational measurement and of validation and other test research.
 e. Professional Counselors should develop procedures for systematically eliminating from data files test score information that has, because of the lapse of time, become obsolete.
 f. Any individual or organization offering test scoring and interpretation services must be able to demonstrate that their programs are based on appropriate research to establish the validity of the programs and procedures used in arriving at interpretations. The public offering of an automated test interpretation service will be considered as a professional-to-professional consultation. In this the formal responsibility of the consultant is to the consultee but his/her ultimate and overriding responsibility is to the client.
 g. Counseling services for the purpose of diagnosis, treatment, or personalized advice are provided only in the context of a professional relationship, and are not given by means of public lectures or demonstrations, newspaper or magazine articles, radio or television programs, mail, or similar media. The preparation of personnel reports and recommendations based on test data secured solely by mail is unethical unless such appraisals are an integral part of a continuing client relationship with a company, as a result of which the consulting Professional Counselor has intimate knowledge of the client's personal situation and can be assured thereby that his written

appraisals will be adequate to the purpose and will be properly interpreted by the client. These reports must not be embellished with such detailed analyses of the subject's personality traits as would be appropriate only after intensive interviews with the subject.

PRINCIPLE 9. PURSUIT OF RESEARCH ACTIVITIES

The decision to undertake research should rest upon a considered judgment by the individual Professional Counselor about how best to contribute to counseling and to human welfare. Professional Counselors carry out their investigations with respect for the people who participate and with concern for their dignity and welfare.

a. In planning a study the investigator has the personal responsibility to make a careful evaluation of its ethical acceptability, taking into account the following principles for research with human beings. To the extent that his appraisal, weighing scientific and humane values, suggests a deviation from any principle, the investigator incurs an increasingly serious obligation to seek ethical advice and to observe more stringent safeguards to protect the rights of the human research participants.

b. Professional Counselors know and take into account the traditions and practices of other professional groups with which they work and cooperate fully with members of such groups when research services, and other functions are shared or in working for the benefit of public welfare.

c. Ethical practice requires investigator to inform the participant of all features of the research that reasonably might be expected to influence willingness to participate, and to explain all other aspects of the research about which the participant inquires. Failure to make full disclosure gives added emphasis to the investigators abiding responsibility to protect the welfare and dignity of the research participant.

d. Openness and honesty are essential characteristics of the relationship between investigator and research participant. When the methodological requirements of a study necessitate concealment or deception, the investigator is required to insure as soon as possible the participant's understanding of the reasons for this action and to restore the quality of the relationship with the investigator.

e. In the pursuit of research, Professional Counselors give sponsoring agencies, host institutions, and publication channels the same respect and opportunity for giving informed consent that they accord to individual research participants. They are aware of their obligation to future research workers and insure that host institutions are given feedback information and proper acknowledgment.

f. Credit is assigned to those who have contributed to a publication, in proportion to their contribution.

g. The ethical investigator protects participants from physical and mental discomfort, harm and danger. If the risk of such consequences exists, the investigator is required to inform the participant of that fact, secure consent before proceeding, and take all possible measures to minimize distress. A research procedure may not be used if it is likely to cause serious and lasting harm to participants.

h. After the data are collected, ethical practice requires the investigator to provide the participant with a full clarification of the nature of the study and to remove any misconceptions that may have arisen. Where scientific or humane values justify delaying or withholding information, the investigator acquires a special responsibility to assure that there are no damaging consequences for the participants.

i. Where research procedures may result in undesirable consequences for the participant, the investigator has the responsibility to detect and remove or correct these consequences, including, where relevant, long-term aftereffects.

j. Information obtained about the research participants during the course of an investigation is confidential. When the possibility exists that others may obtain access to such information, ethical research practice requires that the possibility, together with the plans for protecting confidentiality, be explained to the participants as a part of the procedure for obtaining informed consent.

Note: These regulations were revised in 1981.

Appendix E
Regulations of Virginia Board of Behavioral Science*

POR 8.1: Disciplinary Standards.

The Virginia Board of Behavioral Science is empowered under Section 54-927g of Title 54, Chapter 28 of the Code of Virginia "To revoke, suspend or fail to renew a certificate or license which it has the authority to issue for just causes as are enumerated in regulations of the Board and the appropriate professional board." The professional boards are empowered under Section 54-928g of Title 54, Chapter 28 of the Code of Virginia, "To hold hearings and recommend to the Board (of Behavioral Science), revocation, suspension or nonrenewal of a license or certificate."

To assure uniformity in disciplinary cases, the Board of Behavioral Science has adopted the following disciplinary guidelines for use by the professional boards, hearing officers and itself when hearing disciplinary cases involving licensees of the Board of Behavioral Science against whom charges have been filed.

All section references are to POR 3.3 and 6.2 of the regulations of the Board of Behavioral Science and professional boards, denial of renewal, suspension or revocation of license, and the Ethical Standards of the Board of Behavioral Science and appropriate professional board.

A. *Conviction of a felony.*
   Maximum: Revocation.
   Minimum: Stayed revocation with three years' probation.
   Conditions of Probation:
   1. The conditions depend upon the nature of the conviction and should be tailored to educate the offender to avoid a recurrence. The conditions should include a rehabilitation program tailored to the violation.
   2. In appropriate cases, the order should require treatment as recommended by a qualified professional and approved by the Board.

*covering the practice of counseling, psychology, and social work

B. *Procuring of license by Fraud or Misrepresentation.*
   Revocation — license would not have been issued but for the fraud or misrepresentation.
C. *Misuse of drugs and/or alcohol.*
   Maximum: Revocation.
   Minimum: Stayed revocation with three years' probation.
   Conditions of Probation:
   1. Misuse of drugs:
      a. Successful completion of an education program on drug abuse approved by the Board.
      b. Abstention from use of drugs.
      c. Treatment as recommended by a qualified professional approved by the Board.
      d. Successful completion of an oral examination administered by the Board or its designees.
   2. Misuse of alcohol:
      a. Participation in Alcoholics Anonymous or a similar rehabilitation program approved by the Board.
      b. Treatment as recommended by a qualified professional approved by the Board.
      c. Abstention from use of alcohol.
      d. Successful completion of an oral examination administered by the Board or its designees.
D. *Negligence in conduct of his/her profession or non-conformance with the Code of Ethics.*
   Maximum: Revocation.
   Minimum: One year's suspension, stayed, with three years' probation.
   Conditions of Probation:
   1. Successful completion of a continuing education program related to the worker/client relationship approved by the Board.
   2. Successful completion of an oral examination administered by the Board or its designees.
   3. If deemed appropriate by the trier of fact, practice only in a supervised, structured environment which is approved by the Board.
E. *Performing functions outside the Board certified area of his/her competency.*
   Maximum: One year's suspension with three years' probation.
   Minimum: One year's suspension, stayed, with three years' probation.
   Conditions of Probation:
   1. Successful completion of a continuing education program approved by the Board, which bears a meaningful relationship to the violation.
   2. **If deemed appropriate by the trier of fact, practice only in a supervised, structured environment which is approved by the Board.**
   3. **Successful completion of an oral examination administered by the Board or its designees.**

F. *Mentally, emotionally or physically incompetent to practice profession.*
Maximum: Revocation.
Minimum: Suspension. Application for reinstatement may be made after:
1. Proof of termination of disability to satisfaction of Board.
2. Successful completion of an oral examination administered by the Board or its designees.
3. If reinstated and deemed appropriate by the Board, practice only in a supervised, structured environment which is approved by the Board.

G. *Violates or induces others to violate any provision of Chapter 28, of Title 54, Code of Virginia, any other statute applicable to the practice of the professions so regulated or any provision of the regulations or the Code of Ethics of the Board of Behavioral Science of the applicable professional board or certification committee.*
Maximum: Revocation.
Minimum: One year's suspension, stayed, with three year's probation.
Conditions of Probation:
1. Successful completion of a continuing education program related to the worker/client relationship approved by the Board.
2. Successful completion of an oral examination administered by the Board or its designees.
3. If deemed appropriate by the trier of fact, practice only in a supervised, structured environment which is approved by the Board.

Note: These regulations were revised in 1981.

Appendix F
APGA Convention
Registration Materials
Detroit Michigan, 1982

You'll love Detroit ...

with its wonderful combination of the new and the old. Within easy, safe walking distance of the convention area, with its modern buildings like the Renaissance Center you'll find historic old churches and ethnic neighborhoods. Throughout the Detroit metropolitan area you'll find exciting things to see and do.

How Would You Like to . . .

Visit Greenfield Village and Henry Ford Museum. History book heroes come alive as you visit the authentic homes and workshops of Thomas Edison, Noah Webster, the Wright brothers and many others. Tour the 260-acre Village by horse-drawn carriage, steam locomotive or paddle-wheel river boat that glides past a turn-of-the-century amusement park. Adjacent to the Village is a 14-acre museum housing an endless variety of vintage cars, planes, full-size locomotives and mechanical gadgets. There's a museum theatre and Famous Early Movie Series. The Street of Shops offers demonstrations of crafts such as candle-dipping and book-making.

Go south, yes south to Canada. Our friendly international neighbor Windsor, Ontario, offers fine dining, shopping and recreation only five minutes away by bridge or tunnel. Dieppe Gardens on the riverfront affords an imposing view of the Detroit Skyline. If you have extra time, Jack Miner's Bird Sanctuary and Point Pelee National Park are within a few hours' drive.

Tour the Cultural Center. Just five minutes from Downtown and within walking distance of each other are eighteen museums and educational institutions forming one of America's largest cultural complexes, such as: THE DETROIT INSTITUTE OF ARTS . . . where you can Brunch with

Bach, critique a classic film, hear jazz in a medieval courtyard, see the nation's largest Youtheatre, or roam through 100 galleries, famous for French, Italian and African art. Don't miss the mummies! THE DETROIT PUBLIC LIBRARY, Main Branch . . . houses more than 2 million volumes, art prints, a Rare Book Collection and exhibits. "Please touch" is the unique policy at Detroit's new SCIENCE CENTER . . . take the exciting "Stairway to the Stars" and watch a movie in the domed Space Theatre. THE DETROIT HISTORICAL MUSEUM . . . and the authentically recreated "Streets of Old Detroit" take you back through the history of Detroit under the French, British and American flags. THE CHILDREN'S MUSEUM, INTERNATIONAL INSTITUTE AND YOUR HERITAGE HOUSE, nearby, all have special exhibits and demonstrations . . . call for details.

Take in a performance at one of our theaters. The famous Alvin Ailey Dance group will be at the Music Hall in downtown Detroit during the APGA convention. Other theaters will be featuring excellent local talent as well as national touring groups. If you prefer animal shows, the DETROIT ZOO, the nation's first "natural habitat" environment for more than 5,000 animals is open all year long.

See spectator sports in a great sports town, with action all year long. In March you can see basketball (The Detroit Pistons) or soccer under the 10 acre roof at the Detroit Silverdome. The Detroit Red Wings play hockey in their new downtown location, the 20,000 seat Joe Louis Sports Arena. There's also year-round racing at the Detroit Race Course/Wolverine Harness Raceway, Hazel Park Racetrack and Windsor Raceway.

Eat in one of our many ethnic restaurants. The most famous neighborhood, Greektown, with its delightful, all night restaurants is right downtown. You'll also find Chinese, Middle Eastern, French and Italian restaurants scattered throughout the metropolitan area. Try them, you'll like them!

Registration Information

Advance

You are urged to register in advance by using the registration forms in this booklet. An APGA membership application has also been provided for those who are not members but wish to take advantage of the low member registration fee. When you register in advance, you may pick up your convention materials at the registration desk during the following hours:
Wednesday, March 17—8:00 am-7:00 pm
Thursday, March 18—8:00 am-5:00 pm
Friday, March 19—8:00 am-5:00 pm
Saturday, March 20—8:00 am-12:00 noon

On-Site

If you do not register in advance, you may do so at the registration area at the times listed above. If you wish to take advantage of the lower membership registration fee, please remember that when you arrive at the registration area, visit the membership desk first. Once the membership has been processed, then proceed to the on-site convention registration desk and register as an APGA member.

Pre-Convention Workshops

APGA has planned a series of workshops preceding the opening session of the convention. You may take advantage of a wide variety of subjects which are covered. Information, schedule of fees and registration forms are found in this booklet.

Special Group Discount Rates

We are offering a special group discount rate to members and student members on advance registration only. If three or more registrations are received from your institution, you will be eligible for the special rate. ALL REGISTRATIONS MUST ARRIVE IN THE SAME ENVELOPE. No exceptions to this can be made because of the computerized registration procedures. The special rate applies to MEMBERS only. Including a nonmember as part of your group will result in the return of his or her registration. Remember, you can save $5.00 on each registration if you do a little organizing ahead of time!

Registration Fees

Advance

Member	$ 50
Non-Member	100
Student Member	40
Student Non-Member	45
Spouse (Non-counselor)	15
Exhibitor (Complimentary)	—
Exhibitor (Paid)	20
Special Group Member Rate	45
Special Group Student Member Rate	35

On-Site

Member	$ 60
Non-Member	110
Student Member	50
Student Non-Member	55
Exhibitor (Complimentary)	—
Exhibitor (Paid)	20
Spouse (Non-Counselor)	20

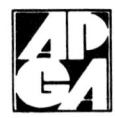

Dear APGA Member:

Service to others is the keystone of our profession and it is imperative that we assist ourselves, as well as those we serve, to meet effectively the changes required by our ever rapidly changing world.

The APGA Convention offers you many opportunities to add to your knowledge and skills through formal content sessions and pre-convention workshops as well as by informal contacts.

The 1982 APGA Convention theme is especially appropriate for the times and conditions we face: "A Renaissance of Responsibility and Responsiveness: Strategies for the Helping Professions". In the spirit of renaissance, historically a time of great creativity and productivity, we seek to work together to make our profession more viable. The theme is intended to spark our enthusiasm and to strengthen our commitment to the helping professions.

I invite you to join us at the Detroit Convention which will be an action arena for self-renewal. Come to learn, to share, to enjoy.

The Convention Committee under the leadership of John R. Webber is planning an exciting Convention. The Detroit community and hundreds of volunteers are planning to welcome us. The Guidepost will provide details.

Please note that on Wednesday, March 17, registration begins at 8:00 A.M., content sessions at 1:00 P.M., and the opening session at 4:00 P.M. Your Officers, Board of Directors, Senators, Division Presidents, Region Chairpersons, and Headquarters Staff look forward to greeting you at the all-APGA-community St. Patrick's Day party at 7:00 P.M.

Sincerely,

Louise B. Forsyth
President, APGA

APPENDIX F

Hotel Information

HOTEL/MOTEL SLEEPING ROOM REQUEST

APGA Housing Bureau
METROPOLITAN DETROIT CONVENTION &
VISITORS BUREAU
100 Renaissance Center, Ste. 1950, Detroit, MI 48243

Telephone reservations will only be
accepted 2 weeks in advance of meeting
General office: (313) 259-4333
Housing office: (313) 259-4424

Hotel/Motel Preference: 1st choice _____

2nd choice _____ 3rd choice _____

Date of Arrival _____ Time _____ **Guarantee: Yes _____ No _____

Date of Departure _____ Credit Card No. _____

Time of Departure _____ Name of Charge & Expiration _____

Type of
Accomodations Requested

Single (no.) _____ Rate Requested _____

AVOID DUPLICATION...
If one or more persons are
requesting accomodations,
only one application is
necessary

Double (no.) _____ Rate Requested _____

Twins (no.) _____ Rate Requested _____

SUITE—Parlor w/1 connecting bedroom _____ Rate Requested _____

SUITE—Parlor w/2 connecting bedrooms _____ Rate Requested _____

NAMES OF OCCUPANTS _____
(Bracket names of persons
occupying same room)
_____

Mail confirmation to: Name _____

Institution _____

Address _____

_____

If accommodations at the hotel/motel of
my choice are not available, I understand
the Housing Bureau will make as good a
reservation as possible elsewhere and that
I will receive confirmation from the
hotel/motel.

**Reservation held regardless of arrival
hour.

**MUST BE MAILED BY
FEBRUARY 17, 1982**

(FOR CONVENTION USE ONLY

Reservation follow through date & initial
Received at Housing Bureau _____

Processed to hotel/motel _____

Received at hotel motel _____

Confirmed to guest _____

Returned to Housing Bureau _____

Advance Registration Form

Detroit, Michigan
1982 APGA Convention
March 17-20, 1981

Registration and Badge Information (Please TYPE or PRINT)

NAME FIRST NAME LAST NAME

ADDRESS

CITY STATE ZIP

PLEASE ATTACH THE LABEL FROM THIS
MAILING FOR NAME AND ADDRESS

MEMBERSHIP NO.

INSTITUTION

CITY & STATE

NAME OF SPOUSE
(IF REGISTERING)

(LEAVE A BLANK BETWEEN WORDS)

Appendix G
1983 APGA Convention
Call for Content Programs

Theme Statement

Our socioeconomic climate reflects a crisis in our national economy. The Federal budget crisis continues. State and local budget crises abound; rural and urban areas are faced with severe inflation, high unemployment, business and industry cutbacks and the consequent human problems. If the helping professions are to remain viable, attention must be focused on assisting ourselves as well as our clients to meet effectively the changes required by an ever more rapidly changing world.

The 1983 APGA Convention theme is especially appropriate for the times and the challenges we face. In order to meet our responsibility to vitalize strategies that assist individuals and groups to develop intrinsic strengths to cope with the adversities of life, counselors help America work through human contributions to productivity and adaption to change. Because the dignity of human existence and achievement are qualities that are inherent in the pursuit of happiness, helping strategies must enhance our efforts to address the prevention of crisis situations which deny human development. These strategies must also recognize the congruency of individuals and their environment in preparation for futuristic projections relevant to careers, employment, technology, leisure, citizenry and positive interpersonal relationships.

The 1983 APGA Convention theme is intended to spark our enthusiasm and strengthen our commitment to the helping professions. The 1983 APGA Convention is planned as an action arena to:
    1. Stimulate responsive and responsible strategies for the helping professions which relate to personal, professional, economic and political survival under present and future conditions.

2. Commit ourselves to strategies that effectively and efficiently serve individuals and groups.
3. Address the crisis of confidence within the helping professions.

Suggested Scope of Proposals

Pre-Convention Workshops. Those wishing to submit proposals for pre-convention fee-charging workshops must write to the APGA Workshop Office, Two Skyline Place, Suite 400, 5203 Leesburg Pike, Falls Church, VA 22041 for the guidelines. Do Not Submit Your Proposal to the Program Coordinator. Proposals must be postmarked July 15, 1982.

Convention Programs: All program proposals, including those for divisional consideration, are submitted to the APGA Program Coordinator and include the following categories:

a. Regular Programs.

Proposals should be planned to remedy gaps in knowledge and to provide skill in innovative methodologies and procedures. Areas in which APGA members have expressed need include: developmental counseling; interdisciplinary approaches to counseling problems; minority needs; career planning and development; counseling of the mature worker and student; counseling handicapped persons; and accountability before the fact. We also hope to see programs that emphasize continuity and completeness of human development and show relationships between agencies, APGA members and the community.

b. Student Programs.

Both graduate and undergraduate students are invited to submit programs related to personnel and guidance practices. Faculty members should encourage students to submit proposals. Please note that the program chairperson must be an APGA member, either student or regular.

c. Research Programs.

We invite submissions of recent research findings and their practical applications. Researchers whose papers are selected will be asked to bring copies of their work for distribution at the sessions. Each researcher will have five minutes to state the research theme, describe the design and hypothesis, and outline the findings and conclusions. Ten minutes will be reserved for questions from the audience. Submit one complete copy of the research paper, and a summary of the report on the form included with the program proposal; two copies of pages 3 and 6 must also be submitted. On the title page of the research paper, please type the name, institution and complete mailing address of the person who will deliver the report at the convention. Mark RESEARCH for item number 1 on the proposal form.

d. Poster Sessions.

An innovation in programming at APGA, you will have one and one-half hours to display graphically your program and chat with individuals who attend the system. You have the option to select a poster session, or the Program Committee may choose to accept some proposals from the general submissions. Please check section 3 on page 3.

e. Extended Time Sessions.
In depth presentations may select the longer time slot. Please be sure you indicate which time period you wish under Section 2 on page 3.

f. Ancillary Programs.
APGA-related groups may schedule committee/commission meetings and/or social events for listing in the convention program. Please use Item 4 on the Program Proposal to give time, length and type of meeting, etc., as appropriate, and return form to the APGA Convention office in Falls Church. Do Not Submit Your Proposal to the Program Coordinator. Be sure to include the complete mailing address of the organizer and/or chairperson.

How to Submit Your Proposal

1. Fill out completely and accurately the forms found on pages 3 and 6. These forms are to be used for all of the above programs except pre-convention workshops. The information on these forms will be used for the final program if your proposal is accepted. Please note that a person may appear as chairperson, speaker, respondent, or any other participant on no more than two programs.

2. Limit the program summary to the space provided on the program proposal form on page 4. In addition all presenters are required to prepare a summary of their presentations on page 5 of the proposal form, duplicated as needed. These summaries must not exceed the space provided. Be sure to include the name, title, institution, and title of presentation for each presenter with the program proposal.

3. Procedures for research program proposals are described earlier; be sure to follow them exactly.

4. A program proposal must also include a letter from each of the participants (including chairperson, recorder, presenters, reactors, and discussants), agreeing to appear on the program in Detroit if the proposal is accepted. This letter should also indicate if the person expects to be on any other programs at the convention and, if so, which ones.

5. Be sure a recorder is named in your proposal. The purpose of the recorder is to check on adequate physical arrangements, secure evaluation forms at the Convention, and conduct the evaluation.

6. Indicate which divisions or committees might sponsor programs submitted. The following groups will consider program proposals:
   American College Personnel Association (ACPA)
   National Vocational Guidance Association (NVGA)
   American School Counselor Association (ASCA)
   American Rehabilitation Counseling Association (ARCA)
   Association for Measurement and Evaluation in Guidance (AMEG)
   National Employment Counselors Association (NECA)

Association for Non-White Concerns in Personnel and Guidance (ANWC)
Association for Religious and Value Issues in Counseling (ARVIC)
Association for Counselor Education and Supervision (ACES)
Association for Humanistic Education and Development (AHEAD)
Association for Specialists of Group Work (ASGW)
Public Offender Counselor Association (POCA)
American Mental Health Counselors Association (AMHCA)
Research Program Committee
Student Program Committee
International Program Committee

7. Use this form for requesting space for ancillary programs, i.e., committee business meetings, board meetings, social functions. Indicate preferred time and date. These may be submitted directly to APGA Headquarters office.

8. Only proposals on the official forms or facsimile will be accepted.

When to Submit Your Proposal

Send the appropriate number of copies of your complete proposal to the Program Coordinator:

> Lee J. Richmond
> Johns Hopkins University
> 105 Whitehead Hall
> Homewood Campus
> Charles and 34th Streets
> Baltimore, MD 21218

All proposals must be received by September 3, 1982. Proposals received after this date will not be considered.

Washington Convention Information

Information on registration, hotel accommodations, placement and preliminary programs will be sent to all APGA members. Convention articles will be published periodically in **Guidepost** and divisional publications. Watch for them.

CONVENTION VOLUNTEER STAFF

APGA PRESIDENT
Helen Washburn
1412 North 13th Street
Boise, ID 83702

CONVENTION COORDINATOR
Martin Gerstein
Virginia Tech
Northern Virginia Graduate Center
2990 Telestar Court
Falls Church, VA 22042

ASSOCIATE CONVENTION COORDINATOR
Dorothy E. Jenkins
District of Columbia Public Schools
415 12th Street, N.W. Suite 906
Washington, D.C. 20004

PROGRAM COORDINATOR
Lee J. Richmond
Johns Hopkins University
105 Whitehead Hall
Homewood Campus
Charles and 34th Streets
Baltimore, MD 21218

PUBLICITY AND PUBLIC RELATIONS COORDINATOR
Grace W. Phillips
1316 Underwood Street, N.W.
Washington, D.C. 20012

CONVENTION SERVICES COORDINATOR
Charles W. Humes
Virginia Tech
Northern Virginia Graduate Center
2990 Telestar Court
Falls Church, VA 22042

SPECIAL ACTIVITIES AND MEALS COORDINATOR
Mary K. Albrittain
Maryland State Department of Education
200 West Baltimore Street
Baltimore, MD 21201

GOVERNMENT RELATIONS COORDINATOR
James P. Stratoudakis
The Social Center
8220 Russell Road
Alexandria, VA 22309

ASSISTANT CONVENTION COORDINATOR
C.D. Johnson
Anne Arundel County
Board of Education
2644 Riva Road
Annapolis, MD 21401

APGA Headquarters Convention Staff
Two Skyline Place, Suite 400
5203 Leesburg Pike
Falls Church, VA 22041

Executive Vice President
Charles L. Lewis
Convention Manager
Nancy P. King

Program Overview

Please type a summary of your program within the lines provided. No summary exceeding the space provided will be accepted. In addition to the program title, and the name, title and institute of the chairperson, this summary should include: (a) objective of the program and any special emphasis, e.g., career development, substance abuse; (b) relevance to the convention theme and (c) summary of content and outcomes for those attending. Research reports should include: statement of purpose, population, methods, and indications of outcomes.

Name:
Institution:
Title of Program:

If program summaries for individual presentations, e.g., experiential, are not needed, please indicate so here and explain why.

CUT ALONG DOTTED LINE

Individual Presentation Summary

Prepare only if needed to explain separate presentations such as panel presentations.

Please type a summary of each presentation within the lines provided, photocopying this form as needed. No summary exceeding the space provided will be accepted. In addition to the program title and the name, title and institution of the chairperson, this summary should include: (a) objective of the program and any special emphasis, i.e., career planning, substance abuse; (b) relevance to the convention theme and (c) summary of content and outcomes for those attending.

Name:
Institution:
Title of Program:

Title of Presentation:

CUT ALONG DOTTED LINE

Organizer _____

Chairperson _____
(Last name only)

Content Program Proposal

INSTRUCTIONS

Please Type

Submit one copy of the proposal for each division you wish to consider your program, plus one complete copy for the master file. A complete program proposal consists of:

1. Proposal form, pages 3 and 6.
2. Letters of acceptance from each participant (including chairperson and recorder) including notation as to what other programs each participant is obligated.
3. Program overview, and summary of individual presentations if these differ substantially from the overview.
4. Complete copy of research paper (research programs only).

Send all program proposals to: Lee J. Richmond, Johns Hopkins University, 105 Whitehead Hall, Homewood Campus, Charles and 34th Streets, Baltimore, MD 21218.

TITLE OF PROGRAM

(Limit of 60 letters. Please leave space between words)

1. **Suggested sponsoring division(s)** (No more than two)
   1st choice _____
   2nd choice _____

2. **Time slots requested** ☐ Regular - 1¼ hours   Circle one   1   2   3
   ☐ Extended - 2½ hours   Circle one   1   2   3

3. **Poster Session** _____ Yes _____ No

4. **Room arrangements** NOTE: All rooms are set with moveable chairs, theater style, with speaker's table.

a. Number at speaker's table	b. Type of lectern	Circle one Table Standing

   c. **Microphones** NOTE: Microphones are not furnished in rooms seating less than 100 and are limited to one in larger rooms.
   Circle one   Table   Lectern   Standing

   d. **Projectors** NOTE: Limit of one projector, although arrangements may be made through the Convention Office to rent additional projectors.
   Circle one
   2 x 2 slide   8mm movie
   Overhead   16mm movie

   e. **Video equipment** No video equipment is furnished. If you wish to use this equipment, you must either bring it with you or rent it in the city of the convention.

   f. **Tape recorders** NOTE: Recorders are playback only.
   Circle one   Cassette   Reel-to-Reel

   g. **Chalkboard**   Yes _____ No _____

5. **For Ancillary Programs Only:**
   ☐ Committee/commission meeting
   ☐ Reception
   ☐ Meal
   Date _____ Time _____

6. **Comments** _____

FOR APGA AND COMMITTEE USE ONLY
Program No. _____
Date _____
Time _____
Time Block _____

Sponsoring Division and No. _____
Ancillary _____ Content _____
Hotel _____
Room _____
Index _____

APGA Washington, D.C. Convention, March 20–23, 1983

APPENDIX G   373

APPENDIX G

CUT ALONG DOTTED LINE

PLEASE TYPE ALL INFORMATION
PROGRAM ORGANIZER†

Name _____
Institution _____
Complete office mailing address _____
zip _____
Office phone (including area code) _____

† Program Organizer will not be listed in convention program

PROGRAM CHAIRPERSON
(Must Be APGA Member)

Name _____
Institution _____

Membership # _____
zip _____
Office phone (including area code) _____

PROGRAM RECORDER

Name _____
Institution _____
Complete office mailing address _____
zip _____

Check membership status:
APGA member Yes____ No____   Office phone (including area code) _____

PROGRAM PARTICIPANT

Check Role:
Reactor _____   Name _____
Discussant _____   Institution _____
Presenter _____   Complete office mailing address _____
Check membership status: zip _____
APGA member Yes____ No____   Office phone (including area code) _____

PROGRAM PARTICIPANT

Check Role:
Reactor _____   Name _____
Discussant _____   Institution _____
Presenter _____   Complete office mailing address _____
Check membership status: zip _____
APGA member Yes____ No____   Office phone (including area code) _____

PROGRAM PARTICIPANT

Check Role:
Reactor _____   Name _____
Discussant _____   Institution _____
Presenter _____   Complete office mailing address _____
Check membership status: zip _____
APGA member Yes____ No____   Office phone (including area code) _____

PROGRAM PARTICIPANT

Check Role:
Reactor _____   Name _____
Discussant _____   Institution _____
Presenter _____   Complete office mailing address _____
Check membership status: zip _____
APGA member Yes____ No____   Office phone (including area code) _____

Name Index

Ackerman, J. M., 72
Adkins, C., 268
Adler, Alfred, 90, 212
Allen, J. W., 90
Alschuler, A. S., 75
Ambron, S. R., 208
Ames, L. B., 196
Andrews, L. M., 72
Anton, J. L., 179, 181, 186
Arbuckle, D. S., 149
Arenberg, D., 259
Arensberg, C. N., 132, 133, 134
Asher, J., 31, 40
Atchley, R., 262, 264, 268
Austin, M. J., 67

Bacon, Francis, 177
Beck, A. T., 90
Benjamin, L., 38
Berensen, B. G., 74, 84
Bergen, A. E., 70
Berry, J. B., 237
Berry, R., 288
Biggs, D. A., 149
Birren, J., 258
Blatt, M., 219
Blocher, D. H., 38, 73
Blum, R., 292
Bocknek, Gene, 232
Bolland, J., 288
Borow, H., 75
Botwinick, J., 259
Boyd, J., 85, 87
Bradley, M. K., 39

Brecher, E. M., 292, 294
Brodsky, A. M., 246
Brophy, J. E., 196
Browne, H., 58
Brubaker, J. D., 126, 129, 230
Burks, H. M., Jr., 148
Burnside, I. M., 98, 257, 266
Busse, E., 258
Butler, R., 253, 264, 267
Butterworth, T. W., 182

Callanan, P., 102, 107, 116
Carkhuff, R. R., 37, 70, 74, 84, 90, 274
Carlson, J., 131
Cattell, R., 259
Coleman, J. S., 224
Conger, J. J., 197, 209
Conroe, R., 244, 245
Corey, G., 96, 97, 102, 107, 116, 118, 119, 148
Corey, M., 96, 102, 107, 116
Cormier, L. S., 88
Cormier, W. H., 88
Cottingham, H. F., 77, 78
Cottle, T. J., 207
Cronbach, L. J., 156, 307
Crutchfield, R. S., 255

Davey, J., 244, 245
Davidson, G. C., 188
DeBlassie, R. R., 203
Dewey, John, 219
Dinkmeyer, D., 131
Dobson, N. H., 120
Dunlop, R., 7

NAME INDEX

Egerton, L. B., 255
Eisdorfer, C., 258
Elkind, D., 216
Elliott, K. P., 37
Ellis, Albert, 52, 85, 86
Engen, H. B., 163
Erikson, E. H., 196, 198, 200, 204, 216, 217, 218, 221, 226, 232, 235, 243
Evans, D. A., 237

Faust, V., 131
Fein, R., 288
Feldstein, P., 288
Fincher, C., 163
Finn, J., 255
Fisher, P., 271
Foner, A., 259
Freud, S., 14, 216, 217, 236
Friedman, H., 255
Frieze, I. H., 240

Gabe, T., 266
Garfield, S. L., 70
Gazda, G. M., 119
Gesell, A., 196
Goffman, E., 281, 282
Goldman, Leo, 156, 185
Goldstein, A., 255
Goodenough, W. G., 132, 133, 134
Gottesman, R., 35, 36
Gould, R. L., 233, 236, 239
Greenwood, E., 7, 8
Greiger, R., 87
Grob, P., 268
Grummon, D. L., 149, 156
Gumaer, J., 97
Gysbers, N. C., 149

Hall, C., 196
Hannum, J. W., 182
Hatcher, H. S., 295
Havighurst, R. J., 17, 196, 199, 200, 204, 212, 213, 233
Hayler, D., 288
Henchert, C. M., 36
Hendricks, C., 260
Hendricks, J., 260
Hoebel, E. A., 209
Hoffman, J. C., 47
Holland, John, 157
Holyroyd, J., 246
Horn, J., 259
Hubbard, D. R., 182
Huber, C. H., 204
Humes, C. W., II, 36
Hurlock, E. B., 208, 222

Ilg, F., 196
Inhelder, B., 196, 197
Ivey, A. E., 75

Jacobson, L., 255
Jayaratne, S., 179
Johnson, P. B., 240
Johnson, V., 257, 266, 291

Kagan, J., 197
Kameen, M. C., 36
Kampwirth, T. J., 36
Kaplan, M., 268, 269
Karlins, M., 72
Keller, K. E., 149
Kelly, J. R., 268
Kerr, N., 284
Kimmel, D. C., 231, 243, 244
Kirkpatrick, J. S., 236
Knowles, M., 259, 271
Kohlberg, L., 196, 199, 200, 204, 218, 219, 226
Kottler, J. A., 48, 49, 51
Kravetz, D., 246
Krech, D., 255
Krouse, J., 36
Krumboltz, J. D., 87, 88
Kurpius, J. D., 126, 129, 130

Lamb, R. R., 163
Laxson, J., 288
Lebsock, M. S., 203
Leiberman, M., 267
Levinson, D., 233, 236, 239, 241
Lewin, K., 208
Levy, R. L., 179
Lincoln, Abraham, 204
Linden, J. D., 171
Lippitt, G., 131
Lippitt, R., 131
Lowenthal, M. F., 235
Lubin, B., 120

MacKay, J. L., 138
Mahoney, M. J., 72, 88, 90, 187
Manaster, G. J., 209, 212, 213, 216, 218, 221, 222
Maples, M. F., 156
Marecek, J., 246
Marino, T. M., 245
Maslow, A., 19
Masters, W., 257, 266
Mayer, G. R., 182
McAlees, D., 27, 28
McArthur, C. C., 233
McCluskey, H., 270, 271
McCully, C. H., 7
McDaniel, J. W., 284
McKain, W., 259
McKelvey, J., 32
Meichenbaum, D., 90
Meyer, G. A., 258
Miles, M., 132, 133, 134
Miller, D. R., 120

NAME INDEX

Moore, W. E., 7, 8
Moreland, J. R., 240
Mussen, P. H., 197

Nelson, R. C., 131
Neugarten, B. L., 241
Newman, B., 242
Nichols, W. C., Jr., 28
Niehoff, A. H., 132, 133, 134
Noble, V. N., 36

Oaklander, V., 97
Oetting, E. R., 186
Osipow, S. H., 76, 88
Overs, R., 268

Paradise, L. V., 55, 57
Parker, L. G., 36
Parsons, Frank, 11, 148
Parsons, J. E., 240
Patterson, C. H., 84, 149, 156
Payton, C. R., 246
Pedersen, 37, 38
Peterson, D., 271
Piaget, J., 196, 197, 200, 204, 213, 214, 219, 226
Pietrofesa, J. J., 49
Prediger, D. J., 163
Protinsky, H., 85

Ralston, N. C., 208
Ramer, B., 85
Raush, H. L., 185
Riegel, K. F., 258
Reigel, R. M., 258
Riley, M. R., 259
Ritchie, M. H., 7, 8
Robertson-Tachabo, E. A., 259
Rockwell, P. J., 178
Rodham, H., 203
Rogers, C. R., 84, 85, 149, 274
Rosenkrantz, P., 246
Rosenthal, R., 255
Ross, P., 179, 181
Rothney, J. W. M., 178, 180, 181
Rousseau, J. J., 196
Rubinstein, E. A., 246
Ruble, D. N., 240
Russell, J. M., 102, 107, 116
Ruzek, S., 8

Sanborn, M., 180
Sax, G., 171
Scarf, M., 241
Scher, M., 245
Schmidt, J. A., 85
Schmuck, R., 132, 133, 134
Schumacher, B., 27, 28
Seligman, N. M., 256
Sells, S. B., 301

Senour, M. N., 151
Sheehy, G., 242
Shelton, J. L., 72
Shepherd, M., 52
Sherman, J., 246
Shertzer, B., 20, 171
Shevlin, M., 7
Shipman, W., 255
Silver, R. J., 120
Skelding, A. H., 67
Smith, P. L., 67
Stefflre, B., 148
Stone, S., 20
Stripling, R. O., 39
Stuart, R. B., 188
Stude, E. W., 32
Swanson, C. D., 28, 31, 39, 50
Sweeney, T. J., 39
Szasz, T. S., 49

Taylor, S., 268
Terry, S., 22
Thomas, G. P., 208
Thoresen, C. E., 72, 88, 182, 188
Tiedt, S. M., 237
Tobin, S., 267
Tolstoy, L., 236
Tosi, D. J., 85
Truax, C. B., 84
Turiel, E., 196, 199

Vaillant, G. E., 233
Van Hoose, W. H., 28, 31, 48, 49, 50, 51, 55, 57
Vogel, F. J., 39
Vriend, J., 49

Walsh, W. B., 88
Walz, G. R., 38
Warner, R. W., 39
Weg, R., 257
Weiss, L., 235
Westling, D. L., 204
White, R. W., 307
Whiteley, J. M., 76
Williams, R. L., 159
Williamson, E. G., 148
Witmer, J. M., 39
Woellner, E. H., 27
Wolfsenberger, W., 281
Wong, M. R., 244, 245
Woodruff, D., 256
Wrenn, C. G., 138
Wright, B. A., 282, 284, 287

Yalom, I. D., 103
Yamamoto, 282

Zell, F., 246
Zellman, G. L., 240
Zytowski, D. G., 163

Subject Index

Abused children, legal issues of, 36
Accountability, 65, 320
   in a group, 115–117
   in consulting, 129
   in counseling, 65
   rehabilitation counselor, 288
Accreditation of Counselor Education
    Programs, 8
Achieving intimacy in adulthood, 235–236
Adolescents
   cognitive development of, 213–216
   counseling adolescents, 221–223
   counselor's role with, 221–223
   cultural effects of, 211–212
   definition of, 208–209
   developmental tasks of, 212–213
   group counseling, 96–97
   handicapped, 225
   issues of, 209
   moral development of, 218–221
   non-traditional students, 224
   personality changes in, 210–211
   physical changes in, 209–210
   psychological development of, 216–218
   specialized studies, 224
   vocational education of, 224
Adulthood, stages of
   early, 233–242
   middle, 242–244
   transition periods, 239, 240–242, 243–244
   young, 233–242
Adults
   achieving intimacy, 235–236
   autonomy, 236–239
   biological changes in, 243

Adults *(continued)*:
   coping with aging parents, 243
   coping with bereavement, 243
   developmental tasks, 230–232, 232–233, 235–239, 243
   early adulthood, 233–242
   female clients, 246–247
   generativity, 243
   group counseling, 97–98
   in higher education, 247–248
   late parenthood, 243
   male clients, 244–246
   middle adulthood, 242–244
   "settling down," 239–240
   sexual concerns, 235, 236
   stages of early and middle adulthood (Chart), 234
   transition periods, 239, 240–242, 243–244
   young adulthood, 233–242
Advantages of group counseling, 99–100
Aging parents, coping with, 243
Alcoholics, 288–292, 300–301
   counselor training, 291–292
   counselor's role with, 290–291
   treatment of, 289–290
Alcoholics Anonymous (AA), 290
American Association of Marriage and
    Family Therapy (AAMFT), 51
American Mental Health Counselors
    Association (AMHCA) regulations, 29–30, 39
American Personnel and Guidance
    Association (APGA), 1, 3, 8, 11–12
   code of ethics, 6, 29, 52, 53, 53–55, 125, 129, 165, 174

SUBJECT INDEX   379

American Personnel and Guidance
  Association (APGA) *(continued):*
    conventions, 326-329
    divisions of, 12
    policy regarding assessment, 165
American Psychological Association (APA)
    ethical codes, 155, 161, 174, 188
    standards for educational and
      psychological tests, 155, 161
American School Counselors Association
      (ASCA), 17
Announcing a group, 101
Anxiety in groups, 110-111
Assessment, 65, 147-148
    competency tests, 160
    criticisms of using tests, 156, 162-165
    errors of difference and predictions,
      161-162
    nonstandardized forms of, 159-160
    purposes of, 156-157
    reliability, 160-162
    role of in counseling, 148-153
    social, ethical and legal issues of, 162-169
    standardized instruments, 155-157
    standardized tests and inventories,
      157-159
    validity, 160-162
Association of Counselor Education and
      Supervision (ACES), 8, 90
Association for Measurement and
      Evaluation in Guidance (AMEG), 163
Association for Specialists in Group Work
      (ASGW), 101-102, 116
    ethical codes, 101-102, 116, 120
Autonomy in adulthood, 236-239

Behavioral approach to counseling, 78, 83,
      87-88
Bereavement, coping with, 243
Berger v. Board of Psychologists
  Examiners, 30
Beyond the couch relationships, 52
Biological changes in adults, 243
Bogust v. Iverson, 28
Buckley Amendment, 33-34, 35, 50, 165, 322
Business and industry counselors, 20, 23

Career counseling, 72, 75-76, 224, 271-272
Categories of information, 153-154
Change theory and innovation, 133-137
Cherry v. Board of Regents of the State of
  New York, 31
Child abuse laws, 36
Childhood, theories of development
    Erikson's theory, 198
    Havighurst's theory, 199-200
    Kohlberg's theory, 199
    Piaget's theory, 196-198
Children
    abused, 36

Children *(continued):*
    cognitive development of, 196-198
    counseling children, 200-203
      group, 96, 201
      individual, 201
    counselor's role with, 200-201
    developmental tasks of, 199-200
    emotional development of, 198
    exceptional, 203-204
    moral development of, 199
    rights of, 203
Claiming expertise not possessed, 51
Classroom group guidance, 201
Client-centered approach to counseling, 78,
      83, 84-85, 149
Cognitive development
    in adolescents, 213-216
    in children, 196-198
Cohesion in groups, 112-114
Collaborative mode in cousulting, 128-129,
      132, 133
College and university counselors, 20, 23
College career planning and placement
      counselors, 6, 15
College student personnel counselors,
      20-21
Community agencies, 23
    counseling adults in, 248
Competency tests, 160
Conducting a pregroup session, 104-105
Confidentiality, 32, 37, 322-323
    violation of, 50-51
Conflicts in groups, 111-112
Constitutional rights of minors and college
      students, 38
Consulting, 65
    accountability, 129
    collaborative mode, 128-129, 132, 133
    definition of, 124, 126, 130-132
    innovation and change theory, 133-137
    mediation mode, 127-128, 131-132
    prescriptive mode, 127, 131
    provisional mode, 127, 130-131
    superordinate goal, 133, 137, 138
    vested interests, 133, 134, 135, 136, 137,
      138
Control of information, 151
Conversation, compared with counseling,
      68-70
Corrections counseling. *See Offenders.*
Council for the Accreditation of Counseling
      and Related Educational Programs
      (CACREP), 8
Counselee misconceptions about
      information, 153
Counseling
    accountability, 65
    adolescents, 221-223
    adult females, 246-247
    adult males, 244-246

SUBJECT INDEX

Counseling *(continued)*:
adults in community agencies, 248
adults in higher education, 247-248
assessment and information giving functions of. *See Assessment and/or Information Giving*
behavioral approach, 78, 83, 87-88
career, 72, 75-76
children, 200-203
children, abused, 36
client-centered approach, 78, 83, 84-85, 149
college and university, 15
consulting function in. *See Consulting.*
conversation compared with counseling, 68-70
developmental, 16-19, 21, 24, 72, 73-75
elderly. *See Elderly.*
evaluation and research in. *See Research and Evaluation.*
goals, 68
"Good Faith Doctrine," 37-38
group. *See Group counseling.*
handicapped, 36, 255
individual, 67, 72-78, 90
legal definitions of, 28-29
malpractice, 38, 48
nontraditional students, 224
personal adjustment, 73, 76-77
psychotherapy compared with counseling, 70-72
rational-emotive approach, 78, 83, 85-87
strategies, 69-70
student personnel services, 15
trait/factor approach, 148-149
Counseling children
abused, 36
classroom group guidance, 201
consultation, 201-203
group, 201
individual, 201
referral services, 203
Counseling Students Association (CSA), 30
Counselor training
alcoholics, 291-292
group leaders, 118-120
offenders, 299
rehabilitation, 287-288, 300
substance abuse, 294-295
Counselors
adult development, 230-232
business and industry, 20, 23
college career planning and placement, 6, 15
college student personnel, 20-21
college and universities, 20, 23
in community agencies, 23
corrections, 20
definition, conventional, 4-6
definition, Dictionary of Occupational Titles, 4-6

Counselors *(continued)*:
definition, Occupational Outlook Handbook, 5-6
definition, professional, 6-8
employment, 5
ethical orientation of, 55-57
incompetent behavior, 49-50
in mental health agencies, 23
of the 1980's, 1-2
in private practice, 20, 23
professional, 23
professional licensure laws, 20, 28-29
professionalization of, 8-11, 27-31
rehabilitation, 5, 20
related professions, 12-16
rights of, 2
school, 5, 20, 23
training, 90
training group leaders, 118-120
unethical conduct, 48-50, 53
Counselor's role
with adolescents, 221-223
with alcoholics, 290-291
with children, 200-201
with the elderly, 273-274
offenders, 297-299
rehabilitation, 286-287, 300
substance abusers, 293-294
Criticisms of research and evaluation, 185-186
Criticisms of using tests, 156, 162-165

Data sources in research and evaluation
observational, 182
questionnaires and inventories, 182-183
tests, 183
Decompetence in the elderly, 256, 261, 264-265
Deductive reasoning, 176
Developmental counseling, 16-19, 21, 24, 73-75
Developmental Disabilities Assistance and Bill of Rights Act of 1978, 34
Developmental tasks
for adolescents, 212-213
for adults, 230-232, 232-233, 235-239, 243
for children, 200
Deviance, 280-283
Dictionary of Occupational Titles (DOT), 4-6, 13, 14, 15, 23, 154
Dying, 265, 273

Education for All Handicapped Children Act, 1975, (PL94-142), 34, 35, 168, 203
Education of the elderly, 269-271, 273
Elderhostel, 271
Elderly
career counseling, 271-272
counselor's role with, 273-274
decompetence, physical and emotional, 256, 261, 264-265

Elderly (continued):
dying, 265, 273
education of, 269-271, 273
employment of, 260-261
expectancy phenomenon, 255
financial issues of, 262-263, 273
group counseling, 98
health of, 256-257, 264-265
incompetence, 256
institutionalization of, 266-267, 273
intellectual capacity of, 258-259
learned helplessness phenomenon, 255-256
learning ability of, 259, 270
leisure and the, 268-269
rehirement of, 271-272, 273
remarriage among, 259-260, 265-266
retirement, 263-264, 267-268
self-fulfilling prophecy, 255
senescence, 254, 261
sexual concerns, 257, 266
stereotyping, 254-255
volunteerism, 261
Emotional development in children, 198
Employee assistance programs, 300-301
Employment counselors, 5
Employment of the elderly, 260-261
Erikson's theory, 198
Errors of difference and predictions, 161-162
Ethical codes, 31, 53-55
  APGA policy regarding assessment, 165
  American Psychological Association, 155, 161, 174, 188
  American Personnel and Guidance Association, 6, 29, 52, 53-55, 125, 129, 165, 174
  Association for Specialists in Group Work, 116, 120
  history of, 2
  other organizations, 29, 55
  self-imposed, 2
Ethical decision making, 57-59
Ethical orientation of counselors, 55-57
Ethics of research and evaluation, 188
Evaluation and research in counseling. See Research and evaluation.
Exceeding professional competency level, 51
Exceptional children, 203-204
Expectancy phenomenon, 255

Family Education Rights and Privacy Act of 1974. See Buckley Amendment.
Federal Privacy Protection Act, 34
Financial issues of the elderly, 262-263, 273
Formation of a group, 100-101, 102-103

Generativity, 243
"Good Faith Doctrine," 37-38
Group counseling, 23, 64
  accountability, 115-117

Group counseling (continued):
for adolescents, 96-97
for adults, 97-98
advantages of, 99-100
announcing a group, 101
anxiety in groups, 110-111
for children, 96
cohesion in groups, 112-114
conducting a pregroup session, 104-105
dealing with conflicts in groups, 111-112
for the elderly, 98
formation of the group, 100-101, 102-103
goals/purposes, 98-99, 108-109
group leader training, 118-120
leader functions, 109-110
leader's competence, 117-118
member functions, 109
postgroup issues, 115-117
purposes/goals, 98-99, 108-109
recruiting group members, 101
screening and selecting group members, 101-102
stages of a group, 105-115
termination of a group, 114-115
trust in groups, 106, 107-108
Group leaders
  competence, 117-118
  functions, 109-110
  training, 118-120
Group member functions, 109
Guidance
  developmental, 17
Guidepost, 12

Handicapped
  adolescents, 225
  counseling the, 36, 225
  Education for All Handicapped Children Act, 1975, (PL94-142), 34, 35, 168, 203
  legal statutes, 36
Havighurst's theory, 199-200
Health of the elderly, 256-257, 264-265
Incompetence, in the elderly, 256
Incompetent behavior, 49-50
Individual counseling, 64
Inductive reasoning, 177
Industry and business counselors, 20, 23
Information giving, 65, 147-148
  categories of information (career, educational, personal/social), 153-154
  control of information, 151
  counselee misconceptions about information, 153
  role of, in counseling, 148-153
  sources of information, 152
Innovation and change theory, 133-137
Institutionalization of the elderly, 266-267, 273
Intellectual capacity of the elderly, 258-259
Intimacy in adulthood, 235-236
Kahan v. Greenfield, 37

SUBJECT INDEX

Knowledge from authority, 174–175
Knowledge from experience, 175–176
Kohlberg's theory, 199
Larry P. v. Wilson Riles, 165
Late parenthood, 243
Learned helplessness phenomenon, 255–256
Learning ability of the elderly, 259, 270
Legal issues
   of abused children, 36
   in assessment, 165
   constitutional rights of minors and college students, 38
   in the future, 38–39
   "Good Faith Doctrine," 37–38
   for the handicapped, 36
   malpractice, 38, 48
   privacy. *See Buckley Amendment.*
   privileged communication, 26, 32–33
Leisure and the elderly, 268–269
Licensure of counselors, 27–28, 90
Lopez v. Williams, 35, 38

Malpractice, 38, 48
Measurement procedure in research and evaluation, 187
Mediation mode in consulting, 127–128, 131–132
Mental health agencies, 23
Methods of research and evaluation, 178–181
   case study, 179
   experimental, 181
   historical, 178–179
   longitudinal, 180–181
   participant observer, 181
   survey, 180
Moral development
   in adolescents, 218–221
   in children, 199

National Vocational Guidance Association (NVGA), 3, 11
Nonstandardized forms of assessment, 159–160
Nontraditional students
   adolescents, 224

Occupational Outlook Handbook, 5–6, 13, 15, 20, 23, 154
Offender Aid and Restoration (OAR), 297
Offenders, 295–299, 301–302
   counselor training, 299
   counselor's role with, 297–299
   treatment of, 296–297

PL 94-142, 34, 35, 168, 203
Perceptions of the researcher, 187–188
Personal adjustment counseling, 73, 76–77
Personality changes in adolescents, 210–211
Personnel and Guidance Journal, 12

Physical changes in adolescents, 209–210
Physically disabled and retarded, 283–284, 300
   treatment of, 285–286
Piaget's theory, 196–198
Placement service, 10–11
Post group issues, 115–117
Pregroup session, conducting a, 104–105
Prescriptive mode in consulting, 127, 131
Private practice, counselors in, 20, 23
Privacy rights. *See Buckley Amendment.*
Privileged communication, 26, 32–33
Professional codes. *See Ethical codes.*
Professional counselors, 23
Professional licensure for counselors, 20, 28–29, 39–40
Professional organizations of interest to counselors, 33
Professionalization of counselors, 8–11, 27–31, 39–40
Provisional mode in consulting, 127, 130–131
Psychological development of adolescents, 216–218
Psychotherapy, compared with counseling, 70–72

Rational-emotive approach to counseling, 78, 83, 85–87
Recruiting group members, 101
Rehabilitation Act of 1973, 286, 299
Rehabilitation counselors
   accountability, 288
   role of, 286–287, 300
   training, 287–288, 300
Rehabilitation Services Administration, 285
Rehirement, 271–272, 273
Reliability
   in assessment, 160–162
   in research, 182
Remarriage among the elderly, 259–260, 265–266
Research and evaluation, 65
   criticisms of, 185–186
   deductive reasoning, 176
   definition of, 174
   ethics, 188
   inductive reasoning, 177
   knowledge from authority, 174–175
   knowledge from experience, 175–176
   measurement procedure, 187
   perceptions of the researcher, 187–188
   reliability, 182
   research design in counseling, 186–187
   scientific method, 177–178
   use of statistics in, 184–185
   validity, 182
Research and evaluation data sources, 182–183
   observational, 182
   questionnaires and inventories, 182–183
   tests, 183

SUBJECT INDEX

Research and evaluation methods. See Methods of research and evaluation.
Research design in counseling, 186-187
Resistance in groups, 110-111
Retarded. See Physically disabled and retarded.
Retirement, 263-264, 267-268
Rights of children, 203
Rights of counselors, 2

School counselors, 5, 20, 23
Scientific method, 177-178
Screening and selecting group members, 101-102
Self-fulfilling prophecy, 255
Senescence, 254, 261
"Settling down," 239-240
Sexual concerns
  adults, 235, 236
  elderly, 257, 266
Sources of information, 152
Special populations
  alcoholics, 288-292, 300-301
  offenders, 295-299, 301-302
  physically disabled and retarded, 283-284, 300
  substance abusers, 292-295, 301
Stages of a group, 105-115
Standardized instruments, 155-157
Standardized tests and inventories, 157-159
Statutory law, 32-36
Stereotyping the elderly, 254-255
Strategies, counseling, 69-70
Student personnel services, 15
Substance abusers, 292-295, 301
  counselor training, 294-295
  counselor's role with, 293-294
  treatment of, 293-294

Superordinate goal, 133, 137, 138

Tarasoff v. The Regents of the University of California, 37, 39
Termination of a group, 114-115
Testing. See Assessment.
Tinker v. DesMoines, 38
Training. See Counselor training.
Trait/factor approach, 148-149
Trust in groups, 106, 107-108

Unethical conduct, 48, 50-53
  beyond the couch relationships, 52
  claiming expertise not possessed, 51
  exceeding professional competency level, 51
  violating confidences, 50-51
Use of statistics in research and evaluation, 184-185

Validity
  in assessment, 160-162
  in research, 182
Vested interests, 133, 134, 135, 136, 137, 138
Violating confidences, 50-51
Virginia Board of Behavioral Sciences, 59
  regulations, 360
Virginia Board of Professional Counselors, 53
  regulations, 350
Virginia Counselors Association (VCA), 55
  ethical responsibilities and procedures, 345
Vocational development of adolescents, 224
Volunteerism, in the elderly, 261

Weldon v. Virginia Board of Psychologists Examiners, 28